BRUCE H. THIERS, MD, Consulting Editor

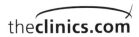

DERMATOLOGIC CLINICS

Internal Malignancy and the Skin: Paraneoplastic and Cancer Treatment-Related Cutaneous Disorders

Valencia D. Thomas, MD
Charles R. Thomas, Jr., MD
Guest Editors

January 2008 • Volume 26 • Number 1

SAUNDERS

An Imprint of Elsevier, Inc.
PHILADELPHIA   LONDON   TORONTO   MONTREAL   SYDNEY   TOKYO

W.B. SAUNDERS COMPANY
A Division of Elsevier Inc.

Elsevier Inc. • 1600 John F. Kennedy Blvd., Suite 1800 • Philadelphia, Pennsylvania 19103-2899

http://www.theclinics.com

DERMATOLOGIC CLINICS
January 2008
Editor: Alexandra Gavenda

Volume 26, Number 1
ISSN 0733-8635
ISBN-13: 978-1-4160-5774-1
ISBN-10: 1-4160-5774-9

The ideas and opinions expressed in *Dermatologic Clinics* do not necessarily reflect those of the Publisher. The Publisher does not assume any responsibility for any injury and/or damage to persons or property arising out of or related to any use of the material contained in this periodical. The reader is advised to check the appropriate medical literature and the product information currently provided by the manufacturer of each drug to be administered to verify the dosage, the method and duration of administration, or contraindications. It is the responsibility of the treating physician or other health care professional, relying on independent experience and knowledge of the patient, to determine drug dosages and the best treatment for the patient. Mention of any product in this issue should not be construed as endorsement by the contributors, editors, or the Publisher of the product or manufacturers' claims.

Dermatologic Clinics (ISSN 0733-8635) is published quarterly by Elsevier Inc., 360 Park Avenue South, New York, NY 10010-1710. Months of publication are January, April, July, and October. Business and editorial offices: 1600 John F. Kennedy Blvd., Suite 1800, Philadelphia, PA 19103-2899. Customer service office: 6277 Sea Harbor Drive, Orlando, FL 32887-4800. Periodicals postage paid at New York, NY, and additional mailing offices. Subscription prices are USD 254 per year for US individuals, USD 392 per year for US institutions, USD 297 per year for Canadian individuals, USD 458 per year for Canadian institutions, USD 327 per year for international individuals, USD 458 per year for international institutions, USD 121 per year for US students, USD 164 per year for Canadian students, and USD 164 per year for international students. International air speed delivery is included in all *Clinics* subscription prices. All prices are subject to change without notice. POSTMASTER: Send address changes to *Dermatologic Clinics*, Elsevier Periodicals Customer Service, 6277 Sea Harbor Drive, Orlando, FL 32887-4800. **Customer Service: 1-800-654-2452 (US). From outside of the US, call 1-407-345-4000. E-mail: hhspcs@harcourt. com.**

Reprints. For copies of 100 or more, of articles in this publication, please contact the Commercial Reprints Department, Elsevier Inc., 360 Park Avenue South, New York, New York 10010-1710. Tel.: (212) 633-3813; Fax: (212) 462-1935; Email: repritns@elsevier.com.

The *Dermatologic Clinics* is covered in *Index Medicus, Current Contents/Clinical Medicine, Excerpta Medica, Chemical Abstracts,* and *ISI/BIOMED*.

Printed in the United States of America.

GUEST EDITORS

VALENCIA D. THOMAS, MD, Assistant Professor, Department of Dermatology, Yale Medical School, New Haven, Connecticut

CHARLES R. THOMAS, Jr., MD, Department of Radiation Medicine, Oregon Health and Science University, Portland, Oregon

CONTRIBUTORS

EDWARD AROUS, BS, Department of Radiation Oncology and the Cancer Center, The University of Massachusetts Medical School and UMass Memorial Health Care, Worcester, Worcester, Massachusetts

JESSE ARONOWITZ, MD, Department of Radiation Oncology; and The Cancer Center, The University of Massachusetts Medical School, UMass Memorial Health Care, Worcester, Massachusetts

SUSAN BALDUCCI, RN, NP, Department of Radiation Oncology; and The Cancer Center, The University of Massachusetts Medical School, UMass Memorial Health Care, Worcester, Massachusetts

MARYANN BISHOP JODOIN, BS, Department of Radiation Oncology; and The Cancer Center, The University of Massachusetts Medical School, UMass Memorial Health Care, Worcester, Massachusetts

MAUREEN BRITTON, BSN, Department of Radiation Oncology, and The Cancer Center, The University of Massachusetts Medical School, UMass Memorial Health Care, Worcester, Massachusetts

M. GIULIA CICCHETTI, MD, Department of Radiation Oncology; and The Cancer Center, The University of Massachusetts Medical School, UMass Memorial Health Care, Worcester, Massachusetts

THERESA S. DEVERE, MD, Assistant Professor of Dermatology, Department of Dermatology, Oregon Health and Science University, Portland, Oregon

LINDA DING, PhD, Department of Radiation Oncology; and The Cancer Center, The University of Massachusetts Medical School, UMass Memorial Health Care, Worcester, Massachusetts

T.J. FITZGERALD, MD, Professor and Chair, Department of Radiation Oncology; and The Cancer Center, The University of Massachusetts Medical School, UMass Memorial Health Care, Worcester, Massachusetts

LISA A. HAMMOND-THELIN, MD, San Antonio, Texas

GINETTE HINDS, MD, Department of Dermatology, Yale Medical School, New Haven, Connecticut

JIAYI HUANG, MD, Department of Radiation Oncology; and The Cancer Center, The University of Massachusetts Medical School, UMass Memorial Health Care, Worcester, Massachusetts

SIDNEY KADISH, MD, Department of Radiation Oncology; and The Cancer Center, The University of Massachusetts Medical School, UMass Memorial Health Care, Worcester, Massachusetts

CAROLINE C. KIM, MD, Instructor, Harvard Medical School; Associate Director, Cutaneous Oncology Program; and Director, Pigmented Lesion Clinic, Department of Dermatology, Beth Israel Deaconess Medical Center, Boston, Massachusetts

ABDEL KADER EL TAL, MD, Department of Dermatology, Oakwood Hospital, Cancer Center Clinic, Wayne State University, Dearborn, Michigan

PETER A. LIO, MD, Instructor in Dermatology, Department of Dermatology, Beth Israel Deaconess Medical Center; and Harvard Medical School, Boston, Massachusetts

Y.C. LO, PhD, Department of Radiation Oncology; and The Cancer Center, The University of Massachusetts Medical School, UMass Memorial Health Care, Worcester, Massachusetts

CHARLES MAYO, PhD, Department of Radiation Oncology; and The Cancer Center, The University of Massachusetts Medical School, UMass Memorial Health Care, Worcester, Massachusetts

SHELAGH McCAULEY, MD, Department of Radiation Oncology; and The Cancer Center, The University of Massachusetts Medical School, UMass Memorial Health Care, Worcester, Massachusetts

KHOSROW MEHRANY, MD, Assistant Clinical Professor of Dermatology, Department of Dermatology, University of California, San Francisco; and Stanislaus Skin Cancer Clinic, Modesto, California

JOSHUA MEYER, MD, Department of Radiation Oncology; and The Cancer Center, The University of Massachusetts Medical School, UMass Memorial Health Care, Worcester, Massachusetts

RACHAEL L. MOORE, MD, Resident, Department of Dermatology, Oregon Health and Science University, Portland, Oregon

CLARE A. PIPKIN, MD, Instructor in Dermatology, Department of Dermatology, Beth Israel Deaconess Medical Center; and Harvard Medical School, Boston, Massachusetts

RICHARD PIETERS, MD, Department of Radiation Oncology; and The Cancer Center, The University of Massachusetts Medical School, UMass Memorial Health Care, Worcester, Massachusetts

GABRIELA ROLZ-CRUZ, MD, Research Fellow, Clinical Unit for Research Trials in Skin, Department of Dermatology, Brigham and Women's Hospital, Boston, Massachusetts

DAVID A. SAUER, MD, Assistant Professor of Medicine, Division of Pathology, Oregon Health and Science University, Portland, Oregon

JOANNA SAWICKA, MD, Department of Radiation Oncology; and The Cancer Center, The University of Massachusetts Medical School, UMass Memorial Health Care, Worcester, Massachusetts

RACHEL E. SANBORN, MD, Assistant Professor of Medicine, Division of Hematology and Medical Oncology, Oregon Health and Science University, Portland, Oregon

BRIAN SOMOANO, MD, Dermatology Resident, Department of Dermatology, Stanford University Medical Center, Stanford, California

ZEINA TANNOUS, MD, Department of Dermatology, Massachusetts General Hospital, Harvard Medical School; and Department of Dermatology, Boston Veteran's Affairs Health Care System, Boston, Massachusetts

VALENCIA D. THOMAS, MD, Assistant Professor, Department of Dermatology, Yale Medical School, New Haven, Connecticut

GAYLE TILLMAN, MD, Department of Radiation Oncology; and The Cancer Center, The University of Massachusetts Medical School, UMass Memorial Health Care, Worcester, Massachusetts

CONTRIBUTORS

HENSIN TSAO, MD, PhD, Associate Professor of Dermatology, Department of Dermatology, Massachusetts General Hospital, Boston, Massachusetts

KENNETH ULIN, PhD, Department of Radiation Oncology; and The Cancer Center, The University of Massachusetts Medical School, UMass Memorial Health Care, Worcester, Massachusetts

MARCIA URIE, PhD, Department of Radiation Oncology; and The Cancer Center, The University of Massachusetts Medical School, UMass Memorial Health Care, Worcester, Massachusetts

ROGER H. WEENIG, MD, MPH, Assistant Professor of Dermatology, Department of Dermatology, Dermatopathology Division, Mayo Clinic, Rochester, Minnesota

CONTRIBUTORS

CONTENTS

FORTHCOMING ISSUES

RECENT ISSUES

THE CLINICS ARE NOW AVAILABLE ONLINE!

Access your subscription at
http://www.theclinics.com

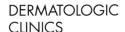

DERMATOLOGIC
CLINICS

Dermatol Clin 26 (2008) xi

Preface

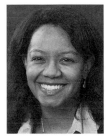 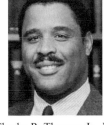

Valencia D. Thomas, MD   Charles R. Thomas, Jr., MD
Guest Editors

Rashes may not just be skin deep. The skin can be a window into the internal workings of the human body, allowing for the elegant and critical diagnosis of internal malignancies and other systemic conditions. As our largest organ, our skin is a complicated structure whose role in barrier function, homeostasis, nutrition, and immune function is indispensable. By focusing a trained eye toward the subtle signs and symptoms of the skin, we can better serve our patients.

The intricate relationship between the skin and internal malignancies is only part of the story, however. The addition of therapeutic interventions further complicates the relationship between the skin and malignancy, challenging the skin in extreme and powerful ways. Both the physician and the patient must understand and address the iatrogenic complications of chemotherapy and radiation therapy to maintain the best health possible for the patient.

This issue of *Dermatologic Clinics* is devoted to the discussion of both the cutaneous manifestations of internal malignancy and the complex relationship between cancer treatment and the integument. The authors of "Internal Malignancy and the Skin: Paraneoplastic and Cancer Treatment-Related Cutaneous Disorders" are some of the leaders in the fields of dermatology, cutaneous oncology, and radiation oncology. The collaboration between these talented individuals has resulted in a comprehensive overview of malignancy and the skin that can provide additional guidance to those treating patients who have cancer.

We would like to thank Dr. Neil Swanson, Alexandra Gavenda, Elsevier Publishing, Oregon Health Sciences University, and the various authors for their hard work and continued support.

Valencia D. Thomas, MD
Section of Cutaneous Oncology
and Dermatologic Surgery
Department of Dermatology
Yale Medical School
40 Temple Street, Suite 5A
New Haven, CT 06510, USA

E-mail address: Valencia.thomas@yale.edu

Charles R. Thomas, Jr., MD
Department of Radiation Medicine
Oregon Health and Science University
M/C L337, 3181 SW Sam Jackson Park Road
Portland, OR 97239-3098, USA

E-mail address: thomasch@ohsu.edu

ELSEVIER
SAUNDERS

Dermatol Clin 26 (2008) 1–15

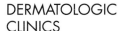

DERMATOLOGIC
CLINICS

Cutaneous Manifestations of Internal Malignancies: An Overview

Clare A. Pipkin, MD[a,b,*], Peter A. Lio, MD[a,b]

[a]Department of Dermatology, Beth Israel Deaconess Medical Center, 330 Brookline Avenue, Boston, MA 02215, USA
[b]Harvard Medical School, Boston, MA 02215, USA

Though it has been said that the eyes are the window to the soul, it may also be said that the skin is the window to within. The skin can provide important clues to systemic diseases, enabling the practitioner to make a tremendous contribution to patient care if a cutaneous disorder associated with malignancy can be identified. This article focuses on the best-described disorders that have cutaneous manifestations associated with internal malignancy or neoplasms (Table 1). In these paraneoplastic disorders, the skin condition generally occurs at a distance from the primary tumor site. Though mechanisms are speculative in most cases, it is hypothesized that mediators such as growth factors, cytokines, or hormones are involved in the pathogenesis of the cutaneous findings. The authors do not address cutaneous metastases of internal tumors, nor do we address genodermatoses with malignant potential in this article. Curth [1] proposed criteria by which a causal relationship between a dermatosis and a malignant internal disease might be evaluated. These requirements include the following: (1) both conditions start at the same time, (2) both conditions follow a parallel course, (3) the condition is not recognized as part of a genetic syndrome, (4) a specific tumor occurs with a certain dermatosis, (5) the dermatosis is not common, and (6) a high percentage of the association is noted. As the authors review each disorder, we will try to address each of her requirements. Recognition of these disorders is important for the practitioner, so that in the best case scenario, he or she may aid in diagnosing a cancer in the early stages of disease.

Acanthosis nigricans and tripe palms

Acanthosis nigricans (AN) was initially reported by Pollitzer and Janovsky separately in the same edition of Unna's famous *International Atlas of Rare Skin Diseases* in 1890 [2]. Pollitzer [3] described a 62-year-old woman who developed characteristic findings, including areas of skin that "project above the general level almost like papillae ... to form a diffuse, discolored warty surface." Although some 80% of AN is associated with benign conditions such as obesity and endocrine abnormalities, Pollitzer's patient died within the year from a presumed "carcinoma occultum," thus setting the stage for AN's paraneoplastic status. AN presents clinically with velvety hyperpigmentation of the skin, sometimes progressing to more thickened verrucous changes with papillary lesions. Intertriginous areas, especially the axillae, neck, and inguinal area, are most commonly affected, although the changes can affect the oral mucosa, lips, and traumatized areas of skin [4]. In 25% of cases, palmar and plantar hyperkeratosis may also be present [5], though there is some disagreement about whether or not this can also occur as a distinct entity [6]. Tripe palm (TP; so named for the rugated appearance of the skin) has also been referred to "acanthosis palmaris," and "acanthosis nigricans of the palms," and thus may represent a variation of AN rather than a separate disease. Indeed, in Pollitzer's initial description, he observes: "The palms are

* Corresponding author. Department of Dermatology, Beth Israel Deaconess Medical Center, 330 Brookline Avenue, Boston, MA 02215.
E-mail address: clarepipkin@gmail.com (C.A. Pipkin).

Table 1
Cutaneous disorders associated with internal malignancy or neoplasms

Disorder	Clinical findings	Associated malignancy or plasma cell disorder
Acanthosis nigricans	Velvety or verrucous hyperpigmentation of intertriginous areas	Gastric adenocarcinoma
Acquired ichthyosis	Fishlike scale on arms and legs	Hodgkin's disease
Pityriasis rotunda	Scaling patches on the trunk	Hepatocellular carcinoma
Acrokeratosis paraneoplastica	Psoriasiform scaling of acral surfaces, ears, nasal bridge, keratoderma	Squamous cell carcinoma of aerodigestive tract
Erythema gyratum repens	Migrating bands of erythema with a wood-grainlike pattern	Lung, esophageal, breast carcinoma
Sign of Leser-Trélat	Diffuse abrupt onset of seborrheic keratoses	Questionable association with adenocarcinoma of stomach, colon, and breast
Erythroderma	Generalized erythema and desquamation	Cutaneous T-cell lymphoma
Hypertrichosis lanuginosa acquisita	Fine, downy hair on face and other areas	Colorectal, lung, and breast carcinoma
Sweet's syndrome	Edematous, mammillated plaques on head and neck	Acute myelogenous leukemia, other hematologic malignancies
Dermatomyositis	Proximal muscle weakness, photodistributed violaceous poikiloderma, nailfold telangiectasia, Gottron's papules	Ovarian, lung, gastrointestinal carcinomas, nasopharyngeal carcinoma in Southeast Asians
Paraneoplastic pemphigus	Stomatitis and other mucosal erosions, flaccid bullae	Non-Hodgkin's lymphoma, chronic lymphocytic leukemia, Castleman's disease
Necrobiotic xanthogranuloma	Yellowish plaques and nodules, especially in periorbital area	Plasma cell dyscrasia, rarely multiple myeloma
Multicentric reticulohistiocytosis	Papulonodular lesions of the hands, arthritis of the hands	No predominant cancer
Primary amyloidosis	Purpura, waxy papules, macroglossia	Plasma cell dyscrasia, multiple myeloma
Scleromyxedema	Symmetric waxy papules that may progress to leonine facies, sclerodermoid changes	Plasma cell dyscrasia
Scleredema	Non-pitting edema around neck and upper back	Lymphomas and multiple myeloma
Vasculitis	Palpable purpura	Hematologic malignancies
Hypertrophic osteoarthropathy	Clubbing of digits, periosteal new bone formation	Lung cancer
Necrolytic migratory erythema	Superficial erosions, vesicles, bullae often in groin	Alpha-cell pancreatic tumors
Carcinoid syndrome	Episodic flushing	Carcinoid tumors
Cushing's syndrome	Hyperpigmentation, edema, proximal muscle weakness	Oat cell carcinoma of lung
Pruritus	No abnormality	Hodgkin's disease

slightly darker than normal, their furrows and folds are strongly marked, and the skin feels dry, hard and thickened" [3]. Histologically, AN shows hyperkeratosis, papillomatosis, and some degree of acanthosis with thickening of the stratum spinosum [4]. The dark color is thought to be from the hyperkeratosis rather than melanin [7]. TP shows very similar histologic features to AN, supporting their possible connection [5]. The malignancy most commonly associated with

AN is adenocarcinoma, most frequently gastric in origin [8]. It seems most commonly to develop simultaneously with the malignancy, but may precede it by years [8]. Because AN and TP tend to closely parallel the underlying cancer, it has been suggested that they may be pathophysiologically related to them via growth factors such as transforming growth factor-α [8]. Beyond treatment of the underlying tumor, treatment suggestions for AN include acitretin [9], tretinoin, and ammonium lactate [10].

Acquired ichthyosis

Acquired ichthyosis clinically resembles ichthyosis vulgaris, and is characterized by numerous symmetrical rhomboidal or fishlike scales, primarily on the arms and legs. The flexural surfaces are relatively spared. Acquired ichthyosis may be associated with a variety of disorders, including malnutrition, hypothyroidism, sarcoidosis, leprosy, acquired immune deficiency, and certain medication use. A subset of acquired ichthyosis may also be associated with an underlying malignancy, most commonly associated with Hodgkin's disease [11]. One series found Hodgkin's disease in 70% to 80% of malignancy-associated cases [12]. Other associated malignancies include multiple myeloma, cutaneous T-cell lymphoma, and other lymphoproliferative disorders. Solid tumors make up a small proportion of cases. Breast, lung, ovary, cervix, leiomyosarcoma, and Kaposi's sarcoma have been reported [12]. The cutaneous changes typically appear several weeks or months after other manifestations of the malignancy [12]. The pathogenesis of ichthyosis is uncertain; however, in patients who have Hodgkin's disease, malabsorption and low levels of vitamin A have been reported [12]. Other studies have implicated impaired lipogenesis as a mechanism [13]. The histology reveals orthokeratosis, a thin or absent granular layer, and mild acanthosis. Treatment consists of topical agents containing salicylic acid, alpha-hydroxy acid, or urea, with the goal being to remove scale and hydrate the skin.

Pityriasis rotunda

Pityriasis rotunda is a rare skin disorder characterized by circular, sharply demarcated scaling patches that are lighter or darker than the surrounding skin. The lesions typically occur on the trunk, are generally multiple, and may become confluent. There is no associated inflammation or pruritus. Some authors believe that pityriasis rotunda may represent a form of localized acquired ichthyosis [14]. The disorder was first described in Japanese patients. In one review, more than one third of patients had an associated disease [15]. This disorder has also been described in West Indian populations, South African blacks, and African-Americans. It is rarely reported in Koreans, Manchurians, and Egyptians [15]. Diseases that have been associated include tuberculosis, leprosy, and liver and pulmonary disease. Malignancies that have been associated include hepatocellular carcinoma, and carcinoma of the stomach, esophagus, palate, and prostate, as well as chronic lymphocytic leukemia and multiple myeloma [15]. This disorder may also be seen as a hereditary disorder in Caucasian patients. Histologically, a decreased granular cell layer is seen [14]. Most topical treatments are unsuccessful [15].

Acrokeratosis paraneoplastica

Acrokeratosis paraneoplastica (APN) was first described by Bazex and colleagues as a marker of malignancy in 1965. Bazex and Griffiths [16] described the progression of disease in three stages. The first stage is characterized by erythema and psoriasiform scaling of the fingers, toes, and margin of the helix, as well as violaceous erythema and pityriasiform scaling over the nasal bridge. Nail changes are frequent and may include tender nailfolds, subungual hyperkeratoses, and onycholysis. In the second stage, the scaling involves the entire hands and feet, producing a keratoderma with a violaceous color. The skin appears edematous and the palms may have a honeycomb appearance. The scaling may progress to involve the entire pinna as well. At this stage, the neoplasm may give either localizing or systemic symptoms. In the third stage, additional areas may be involved, such as the knees, legs, arms, and scalp. Bullous lesions have been described primarily on the hands and feet [17]. Several patients have had associated paraneoplastic phenomena of acquired ichthyosis, pruritus, dermatomyositis, the sign of Léser-Trelat, and clubbing [17]. APN is highly correlated with malignancy. One review found that all cases of APN have had an associated underlying malignancy [18]. In a review of 113 cases [17], the psoriasiform lesions preceded the diagnosis of the associated malignancy in 67% of the cases. The skin lesions were present on average 12 months before the diagnosis. In only 15% of cases, the skin manifestations occurred after the diagnosis. Ninety-three percent of cases that were adequately described improved significantly when the underlying malignancy was treated. Occasional reappearance of the skin lesions may herald the recurrence of disease [17]. The majority of cases are associated with a squamous cell carcinoma of the upper aerodigestive tract. The histopathology of skin lesions show significant overlap with those of psoriasis, and include hyperkeratosis, acanthosis, parakeratosis, and perivascular lymphohistiocytic infiltrate [17]. Diagnostic testing may initially include chest radiograph, complete blood count, serum transaminases, upper endoscopy, and CT of the chest and abdomen. It is rare for the skin lesions to clear spontaneously without adequate treatment of the underlying cancer [17]. Etretinate has been used with variable success.

Erythema gyratum repens

Erythema gyratum repens (EGR) is a rare disorder and is considered to be highly specific as paraneoplastic syndrome [19]. It was first described in 1952 by Gammel [20], who reported a female who had an eruption consisting of "erythema in irregular wavy bands with ... marginal desquamation." He likened the pattern of the erythema to that of graining of a knotty cypress board, and noted that the bands moved constantly at the rate of about 1 cm per day [20]. Hands and feet were spared. The rash cleared rapidly following the removal of a breast cancer discovered during evaluation. In one review of 49 cases, 84% of the patients had an associated malignancy [21]. The male-to-female ratio was 2:1, with an average onset age of 63 years. Most patients had their eruption on average 9 months before the cancer diagnosis [21]. The most commonly associated cancer was lung cancer, followed by esophageal cancer and breast cancer. In rare instances, a primary malignancy could not be identified [21]. The course of the rash closely follows that of the underlying illness [22]. Nonmalignant EGR has been rarely associated with a variety of conditions, including tuberculosis and calcinosis, Raynaud's phenomenon, esophageal dysmotility, sclerodactyly, and telangiectasia (CREST) syndrome [19,21]. Patients who develop the classic eruption should be assumed to have an underlying malignancy and screened aggressively [21]. Less common additional skin manifestations may include palmoplantar hyperkeratosis, onychodystrophy, and ichthyosis of

the extremities [19]. The most common associated symptom is intense pruritus [19]. A peripheral eosinophilia may be seen [21], though this may represent a nonspecific abnormality in the setting of an underlying malignancy [23]. The histology is nonspecific. Mild to moderate hyperkeratosis, parakeratosis, and spongiosis of the epidermis may be seen, as well as a perivascular lymphocytic infiltrate [21]. The etiology remains unclear, but it is speculated that it involves an immunologic mechanism. There have been reports of granular deposits of immunoglobulin G (IgG) and C3 protein found at the basement membrane zone of involved skin [23,24]; however, these results have not been a consistent finding [25]. Treatment of the EGR is achieved by optimally treating the underlying malignancy. After the tumor is treated, the erythema and pruritus will begin to resolve [19]. In the absence of successful tumor clearance, antihistamines and topical steroids have been tried, generally without success [20,22].

The sign of Leser-Trélat

The sign of Leser-Trélat refers to the abrupt onset of and rapid increase in size and number of seborrheic keratoses. As a historical note, both Leser and Trélat made their observations about a link between angioma and malignancy [26]. De Bersaques [26] reports that Holländer was the first to note an association between seborrheic keratoses and malignancy. Because both seborrheic keratoses and malignancy are more common with increasing age, many have doubted the existence of this sign [27], and another large study failed to support the validity of this sign [28]. In approximately 20% of patients, acanthosis nigricans has also been noted [29]. In these instances, the sign may be regarded as part of a disease spectrum [27]. Pruritus and inflammation of the seborrheic keratoses are inconsistent features [27]. The sign of Leser-Trélat has been associated with adencarcinoma, most frequently of the stomach, colon, and breast. Lymphoproliferative disorders compose an additional 20% of cases [30]. In cases of concurrent Leser-Trélat and AN, elevated transforming growth factor-a has been hypothesized to cause both findings [31]. Elevation of urine epidermal growth factor and insulinlike growth factor have also been found in patients who have the sign of Leser-Trélat [30]. The relevance of these findings has not been established. The pathology of a lesion is that of a seborrheic keratosis. No specific treatment is required for such lesions.

Erythroderma

Erythroderma is a condition characterized by generalized erythema and desquamation. Generalized adenopathy, hypothermia, high-output cardiac failure, and hypoalbuminemia may be present. Though most cases are related to medications or pre-existing skin conditions such as atopic dermatitis, a subset is also linked to malignancy. In one series of 82 cases [32], 20% were related to lymphoreticular neoplasm, primarily cutaneous T-cell lymphoma (CTCL). In this series, CTCL was more likely to be the underlying cause if the erythroderma had an insidious onset and a chronic course [32]. Other lymphoreticular disorders and solid tumors have also rarely been associated [33]. In patients who have CTCL, the erythroderma may be considered more of a direct result of tumor invasion rather than a paraneoplastic phenomenon [34].

Hypertrichosis lanuginosa acquisita

Hypertrichosis lanuginosa acquisita (HLA) was first described in 1865 in a patient who had a "thick crop of short and white downy hair" suffering from breast cancer [35]. Since that time, approximately fifty additional cases have been described in the literature [36]. The disorder was termed "malignant down" by Fretzin [37], and later given the current name based on the resemblance of the observed hair to the lanugo hair present during fetal development [38]. In 73% of cases, the disorder has been reported in females [39]. In females, the most commonly associated neoplasms are colorectal, lung, and breast cancer. In males, lung and colorectal carcinoma are most common [39]. Although HLA may appear up to 2.5 years before the diagnosis of the tumor [30], the majority of cases are seen in the later stages of disease, when the tumor has become metastatic [40]. Most patients live less than 3 years after the diagnosis [39]. HLA is strongly associated with malignancy [5]. The syndrome is characterized by the abrupt onset of fine, downy hair, typically on the face, and has been reported to follow a craniocaudal spread [38]. The hair may appear elsewhere on the body as well; however, it typically spares the palms and soles [36]. Associated findings commonly include glossitis, papillary hypertrophy of the tongue, and disturbances of taste

[39]. Weight loss, lymph node enlargement, and diarrhea are less commonly seen [39]. Some authors have postulated that the glossitis may be secondary to a manifestation of vitamin deficiency [4]. It has been hypothesized that the hair growth is stimulated by an as yet unidentified growth factor secreted by the tumor [36]. No consistent hormonal or biochemical abnormality has been identified to date [40]. Like vellus hairs, the hairs of HLA have a fine texture, are pale or colorless, and are nonmedullated [40]. Histologically, the hairs of HLA have been described as small, and are often found implanted in a horizontal or parallel position to the epidermis, in contrast to normal vertical position seen in terminal and vellus hairs [36,41,42]. Follicles have been noted to be surrounded by small mantles representing immature sebaceous ducts [42]. Treatment for HLA, if desired, consists of standard hair removal techniques such as electrolysis, depilatories, or shaving [30].

Sweet's syndrome

Sweet's syndrome was first described in 1964 as "acute febrile neutrophilic dermatosis" in a series of eight patients with the features of fever, neutrophilia, painful plaques on the limbs, face, and neck, and histologically a dense dermal infiltrate of neutrophils [43]. Since then more than 500 cases have been described, with a female predominance of 4 to 1 [44]. The associated conditions are varied and include many systemic disorders [45]. In most series, approximately 20% of cases are secondary to malignancy [46]; however, one review of 48 cases showed an unusually high percentage (54%) of malignancy-related Sweet's syndrome [45]. The majority of cases are associated with acute myelogenous leukemia, additional hematologic malignancies, and rarely, solid tumors (genitourinary, breast, gastrointestinal carcinomas) [47,48]. Initial series showed that in malignancy-associated Sweet's syndrome, male-to-female incidence was roughly equal [47]; however, not all series have supported this finding [45,46]. Risk factors for malignancy include concomitant anemia and thrombocytopenia [45,46]. The onset of Sweet's syndrome either precedes or is concurrent with the discovery of a previously undiagnosed cancer in more than 60% of patients [47]. Recurrences are more common in cancer-related cases and reappearance of lesions may represent recurrent malignancy [48]. In malignancy-associated cases, fever may be absent [49].

Erythematous tender papules or plaques are present on the head, neck, and upper extremities. because of the intense edema within the dermis, the skin surface may have a mammillated appearance. Some lesions may even develop vesiculation, pustules, or bullae [44]. The evolution to bullae or even ulceration has been associated with malignancy [49]. Mucosal involvement, though rare, has been strongly correlated with malignancy [45]. Extracutaneous sites of involvement are many, and include eyes, joints, and lungs. The pathogenesis of Sweet's syndrome is still poorly understood [50]. Histologically, the hallmark is a dense infiltrate composed of mature neutrophils, usually in the upper half of the dermis, with a variable degree of edema. True leukocytoclastic vasculitis is absent [50]. More recently, in some cases of hematologic malignancy-associated Sweet's syndrome, skin lesions have shown concurrent leukemia cutis [48]. As in idiopathic Sweet's syndrome, first-line treatment consists of corticosteroids [45]. Recommended evaluation includes a detailed physical examination, complete blood count with differential, serum chemistries, Pap smear in women, stool guaiac, urinalysis and urine culture, chest radiograph, sigmoidoscopy if older than 50, and endometrial biopsy in selected individuals. Complete blood count should be repeated every 6 to 12 months [49].

Additionally, atypical pyoderma gangrenosum has been also associated with myeloproliferative disorders, particularly acute myelogenous leukemia [51]. It has been suggested that Sweet's syndrome and pyoderma gangrenosum may represent different ends of the spectrum of the same disease process [42].

Dermatomyositis

Dermatomyositis (DM) is characterized by clinical and laboratory signs of a proximal muscle extensor inflammatory myopathy and a photodistributed violaceous poikiloderma involving scalp, periocular, and extensor skin sites with nailfold telangiectasias [52]. When lesions occur on the knuckles and become lichenified, they are called Gottron's papules. Subsets of the disease include polymyositis (PM), in which the cutaneous features are absent, and amyopathic dermatomyositis, where the muscles are unaffected. The first case of malignancy-associated DM was reported by Stretz [5] in 1916 in a patient who had gastric carcinoma. Since that time, many reviews have been conducted, primarily in Scandinavia and East Asia, to ascertain the link between adult DM and malignancy. Most studies demonstrate a significant increase in the risk of cancer in DM (range from 6%–60%, though probably closest to 25%) and a modest increase in PM [5,53,54]. Whether the increased risk in PM reflects a detection bias has been asked [55]. It has been shown that patients who have DM have an increase in malignancy-related mortality, whereas patients who have PM do not [56]. There are insufficient data to determine if amyopathic DM also has an increased risk of malignancy [56]. Malignancies may occur prior to, concurrent with, or after the onset of DM, and treatment of the malignancy may or may not improve the symptoms of DM [57]. The most closely associated malignancies include ovarian, lung, pancreatic, stomach, colorectal, and lymphomas. Studies involving primarily ethnically Chinese patients from Southeast Asia have demonstrated an increase in nasopharyngeal carcinoma [53,58]. Indicators that may favor malignancy include rapid onset of disease, cutaneous necrosis, absence of Raynaud's phenomenon, and elevated erythrocyte sedimentation rate [59]. The presence of interstitial lung disease has been noted to be correlated with non–malignancy-related DM [53]. Histologically, the hallmark of this disorder is a vacuolar interface dermatitis. There may be epidermal atrophy, interstitial mucin deposition, and a sparse lymphocytic infiltrate. Muscle biopsy specimens show a combination of Type II muscle fiber atrophy, necrosis, regeneration ,and hypertrophy, with centralized sarcolemmal nuclei and lymphocytes in both perifascicular and perivascular distribution [52]. Though there is a great variation as to how aggressively screen patients who have DM, it has been recommended that all patients who have DM have an evaluation that includes complete blood count, metabolic panel, fecal blood examination, and CT scans of chest and abdomen. In women, additional tests should include mammogram, pelvic CT scan, and gynecologic examination [55]. Southeast Asian patients should also have a careful ear, nose, and throat examination [56]. All patients should be up-to-date on age-appropriate screening tests. Because the risk of malignant disease remains elevated for many years after diagnosis, vigilance must be maintained and any new symptom should be evaluated thoroughly [55]. Treatment of malignancy-related DM is the same as nonmalignancy DM: oral prednisone is the mainstay of treatment. Other systemic treatments include methotrexate and azathioprine. For cutaneous lesions, treatments include sunscreen, topical corticosteroids, and hydroxychloroquine [56].

Paraneoplastic pemphigus

The concept of paraneoplastic pemphigus (PNP) has evolved from an initial observation that pemphigus occurred more frequently in patients who had known malignancy. This led to the recognition in 1990 by Anhaltz of a unique bullous disease with a characteristic autoantibody profile. Since that time, additional autoantibodies have been detected [60]. Although the presentation can be quite variable, the most constant feature is the development of painful and persistent stomatitis [61]. Other mucosal surfaces, including conjunctiva and genitalia, may be involved. There may be blistering and erosions of the trunk and extremities. In some cases, lichenoid lesions may predominate. Surrounding erythema of some lesions may resemble erythema multiforme, and confluent lesions may mimic toxic epidermal necrolysis. In contrast to pemphigus vulgaris, acral and paronychial involvement is common [61]. The average age of onset is 59 years, and there is no gender predominance [5]. In two thirds of patients, the neoplasm is recognized before diagnosis. The most common neoplasms include non-Hodgkin's lymphoma, chronic lymphocytic leukemia, and Castleman's disease. Less common associations include retroperitoneal sarcoma, thymoma, and Waldenstrom's disease [61]. In the pediatric population, Castleman's disease is the underlying disease in almost all cases [61]. Evolution of the disease differs according to whether the neoplasm is benign or malignant [61,62]. When PNP is associated with a malignancy, 90% of patients will die between 1 month to 2 years after diagnosis [63]. Respiratory failure is a common terminal event. Because of variation in clinical presentation, histology is correspondingly heterogeneous.

Biopsy of lesional skin may show epidermal suprabasilar acantholysis, lichenoid, or interface change. Inflammation may be present in contrast to other types of pemphigus [64]. Perilesional direct immunofluorescence (IF) will demonstrate IgG and complement in epidermal intercellular areas as well as a granular-linear pattern at the basement membrane zone; however, direct IF is frequently negative, and serologic markers should be obtained. The key serologic marker for this disorder is the presence of antiplakin antibodies, including periplakin or envoplakin [61]. Serum

from patients will react with transitional epithelium (in contrast to other blistering disorders), and for this reason, a positive test for IgG autoantibodies by indirect IF on rodent bladder may confirm the diagnosis. Immunochemical techniques can most precisely characterize the antibodies present in the serum, however. Additional antibodies may include those directed at: desmoglein 3, desmoglein 1, bullous pemphigoid antigen 1, desmoplakin I, desmoplakin II, plectin, and plakoglobin [61]. The evaluation for malignancy should include a thorough physical examination of the liver, spleen, and lymph nodes. Laboratory investigation should include complete blood count, serum protein electrophoresis, and CT of the chest, abdomen, and pelvis [63]. First-line treatment for PNP is oral corticosteroids. A variety of other treatments often used in combination with corticosteroids, includes cyclophosphamide, azathioprine, gold, dapsone, plasmapheresis, high-dose intravenous immunoglobulin, and rituximab [61].

Necrobiotic xanthogranuloma

Necrobiotic xanthogranuloma (NXG) was first described in 1980 by Kossard and Winkelmann [65]. This disease is characterized by multiple yellowish or xanthomatous plaques and subcutaneous nodules, often found in a periorbital distribution. A subset of lesions may ulcerate, and there is a predilection for lesions to develop in scars. Most cases are asymptomatic. In one review of 48 cases, 80% of cases in which protein electrophoresis was performed revealed an abnormality [66]. The majority had an IgG-kappa paraprotein, and the remainder had either IgG-lambda paraprotein or an unspecified IgG paraprotein [66]. A small percentage of patients also had cryoglobulinemia. Other features that have been seen include leucopenia and hypocomplementemia [66]. Rare progression to multiple myeloma or myelodysplastic syndrome was observed in this series. In one small series, malignancy was shown to occur up to 8 years before and 11 years after the skin lesions developed [67]. Chronic lymphocytic leukemia, Hodgkin's disease, and non-Hodgkin's lymphoma are also rarely associated [5]. The pathogenesis is not well understood. Histologically, there are large areas of necrobiosis and granulomatous foci composed of histiocytes, foam cells, and multinucleate giant cells. Giant cells may be both Touton and foreign-body type [42]. Cholesterol clefts may sometimes be seen [42]. Various treatments have been tried with limited success, including local corticosteroid injection, plasmapheresis, methotrexate, azathioprine, melphalan, chlorambucil, cyclophosphamide, nitrogen mustard, prednisone, and interferon alpha-2b [67]. Radiation has occasionally been used. Excision of lesions is associated with a high recurrence rate (42% in one study) and the development of lesions larger than original surgical scars [67].

Multicentric reticulohistiocytosis

Multicentric reticulohistiocytosis (MR) is a rare disorder characterized by joint symptoms and papulonodular skin lesions. Fewer than 200 cases have been published [68]. About 40% of cases present with joint symptoms first [68]. A symmetric arthritis typically affects the hands. The skin lesions are typically skin-colored, dome-shaped, symmetrical papules or nodules. They are found on the upper half of the body, with hands being the most common site, followed by the face. The characteristic "coral bead" sign refers to papules found along the nailfold. Vermicular erythematous lesions bordering the nostrils and lesions clinically resembling eyelid xanthelasmas, though uncommon, are also characteristic. Other rare presenting symptoms may be dysphagia caused by involvement of the esophagus with nodules [68]. Weight loss and fever may also been seen in a minority of patients [68]. Progression to arthritis mutilans occurs in about half of patients [34]. The association with malignancy has been found to vary between 20% and 31% [68]. In 75% of cases, the MR preceded the diagnosis of cancer [34]. No predominant cancer has been seen in this disorder, and MR does not usually run a course parallel to neoplasm [68]. An evaluation for malignancy is recommended, though not targeted at any specific organ or disease. Pathologically, a well-circumscribed nodular infiltrate of histiocytic cells and multinucleated giant cells with a ground glass cytoplasm are seen. There may be collagen phagocytosis activity of the histiocytes [68]. For treatment, cyclophasamide and methotrexate are often used; however, no therapy has been shown to have a consistent benefit. The disease tends to remit spontaneously after 8 years on average [34].

Amyloidosis

Amyloidosis represents a diverse group of disorders that share the common feature of extracellular deposition of pathologic fibrillar proteins. The classificiation of amyloidosis is based on the nature of the precursor protein. In primary amyloidosis, clonal plasma cells produce immunoglobulins, usually lambda light chains that are amyloidogenic. The clinical features vary on the organs primarily affected. Renal failure is reported in 28% of cases, congestive heart failure in 17%, carpal tunnel syndrome in 21%, polyneuropathy in 17%, and orthostatic hypotension in 11% [69]. Cutaneous involvement occurs in 29% to 40% of cases [70]. Purpura, particularly in the periorbital area and often called "pinch purpura," is present in about 15% of cases [69]. Other findings include waxy papules and plaques in flexural areas, around the eyes and retroauricular areas. When these lesions are widespread, they may resemble xanthomas [70]. Other findings include accumulation of amyloid around the shoulders, leading to the "shoulder pad sign" [71]. Macroglossia may be present. Primary amyloidosis is usually associated with a monoclonal gammopathy of uncertain significance, and less commonly multiple myeloma [30]. About 12% to 15% of patients who have multiple myeloma will develop clinical manifestations of amyloidosis [72]. In most patients, immunofixation of serum and urine will detect a monoclonal protein [73]. Demonstration of amyloid in tissue is also required for diagnosis. The amyloid will stain positively with a Congo red stain, and will demonstrate apple green birefringence under polarized light. Subcutaneous fat pad aspirate and bone marrow are the preferred biopsy sites [73]. The mainstay of treatment has been melphalan and prednisone. Newer treatment modalities include autologous stem cell transplant, and for those cases associated with multiple myeloma, lenalomide and bortezomid show promise [73].

Scleromyxedema

Scleromyxedema or lichen myxedematosus was first reported by Dubreuilh in 1906 under the name "fibromes militaries folliculares" [5]. Specifically, scleromyxedema refers to the generalized variant of lichen myxedematosus with four features: (1) papular and sclerodermoid lesions, (2) mucin deposition and fibrosis with fibroblast proliferation, (3) monoclonal gammopathy, and (4) the absence of thyroid disease [74]. It is an uncommon disease with no gender predilection, which presents as a widespread symmetric eruption of small waxy papules, with a predilection for the head and neck, arms, and upper trunk

[75]. Erythema and edema with pigmentary alteration may also occur. Frequently the glabella shows deep longitudinal furrowing that may progress to more diffuse involvement of the face, leading to leonine facies [5,76]. Over time, sclerodermoid changes may occur, resulting in the loss of joint mobility and skin stiffening. Unlike scleroderma, however, calcinosis and telangeictasia are absent [76]. Systemic manifestations may include dysphagia, proximal muscle weakness, and peripheral neuropathies, carpal tunnel syndrome, or a scleroderma-like renal disease [5,75]. Histologically, scleromyxedema is characterized by diffuse mucin deposition in the dermis, increased collagen, and proliferation of irregular fibroblasts [75]. Scleromyxedema is associated with a monoclonal gammopathy, generally IgG-delta type, but usually these are of unclear significance and are not clearly malignant. The pathophysiology remains unclear [77]. Therapy is generally unsatisfactory, and much of the evidence is anecdotal, with reports of responses to corticosteroids, melphalan, methotrexate, extracorporeal photochemotherapy, plasmapheresis, thalidomide, intravenous immunoglobulin, and even autologous peripheral blood stem cell transplant [77].

Scleredema

Scleredema adultorum of Buschke is an uncommon dermatosis most frequently associated with diabetes mellitus; however, it has been reported to be a paraneoplastic syndrome in lymphomas and myeloma [78–81]. Initially described in 1752 by Curzio, it was formalized in 1902 when Buschke described a patient who had progressive skin hardening that began at the neck after influenza [78]. It presents as firm, indurated non-pitting edema around the neck and upper back, and can progress to woody sclerosis over larger areas of the body. Three variants exist: (1) following an acute febrile illness (Buschke's original description), (2) progressive type with or without underlying disease, and (3) associated with diabetes mellitus (Krakowski type) [82]. Clinically, it must be distinguished from scleromyxedema and scleroderma. On biopsy, the dermis is greatly expanded. There is usually abundant thickened collagen with mucin between the bundles in edematous spaces. Unlike in scleromyxedema, there is no increase in the number of fibroblasts [83]. Other organ systems can be involved, including the heart, bone, and liver, as well as the eyes [84]. As in scleromyxedema,

treatments are highly variable, with no clear consensus [78]. Therapies include systemic corticosteroids, antibiotics, cyclosporine, electron beam therapy, and ultraviolet A-1 (UVA-1) [85,86]. Of these, electron beam therapy and UVA-1 seem very promising, but require further study.

Vasculitis and cryoglobulinemia

Purpura, which manifests as non-blanching violaceous or erythematous lesions secondary to red blood cell extravasation, may be rarely associated with underlying malignancy. The purpura may either be caused by vasculitis or cryoglobulinemia. According to a review by Wooten and Jasin [87], 1% of cases of vasculitis were associated with a lymphoproliferative disorder. The most common association is a leukocytoclastic vasculitis, of which palpable purura, particularly of the lower extremities, is the hallmark. A variety of disorders have been associated, including lymphocytic lymphoma, cutaneous T-cell lymphoma, Hodgkin's disease, chronic lymphocytic leukemia, and hairy cell leukemia [87]. Hairy cell leukemia has also been associated with polyarteritis nodosa [87].

Cryoglobulenemia is characterized by a cold-induced precipitation of immunoglobulin or cryoglobulin in blood vessels of the skin and internal organs [64]. Type I cryoglobulinemia is the result of a monoclonal cryoglobulin. This is frequently associated with multiple myeloma, Waldenstrom's macroglobulenemia, and other B-cell malignancies. In addition to purpura, ischemic ulceration, livedo reticularis, acrocyanosis, Raynaud's phenomenon, and arterial thrombosis may be seen. The histology of a pupuric lesion will show small vessels in the upper dermis filled with homogenous, eosinophilic material that is periodic acid and Schiff's reagent (PAS)-positive. No vasculitis is present [42]. Types II and III cryoglobulinemia are categorized as mixed cryoglobulenemias. They are more commonly associated with chronic inflammatory disorders, such as hepatitis C and collagen vascular disease. Type II, which has a monoclonal rheumatoid factor, is rarely associated with B-cell malignancies [64]. Additional features may include arthritis, arthralgias, renal disease, and neuropathy. The primary histologic feature is one of leukocytoclastic vasculitis.

Hypertrophic osteoarthropathy

Clubbing refers to focal enlargement of the connective tissue in the terminal phalanges of the digits, especially on the dorsal surfaces. Clubbing is associated with a variety of underlying cardio-pulmonary diseases. Hypertrophic osteoarthropathy (HOA) is a systemic disorder of the bones, joints, and soft tissues. It is characterized by clubbing of the digits, periosteal new bone formation, particularly of the distal extremities, and symmetric arthritis-like changes in the joints and periarticular tissues, most commonly affecting the ankles, knees, wrists, and elbows [88]. In those cases associated with an underlying neoplasm, the new bone formation is usually monolayered and spares the epiphyses [89]. Bone scintigraphy has emerged as the most sensitive test for HOA [88]. In adults, more than 80% of cases have been associated with lung cancer, usually bronco-genic carcinoma [89]. Other associations include metastatic disease to the lung (often sarcoma) and mesothelioma. The most effective treatment for HOA is treatment of the underlying condition. Nonsteroidal anti-inflammatory agents have been found to be effective for joint and bone pain [88].

Necrolytic migratory erythema

Necrolytic migratory erythema (NME), or the cutaneous manifestation of the glucagonoma syndrome, was first described in 1942 by Becker and colleagues [5]. It is a widespread eruption that presents as irregular patches of erythema with superficial erosions, vesicles, and bullae. These lesions may have arcuate or polycyclic forms, and tend to be more prominent on the central areas of the body, often concentrating on the groin [90]. NME may also show lesions around the mouth, and patients may have frank glossitis as well. In addition to the skin lesions, systemic symptoms are common including hyper-glycemia, weight loss, and diarrhea, all seemingly related to increased glucagon levels produced by the α-cell pancreatic tumor [91]. Because of similarities to the eruption of zinc deficiency and other dermatoses, particularly nutritional deficiencies, however, it is frequently misdiagnosed, and diagnosis is often delayed [92]. Interestingly, it has been hypothesized that zinc, essential fatty acids, or amino acids may be deficient, either primarily or secondarily, and this may explain the clinical similarities to these disorders. The fact that NME has been seen in the setting of malabsorption syndromes, hepatic failure, inflammatory bowel disease, and celiac disease without evidence of glucagonoma supports this [93]. Necrolytic acral erythema is a closely related dermatosis that is associated with hepatitis C infection, and may simply represent part of a spectrum of disease [94,95]. Histology may be nonspecific and may show different features, depending on the stage of the eruption [5]. Psoriasiform hyperplasia and parakaratosis with epidermal vacuolization and necrosis are commonly described, along with spongiosis and dyskeratotic cells in the epidermis [5,96]. Successful treatment of NME has been reported with somatostatin analogs [97], resection of the tumor [91], liver transplant [98], interferon [99], ribavirin [100], and zinc [101].

Carcinoid syndrome

Carcinoid tumors are derived from neuroen-docrine cells most commonly found in the small intestine. Carcinoid tumors located within the gastrointestinal tract rarely cause cutaneous manifestations unless the tumor is metastatic to the liver. Carcinoid tumors outside of the gastrointestinal tract may produce symptoms in the absence of metastasis. In patients who have carcinoid syndrome, approximately 85% will have episodic flushing of the face, neck, and upper chest [102]. Over time, with repeated flushing, telangiectasias may develop. The other cardinal features of the syndrome are diarrhea and bronchial constriction, resulting in asthma attacks. The cause of the symptoms is an overproduction of serotonin by the tumor. As tryptophan is consumed in producing serotonin, a pellagra-like eruption may also be seen. The diagnosis is made by demonstrating an elevated 5-hydroxyin-dolacetic acid level in the urine. Removal of the tumor will cause symptoms to cease. In the event of nonresectable disease, somatostatin analogs are used.

Cushing's syndrome

Cushing's syndrome is seen in the setting of either endogenous or exogenous elevated gluco-corticoids. The majority of cases of endogenous glucocorticoid excess are caused by an anterior pituitary tumor; however, a small proportion are caused by tumors, which ectopically produce adrenocorticotropin hormone. Typical features of Cushing's syndrome include altered subcutaneous fat distribution leading to a "buffalo hump" over the dorsal neck and "moon facies," as well as central obesity. In patients who have underlying malignancy, however, it has been noted that obesity may be absent [4]. Hyperpigmentation, typically a rare finding, is more common in patients who have associated underlying malignancy [6]. Other findings include proximal muscle weakness, edema, mental confusion, hypertension, hyperglycemia, and hypokalemia [6]. The most commonly associated malignancy is oat cell carcinoma of the lung. Other reported causes include carcinoid tumors, carcinoma of the thymus, pancreatic carcinoma, pheochromocytoma, medullary thyroid carcinoma, and cancers of the male and female reproductive organs [64,103].

Pruritus

When the lengthy list of nonmalignant causes is carefully eliminated, cancer as a cause of itch must be sought. Numerous malignancies are associated with pruritus as a paraneoplastic manifestation, including breast carcinoma, carcinoid syndrome, cutaneous T-cell lymphoma, and gastrointestinal cancers [104]; however, generalized itching without an associated eruption has most frequently been associated with Hodgkin's disease and may occur in more than 25% of these patients [105]. The etiology of paraneoplastic pruritus is poorly understood and may be refractory to standard treatments [104]. In an interesting recent paper, the incidence of eczematous eruptions and cutaneous T-cell lymphoma in patients who had Hodgkin's disease was found to be significantly higher than in the general population [106]. This prompted the authors to hypothesize that there may be a similar T-cell dysregulation and increased Th2 cytokine profiles pushing these patients toward atopy, perhaps explaining some of the pruritus. Alternatively, they suggested, reduced pre-existing cell-mediated Th1 immunity in these patients may also play a role in the development of a lymphoid malignancy [106]. Management of these patients can be very difficult because many of them have incurable underlying malignancies [104]. In addition to standard, nonspecific antipruritic treatments such as good moisturization, topical camphor, menthol, topical pramoxine, and calamine, many systemic treatments have been reported to be helpful.

Low-sedative antihistamines are often ineffective, and thus some of the following have been recommended: opioid antagonists (eg, naltrexone), ondansetron, colestyramine, thalidomide, corticosteroids, aspirin, and mirtazapine [107]. Paroxetine at a dose of 20 mg daily was more effective than placebo in one study for severe pruritus of multiple etiologies, including some hematologic

malignancies [108]. In another study, the combination of mirtazapine and gabapentin was shown to be helpful in treating the pruritus in patients who have cutaneous T-cell lymphoma [109].

Summary

This article summarizes the clinical and histologic features of many cutaneous disorders that may be associated with underlying malignancies. For some of these conditions, such as erythema gyratum repens, the likelihood of malignancy can be quite high. For others, such as acquired ichthyosis, the strength of association is considerably weaker. Recognition of any of the paraneoplastic skin disorders reviewed here should raise suspicion for an occult malignancy. The decision to pursue further evaluation can be made based on the likelihood of malignancy (Box 1) and through consultation with the patient's internist. In certain cases, a high level of suspicion for

---

Box 1. Likelihood of associated underlying malignancy/plasma cell disorder

Very likely
Acrokeratosis paraneoplastica
Hypertrichosis lanuginosa acquisita
Erythema gyratum repens
Paraneoplastic pemphigus
Hypertrophic osteoarthropathy
Necrobiotic xanthogranuloma
Primary amyloidosis
Scleromyxedema
Necrolytic migratory erythema
Carcinoid syndrome

Somewhat likely
Sweet's syndrome
Dermatomyositis
Pityriasis rotunda
Multicentric reticulohistiocytosis

Less likely
Acanthosis nigricans
Acquired ichthyosis
Erythroderma
Sign of Leser-Trélat
Scleredema
Vasculitis
Cushing's syndrome
Pruritus

occult malignancy must be maintained for many years. It is hoped that recognition of these disorders may lead to a rapid diagnosis and treatment of underlying malignancy.

References

[1] Curth HO. Skin lesions and internal carcinoma. In: Andrade R, editor. Cancer of the skin: biology, diagnosis, management. Philadelphia: Saunders; 1976.

[2] Mekhail TM, Markman M. Acanthosis nigricans with endometrial carcinoma: case report and review of the literature. Gynecol Oncol 2002; 84(2):332–4.

[3] Shelley WB, Crissey JT. Classics in clinical dermatology, with biographical sketches. 50th anniversary. 2nd edition. New York: Parthenon Pub. Group; 2003.

[4] Callen JP. Skin signs of internal malignancy. In: Callen JP, editor. Dermatological signs of internal disease. 3rd edition. Philadelphia: W.B. Saunders; 2003. p. 95–110.

[5] Chung VQ, Moschella SL, Zembowicz A, et al. Clinical and pathologic findings of paraneoplastic dermatoses. J Am Acad Dermatol 2006;54(5): 745–62; Quiz 63–6.

[6] Braverman IM. Skin manifestations of internal malignancy. Clin Geriatr Med 2002;18(1):1–19, v.

[7] Stuart CA, Driscoll MS, Lundquist KF, et al. Acanthosis nigricans. J Basic Clin Physiol Pharmacol 1998;9(2–4):407–18.

[8] Pentenero M, Carrozzo M, Pagano M, et al. Oral acanthosis nigricans, tripe palms and sign of Leser-Trelat in a patient with gastric adenocarcinoma. Int J Dermatol 2004;43(7):530–2.

[9] Ozdemir M, Toy H, Mevlitoglu I, et al. Generalized idiopathic acanthosis nigricans treated with acitretin. J Dermatolog Treat 2006;17(1):54–6.

[10] Blobstein SH. Topical therapy with tretinoin and ammonium lactate for acanthosis nigricans associated with obesity. Cutis 2003;71(1):33–4.

[11] Van D. Ichthyosiform atrophy of the skin associated with internal malignant diseases. Dermatologica 1963;127:413–28.

[12] Aram H. Acquired ichthyosis and related conditions. Int J Dermatol 1984;23(7):458–61.

[13] Cooper MF, Wilson PD, Hartop PJ, et al. Acquired ichthyosis and impaired dermal lipogenesis in Hodgkin's disease. Br J Dermatol 1980;102(6): 689–93.

[14] DiBisceglie AM, Hodkinson HJ, Berkowitz I, et al. Pityriasis rotunda. A cutaneous marker of hepatocellular carcinoma in South African blacks. Arch Dermatol 1986;122(7):802–4.

[15] Grimalt R, Gelmetti C, Brusasco A, et al. Pityriasis rotunda: report of a familial occurrence and review

of the literature. J Am Acad Dermatol 1994;31 (5 Pt 2):866–71.

[16] Bazex A, Griffiths A. Acrokeratosis paraneoplastica—a new cutaneous marker of malignancy. Br J Dermatol 1980;103(3):301–6.

[17] Bolognia JL. Bazex syndrome: acrokeratosis paraneoplastica. Semin Dermatol 1995;14(2):84–9.

[18] Valdivielso M, Longo I, Suarez R, et al. Acrokeratosis paraneoplastica: Bazex syndrome. J Eur Acad Dermatol Venereol 2005;19(3):340–4.

[19] Eubanks LE, McBurney E, Reed R. Erythema gyratum repens. Am J Med Sci 2001;321(5):302–5.

[20] Gammel JA. Erythema gyratum repens; skin manifestations in patient with carcinoma of breast. AMA Arch Derm Syphilol 1952;66(4):494–505.

[21] Boyd AS, Neldner KH, Menter A. Erythema gyratum repens: a paraneoplastic eruption. J Am Acad Dermatol 1992;26(5 Pt 1):757–62.

[22] Appell ML, Ward WQ, Tyring SK. Erythema gyratum repens. A cutaneous marker of malignancy. Cancer 1988;62(3):548–50.

[23] Caux F, Lebbe C, Thomine E, et al. Erythema gyratum repens. A case studied with immunofluorescence, immunoelectron microscopy and immunohistochemistry. Br J Dermatol 1994;131(1):102–7.

[24] Holt PJ, Davies MG. Erythema gyratum repens—an immunologically mediated dermatosis? Br J Dermatol 1977;96(4):343–7.

[25] Kurzrock R, Cohen PR. Erythema gyratum repens. JAMA 1995;273(7):594.

[26] De Bersaques J. Sign of Leser-Trelat. J Am Acad Dermatol 1985;12(4):724.

[27] Rampen HJ, Schwengle LE. The sign of Leser-Trelat: does it exist? J Am Acad Dermatol 1989; 21(1):50–5.

[28] Lindelof B, Sigurgeirsson B, Melander S. Seborrheic keratoses and cancer. J Am Acad Dermatol 1992;26(6):947–50.

[29] Yeh JS, Munn SE, Plunkett TA, et al. Coexistence of acanthosis nigricans and the sign of Leser-Trelat in a patient with gastric adenocarcinoma: a case report and literature review. J Am Acad Dermatol 2000;42(2 Pt 2):357–62.

[30] Kurzrock R, Cohen PR. Cutaneous paraneoplastic syndromes in solid tumors. Am J Med 1995;99(6): 662–71.

[31] Heaphy MR Jr, Millns JL, Schroeter AL. The sign of Leser-Trelat in a case of adenocarcinoma of the lung. J Am Acad Dermatol 2000;43(2 Pt 2):386–90.

[32] King LE Jr, Dufresne RG Jr, Lovett GL, et al. Erythroderma: review of 82 cases. South Med J 1986;79(10):1210–5.

[33] Cohen PR, Kurzrock R. Mucocutaneous paraneoplastic syndromes. Semin Oncol 1997;24(3):334–59.

[34] Kurzrock R, Cohen PR. Mucocutaneous paraneoplastic manifestations of hematologic malignancies. Am J Med 1995;99(2):207–16.

[35] Turner M. Case of a woman whose face and body in two or three weeks became covered with a thick

crop of short and white downy hair. Medical Times Gazette 1865;2:507.

[36] Farina MC, Tarin N, Grilli R, et al. Acquired hypertrichosis lanuginosa: case report and review of the literature. J Surg Oncol 1998;68(3):199–203.

[37] Fretzin DF. Malignant down. Arch Dermatol 1967;95(3):294–7.

[38] Jemec GB. Hypertrichosis lanuginosa acquisita. Report of a case and review of the literature. Arch Dermatol 1986;122(7):805–8.

[39] Perez-Losada E, Pujol RM, Domingo P, et al. Hypertrichosis lanuginosa acquisita preceding extraskeletal Ewing's sarcoma. Clin Exp Dermatol 2001;26(2):182–3.

[40] Hovenden AL. Acquired hypertrichosis lanuginosa associated with malignancy. Arch Intern Med 1987;147(11):2013 8.

[41] Samson MK, Buroker TR, Henderson MD, et al. Acquired hypertrichosis languiginosa. Report of two new cases and a review of the literature. Cancer 1975;36(4):1519–21.

[42] Weedon D. Skin pathology. 2nd edition. London; New York: Churchill Livingstone; 2002.

[43] Sweet RD. An acute febrile neutrophilic dermatosis. Br J Dermatol 1964;76:349–56.

[44] Moschella SL. Neutrophilic dermatoses. In: Bolognia J, Jorizzo JL, Rapini RP, editors. Dermatology. London; New York: Mosby; 2003. p. 411–23.

[45] Fett DL, Gibson LE, Su WP. Sweet's syndrome: systemic signs and symptoms and associated disorders. Mayo Clin Proc 1995;70(3):234–40.

[46] Bourke JF, Keohane S, Long CC, et al. Sweet's syndrome and malignancy in the UK. Br J Dermatol 1997;137(4):609–13.

[47] Cohen PR, Talpaz M, Kurzrock R. Malignancy-associated Sweet's syndrome: review of the world literature. J Clin Oncol 1988;6(12):1887–97.

[48] Cohen PR, Kurzrock R. Sweet's syndrome revisited: a review of disease concepts. Int J Dermatol 2003;42(10):761–78.

[49] Sweet's syndrome. 2003. Available at: http://www.orpha.net/data/patho/GB/uk-Sweet.pdf. Accessed October 1, 2006.

[50] Cohen PR, Kurzrock R. Sweet's syndrome and malignancy. Am J Med 1987;82(6):1220–6.

[51] Caughman W, Stern R, Haynes H. Neutrophilic dermatosis of myeloproliferative disorders. Atypical forms of pyoderma gangrenosum and Sweet's syndrome associated with myeloproliferative disorders. J Am Acad Dermatol 1983;9(5):751–8.

[52] Jorizzo JL. Dermatomyositis. In: Bolognia J, Jorizzo JL, Rapini RP, editors. Dermatology. London; New York: Mosby; 2003. p. 615–23.

[53] Chen YJ, Wu CY, Shen JL. Predicting factors of malignancy in dermatomyositis and polymyositis: a case-control study. Br J Dermatol 2001;144(4):825–31.

[54] Wakata N, Kurihara T, Saito E, et al. Polymyositis and dermatomyositis associated with malignancy: a 30-year retrospective study. Int J Dermatol 2002;41(11):729–34.

[55] Hill CL, Zhang Y, Sigurgeirsson B, et al. Frequency of specific cancer types in dermatomyositis and polymyositis: a population-based study. Lancet 2001;357(9250):96–100.

[56] Callen JP. When and how should the patient with dermatomyositis or amyopathic dermatomyositis be assessed for possible cancer? Arch Dermatol 2002;138(7):969–71.

[57] Callen JP. Dermatomyositis. In: Callen JP, editor. Dermatological signs of internal disease. 3rd edition. Philadelphia: W.B. Saunders; 2003. p. 11–6.

[58] Leow YH, Goh CL. Malignancy in adult dermatomyositis. Int J Dermatol 1997;36(12):904–7.

[59] Sparsa A, Liozon E, Herrmann F, et al. Routine vs extensive malignancy search for adult dermatomyositis and polymyositis: a study of 40 patients. Arch Dermatol 2002;138(7):885–90.

[60] Wade MS, Black MM. Paraneoplastic pemphigus: a brief update. Australas J Dermatol 2005;46(1):1–8; Quiz 9–10.

[61] Anhalt GJ. Paraneoplastic pemphigus. J Investig Dermatol Symp Proc 2004;9(1):29–33.

[62] Barnadas M, Roe E, Brunet S, et al. Therapy of paraneoplastic pemphigus with rituximab: a case report and review of literature. J Eur Acad Dermatol Venereol 2006;20(1):69–74.

[63] Anhalt GJ. Paraneoplastic pemphigus. Adv Dermatol 1997;12:77–96 [discussion: 7].

[64] Boyce S, Harper J. Paraneoplastic dermatoses. Dermatol Clin 2002;20(3):523–32.

[65] Kossard S, Winkelmann RK. Necrobiotic xanthogranuloma. Australas J Dermatol 1980;21(2):85–8.

[66] Mehregan DA, Winkelmann RK. Necrobiotic xanthogranuloma. Arch Dermatol 1992;128(1):94–100.

[67] Ugurlu S, Bartley GB, Gibson LE. Necrobiotic xanthogranuloma: long-term outcome of ocular and systemic involvement. Am J Ophthalmol 2000;129(5):651–7.

[68] Luz FB, Gaspar TAP, Kalil-Gaspar N, et al. Multicentric reticulohistiocytosis. J Eur Acad Dermatol Venereol 2001;15(6):524–31.

[69] Muller AM, Geibel A, Neumann HP, et al. Primary (AL) amyloidosis in plasma cell disorders. Oncologist 2006;11(7):824–30.

[70] Breathnach SM. Amyloid and amyloidosis. J Am Acad Dermatol 1988;18(1 Pt 1):1–16.

[71] Falk RH, Comenzo RL, Skinner M. The systemic amyloidoses. N Engl J Med 1997;337(13):898–909.

[72] Bahlis NJ, Lazarus HM. Multiple myeloma-associated AL amyloidosis: is a distinctive therapeutic approach warranted? Bone Marrow Transplant 2006;38(1):7–15.

[73] Roy A, Roy V. Primary systemic amyloidosis. Early diagnosis and therapy can improve survival rates and quality of life. Postgrad Med 2006;119(1):93–9.

[74] Lin YC, Wang HC, Shen JL. Scleromyxedema: an experience using treatment with systemic corticosteroid and review of the published work. J Dermatol 2006;33(3):207–10.

[75] Rongioletti F. Lichen myxedematosus (papular mucinosis): new concepts and perspectives for an old disease. Semin Cutan Med Surg 2006;25(2): 100–4.

[76] Rongioletti F, Rebora A. Updated classification of papular mucinosis, lichen myxedematosus, and scleromyxedema. J Am Acad Dermatol 2001; 44(2):273–81.

[77] Lacy MQ, Hogan WJ, Gertz MA, et al. Successful treatment of scleromyxedema with autologous peripheral blood stem cell transplantation. Arch Dermatol 2005;141(10):1277–82.

[78] Beers WH, Ince A, Moore TL. Scleredema adultorum of Buschke: a case report and review of the literature. Semin Arthritis Rheum 2006;35(6):355–9.

[79] Santos-Juanes J, Osuna CG, Iglesias JR, et al. Treatment with chemotherapy of scleredema associated with Ig A myeloma. Int J Dermatol 2001; 40(11):720–1.

[80] Sansom JE, Sheehan AL, Kennedy CT, et al. A fatal case of scleredema of Buschke. Br J Dermatol 1994;130(5):669–70.

[81] Salisbury JA, Shallcross H, Leigh IM. Scleredema of Buschke associated with multiple myeloma. Clin Exp Dermatol 1988;13(4):269–70.

[82] Bowen AR, Smith L, Zone JJ. Scleredema adultorum of Buschke treated with radiation. Arch Dermatol 2003;139(6):780–4.

[83] Basarab T, Burrows NP, Munn SE, et al. Systemic involvement in scleredema of Buschke associated with IgG-kappa paraproteinaemia. Br J Dermatol 1997;136(6):939–42.

[84] Angeli-Besson C, Koeppel MC, Jacquet P, et al. Electron-beam therapy in scleredema adultorum with associated monoclonal hypergammaglobulinaemia. Br J Dermatol 1994;130(3):394–7.

[85] Tamburin LM, Pena JR, Meredith R, et al. Scleredema of Buschke successfully treated with electron beam therapy. Arch Dermatol 1998;134(4): 419–22.

[86] Janiga JJ, Ward DH, Lim HW. UVA-1 as a treatment for scleredema. Photodermatol Photoimmunol Photomed 2004;20(4):210–1.

[87] Wooten MD, Jasin HE. Vasculitis and lymphoproliferative diseases. Semin Arthritis Rheum 1996; 26(2):564–74.

[88] Hansen-Flaschen J, Nordberg J. Clubbing and hypertrophic osteoarthropathy. Clin Chest Med 1987;8(2):287–98.

[89] Cohen PR. Hypertrophic pulmonary osteoarthropathy and tripe palms in a man with squamous cell carcinoma of the larynx and lung. Report of a case and review of cutaneous paraneoplastic syndromes associated with laryngeal and lung malignancies. Am J Clin Oncol 1993;16(3):268–76.

[90] Callen JP. Dermatological signs of internal disease. 3rd edition. Philadelphia: Saunders; 2003.

[91] Kovacs RK, Korom I, Dobozy A, et al. Necrolytic migratory erythema. J Cutan Pathol 2006;33(3): 242–5.

[92] Cruz-Bautista I, Lerman I, Perez-Enriquez B, et al. Diagnostic challenge of glucagonoma: case report and literature review. Endocr Pract 2006;12(4): 422–6.

[93] Nakashima H, Komine M, Sasaki K, et al. Necrolytic migratory erythema without glucagonoma in a patient with short bowel syndrome. J Dermatol 2006;33(8):557–62.

[94] Kitamura Y, Sato M, Hatamochi A, et al. Necrolytic migratory erythema without glucagonoma associated with hepatitis B. Eur J Dermatol 2005; 15(1):49–51.

[95] Nofal AA, Nofal E, Attwa E, et al. Necrolytic acral erythema: a variant of necrolytic migratory erythema or a distinct entity? Int J Dermatol 2005;44(11):916–21.

[96] Hunt SJ, Narus VT, Abell E. Necrolytic migratory erythema: dyskeratotic dermatitis, a clue to early diagnosis. J Am Acad Dermatol 1991;24(3):473–7.

[97] Appetecchia M, Ferretti E, Carducci M, et al. Malignant glucagonoma. New options of treatment. J Exp Clin Cancer Res 2006;25(1):135–9.

[98] Radny P, Eigentler TK, Soennichsen K, et al. Metastatic glucagonoma: treatment with liver transplantation. J Am Acad Dermatol 2006;54(2):344–7.

[99] Hivnor CM, Yan AC, Junkins-Hopkins JM, et al. Necrolytic acral erythema: response to combination therapy with interferon and ribavirin. J Am Acad Dermatol 2004;50(5 Suppl):S121–4.

[100] Khanna VJ, Shieh S, Benjamin J, et al. Necrolytic acral erythema associated with hepatitis C: effective treatment with interferon alfa and zinc. Arch Dermatol 2000;136(6):755–7.

[101] Abdallah MA, Hull C, Horn TD. Necrolytic acral erythema: a patient from the United States successfully treated with oral zinc. Arch Dermatol 2005; 141(1):85–7.

[102] Krause W. Skin diseases in consequence of endocrine alterations. Aging Male 2006;9(2):81–95.

[103] Malchoff CD, Orth DN, Abboud C, et al. Ectopic ACTH syndrome caused by a bronchial carcinoid tumor responsive to dexamethasone, metyrapone, and corticotropin-releasing factor. Am J Med 1988;84(4):760–4.

[104] Fleischer AB. The clinical management of itching. New York: Parthenon; 2000.

[105] Cohen PR. Cutaneous paraneoplastic syndromes. Am Fam Physician 1994;50(6):1273–82.

[106] Rubenstein M, Duvic M. Cutaneous manifestations of Hodgkin's disease. Int J Dermatol 2006; 45(3):251–6.

[107] Twycross R, Greaves MW, Handwerker H, et al. Itch: scratching more than the surface. QJM 2003;96(1):7–26.

[108] Zylicz Z, Krajnik M, Sorge AA, et al. Paroxetine in the treatment of severe non-dermatological pruritus: a randomized, controlled trial. J Pain Symptom Manage 2003;26(6):1105–12.

[109] Demierre MF, Taverna J. Mirtazapine and gabapentin for reducing pruritus in cutaneous T-cell lymphoma. J Am Acad Dermatol 2006; 55(3):543–4.

ELSEVIER SAUNDERS

Dermatol Clin 26 (2008) 17–29

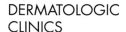

DERMATOLOGIC CLINICS

Epidermal Manifestations of Internal Malignancy

Rachael L. Moore, MD, Theresa S. Devere, MD*

Department of Dermatology, Oregon Health and Science University, 3303 SW Bond Avenue, CH16D, Portland, OR 97239, USA

In this article paraneoplastic syndromes with cutaneous findings localized to the epidermis are discussed. A paraneoplastic syndrome is a condition that arises in association with a malignancy elsewhere in the body but, in itself, is not cancerous. Generally, the onset and course of the disease will closely correlate with the malignancy, as described in Curth's original criteria for paraneoplastic syndromes [1], although this is not always the case. Subjects discussed include malignant acanthosis nigricans, the sign of Leser-Trélat, tripe palms, palmoplantar keratodermas, Bazex syndrome, and acquired ichthyosis (see Table 1 for summary).

Malignant acanthosis nigricans, the sign of Leser-Trélat, and tripe palms

Malignant acanthosis nigricans (MAN), the sign of Leser-Trélat (LT), and tripe palms (TP) are related and often found together. Andreev [2] described TP and the sign of LT as clinical variations of MAN; however, they have occurred in patients without other symptoms of acanthosis nigricans [3,4]. Malignancy-associated TP was reported with acanthosis nigricans and the sign of LT in 72% and 10% of cases, respectively [3]. In another study, the sign of LT was found to coexist with acanthosis nigricans approximately 29% of the time [5]. Perhaps a better understanding of these entities, as described by Schwartz [6], is that they are separate, but exist on a continuum, a concept supported by similar proposed etiologies. For the purposes of this chapter, we will discuss them as separate markers for paraneoplasia

and present their etiologies and prognoses together.

Malignant acanthosis nigricans

History and epidemiology

Acanthosis nigricans can broadly be categorized into benign or malignant types [7]. More recently, however, it has been divided into eight subtypes, including (1) benign, (2) obesity-associated, (3) syndromic, (4) malignant, (5) acral, (6) unilateral, (7) medication-induced, and (8) mixed-type acanthosis nigricans [6]. The malignant version will be the focus in this section.

The benign versions of acanthosis nigricans are relatively common, affecting 7% of school-aged children in one study [8]. In contrast, MAN is rare, with approximately 1000 reported cases in the world literature [9]. It occurs in men and woman equally and has no racial predilection or known familial association [7,10,11]. It primarily affects adults over age 40, although cases have been reported in children.

Clinical manifestations

Clinically, acanthosis nigricans presents as symmetric, hyperpigmented plaques with variable amounts of epidermal hypertrophy, creating a velvety texture (Fig. 1A) [6,10]. The plaques range in color from yellow to brown and/or gray to black and often have overlying skin tags or papillomas [7]. The process is progressive, beginning with increased pigmentation and advancing to hypertrophy with accentuation of skin lines [2]. Although any body surface can be involved, the most common affected sites include body flexures and the posterior neck [6]. Unusual locations have been reported, such as the nipple/areola area [12] and the skin surface overlying cutaneous metastases [6]. Generalized pruritus is frequently described

* Corresponding author.

E-mail address: deveret@ohsu.edu (T.S. Devere).

Table 1
Epidermal paraneoplastic syndromes and their most
common associated malignancies

Paraneoplastic syndrome	Most common associated malignancies
Malignant acanthosis nigricans	Adenocarcinoma of the gut (usually gastric)
Tripe palms	Gastric and pulmonary carcinoma
Sign of Leser-Trélat	Adenocarcinoma of the gut and lymphoproliferative disorders
Palmoplantar keratoderma	Esophageal carcinoma (Howel-Evans Syndrome)
	Squamous cell carcinoma of skin (other PPK variants)
Bazex syndrome	Squamous cell carcinoma of the upper aerodigestive tract
Acquired ichthyosis	Hodgkin's disease and other lymphoproliferative disorders

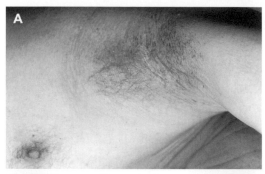

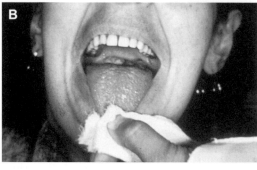

Fig. 1. Malignant acanthosis nigricans in (*A*) the axilla and (*B*) the mouth.

with the characteristic skin changes, occurring in 41% of affected individuals with MAN [10].

Mucosal surface involvement is frequent [6] and may be the only clinical symptom present (Fig. 1B). Brown and Winkelmann [10] reported 35% of patients with MAN had mucosal involvement. It commonly has a more papillated, or wart-like, appearance without associated hyperpigmentation [2]. Any mucosal surface can be involved, including the eyes, oral cavity, and anal and genital mucosa [6]. Eyelid margins can have extensive papillations causing visual obstruction [13]. Within the mouth, disease affecting the lips, tongue, buccal mucosa, palate, gingival, and esophagus [14] has been reported, as well as involvement of the larynx [15].

Acral sites are involved in approximately one quarter of cases [10]. The palms and soles may have yellow, hyperkeratotic plaques with accentuation of skin lines, a condition known as tripe palms [3]. MAN can also be associated with eruptive seborrheic keratoses (the sign of LT) and extensive wart-like growths. The latter condition has been termed florid cutaneous papillomatosis to distinguish it from basic warts (Fig. 2) [16]. Although some may argue florid cutaneous papillomatosis is a separate entity, it almost never, if at all, exists without acanthosis nigricans, and is therefore more likely a clinical variation of MAN.

Histopathology

Histologically, MAN is characterized by hyperkeratosis and papillomatosis with minimal acanthosis [11]. The epidermis often has alternating acanthosis and atrophy, which may become more prevalent with progression of the malignancy. Usually, there is increased basal layer pigmentation.

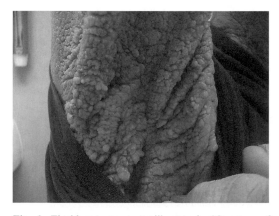

Fig. 2. Florid cutaneous papillomatosis (*Courtesy of* Kevin White, MD).

There is no significant inflammatory infiltrate. In addition to the hyperkeratosis and papillomatosis, mucosal surfaces show mild parakaratosis and are usually devoid of the increased pigmentation [6].

Associated malignancies

In general, the cutaneous findings for each of these conditions can precede or appear simultaneously or after the diagnosis of the cancer [3,4,17]. In one review of acanthosis nigricans, this occurred 58%, 13%, and 29% of the time, respectively [17]. Similar statistics have been reported for TP [3] and the sign of LT [4].

MAN is primarily associated with adenocarcinoma originating in the abdominal cavity. Curth [7], in her 1943 review of the literature, reported 70% of the cancers were of gastric origin. The remainder included uterine, liver, intestinal, ovarian, renal, breast, and lung cancers, with the overwhelming majority representing adenocarcinomas. Cases of MAN-associated pancreatic [18], bladder [19], adrenal [20], and gallbladder [14] cancers, among others, have also been observed. There are also reports of MAN-associated epidermal carcinomas and sarcomas such as lymphoma [21] and various squamous cell carcinomas, such as those originating from the lung [13,22] and cervix [23].

Having both acanthosis nigricans and cancer does not always make them associated. There are some general observations that can aid in this distinction [7]. MAN tends to parallel the course of the cancer—that is, it will spread and worsen with progression of the neoplasm, subside with treatment, and resurface with recurrence and metastases. In this way, MAN can often serve as a marker for neoplasm progression or recurrence. Additionally, MAN usually appears in adulthood and later, has a more sudden onset often with extensive involvement, is symmetrical in presentation, and has no familial association. The benign versions, on the other hand, usually present earlier in life (birth to puberty) and can be unilateral and have a genetic component.

Tripe palms

History and epidemiology

The term "tripe" palms was first used by a patient of Breathnach and Wells [24] who likened the condition of his hands unto tripe, the edible lining of a bovine foregut. It was later reported by Clarke [15] to describe a similar condition in a patient with malignant acanthosis nigricans and was popularized by Breathnach and Wells [24] in their description of five patients with the condition. Other terminology synonymous with tripe palms in the literature includes acanthosis palmaris [25], acanthosis nigricans of the palms [2], palmar hyperkeratosis [26], palmar keratoderma [24], and pachydermatoglyphy [22,24].

Tripe palms is rare with less than 100 reported cases and is usually associated with malignant acanthosis nigricans [3]. It affects men more than women (63% versus 37%, respectively). This difference becomes more pronounced when tripe palms is seen without acanthosis nigricans, where 86% of affected individuals are men. It appears almost exclusively in adults (median age = 62 years). There appears to be no familial association or racial predilection [27].

Clinical manifestations

Clinically, tripe palms presents as hypertrophy of the palms, and often the soles, with papillations, creating a velvety, or rugose, appearance often with a yellow hue (Fig. 3A, B) [3,24]. There is exaggeration of the skin lines; however, the dermatoglyphics can become distorted with extensive epidermal hyperkeratosis [26,28]. A variant of

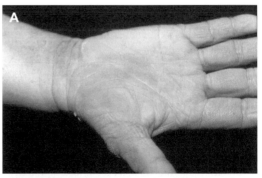

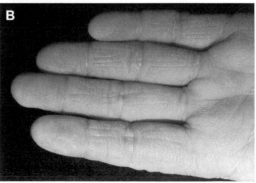

Fig. 3. (A, B) Tripe palms.

tripe palms has been described where a pitted hyperkeratosis is present, giving a "honeycomb" appearance [24]. Clinically, tripe palms differs from other keratodermas, which are usually distinguished by a more diffuse hyperkeratosis without significant papillations [29]. Tripe palms can be associated with clubbing of the nails and pruritus (18% and 25% of the time, respectively) [3]. When clubbing is present, a pulmonary carcinoma is overwhelmingly the underlying malignancy.

Histopathology

Histologically, tripe palms is characterized by hyperkeratosis and acanthosis [3]. Papillations, dermal mucinosis, and increased mast cells in the dermis can also be present. The latter findings do not appear to be tumor-specific.

Associated malignancies

Tripe palms is associated with an underlying neoplasm over 90% of the time [3]. The malignancies associated with tripe palms are primarily gastric and pulmonary carcinomas, each occurring approximately one quarter of the time. In tripe palms without acanthosis nigricans, lung carcinomas account for over 50% of the malignancies. Other tumors associated with tripe palms include those of the genitourinary tract (bladder, cervix, kidney, ovary, uterus, and prostate) and breast with rare reports of associated lymphoma and brain and tongue malignancies, among others. Bullous pemphigoid [25], psoriasis [24], exfoliative dermatitis [24], and pruritus [30] have been described with non–malignancy-associated tripe palms.

The sign of Leser-Trélat

History and epidemiology

The sign of Leser-Trélat (LT) is the sudden increase in the size and number of seborrheic keratoses that coincides with an internal malignancy [31]. The name is attributed to Edmund Leser and Ulysse Trélat, two European surgeons who first independently associated internal malignancies with these skin lesions in 1890. However, it is now thought that Leser and Trélat both described vascular angiomas and it was Hollander who first associated "verrucae seborrheicae" with internal malignancy in 1900 [32].

The sign of Leser-Trélat is rare, with only 75 cases described in the literature in 1994 [33]. It primarily affects older individuals, with a median age of 61 (range 22 to 87) [4]. There is no significant gender preference [33] and no reported racial predilection.

There is significant debate over the validity of this sign. Both seborrheic keratoses and internal malignancy are relatively common in the elderly population, making it difficult to separate this sign from a mere coincidence [34]. Small case-control studies comparing those patients with (1) seborrheic keratoses alone and (2) seborrheic keratoses with malignancies showed no significant association between the two [35,36]. Additionally, the definition of "sudden appearance" of seborrheic keratoses is vague and interpreted differently in the literature. In a review of 29 cases, the development of seborrheic keratoses took an average of 15 weeks, ranging from a few days to as long as 52 weeks [4].

Rampen and Schwengle [34], arguing against the sign of LT as being a useful marker for malignancy, made the following points: (1) the sign of LT may not be an entity alone but part of acanthosis nigricans (indeed, Andreev [2] considered the sign of LT to be a more generalized form of MAN); (2) there are questionable seborrheic keratosis diagnoses (versus verrucae or papillomas) in reported cases due to lack of histologic evaluation; (3) the sign of LT can be associated with disease processes unrelated to malignancy. Opposing his argument, however, is that the sign of LT only coexists with acanthosis nigricans approximately 29% of the time, supporting its existence as a separate entity [5]. Second, Holdiness [4] stressed the importance of histologic evaluation as well, but held the validity of the sign. He reported 34 of 60 cases had histologic evaluation and of those 34, 91% were consistent with seborrheic keratoses.

Finally, multiple eruptive seborrheic keratoses can be associated with other, nonmalignant, conditions including HIV [37], a heart transplant [38], acromegaly [39] and erythroderma [40]. Other diseases can mimic the sign of LT, such as a case of pemphigus foliaceus described by Bruckner and colleagues [41]. Despite these other associations, some would still argue it is a useful, albeit rare, marker for malignancy, and if present, should warrant a workup [4].

Clinical manifestations

Clinically, it presents as multiple, eruptive seborrheic keratoses primarily on the trunk and extremities [5,31]. Ellis and Yates [5], in his review of 68 cases, found involvement on the back/chest and extremities 76% and 38% of the time, respectively. The eruption has been described as a "Christmas-tree" pattern [38]. Pruritus is a prominent feature, found 26% [31] to 51% [5] of the time.

Histopathology

Microscopically, seborrheic keratoses show varying degrees of hyperkeratosis, papillomatosis, and acanthosis [4]. There are often pseudo-horned cysts within the epidermis.

Associated malignancies

Approximately half of the cancers associated with the sign of LT are adenocarcinomas, with 32% of those occurring in the gastrointestinal tract [5]. This is a similar pattern to that seen in malignant acanthosis nigricans [7]. However, unlike malignant acanthosis nigricans, lymphoproliferative disorders are the next most common associated malignancy, occurring 21% of the time [5]. There are rare reports of the sign of LT occurring with many other cancers, such as transitional cell bladder cancer [33], renal cell carcinoma [42], and melanoma [43].

Pathogenesis

The exact etiology of malignant acanthosis nigricans, tripe palms, and the sign of Leser-Trélat is unknown but may result from release of tumor products that act on epidermal growth factor receptors. Epidermal growth factor receptors (EGFR) are found primarily in the basal layer of keratinocytes in the epidermis and are increased in number throughout the entire epidermis in hyperproliferative disorders, such as psoriasis [44]. Epidermal growth factor (EGF), a ligand for EGFR, promotes proliferation and differentiation of the cells. Indeed, growth hormone levels have been shown to be increased in patients with malignancy-associated TP and the sign of LT [26,45] with return to near-normal levels after the cancer was treated [45]. However, some patients with malignancy-associated TP and the sign of LT [15] and the sign of LT alone [46] have not shown elevated growth hormone levels.

Tumors may secrete transforming growth factor alpha (TGF-alpha), a protein structurally similar to EGF, which binds to the EGFR and stimulates keratinocyte growth [43,47]. High levels of urinary TGF-alpha and increased epidermal staining of EGFRs was found in biopsy specimens of seborrheic keratoses and acanthosis nigricans in a patient with the sign of LT, MAN, and a melanoma [43]. Epidermal staining and urinary TGF-alpha levels decreased when the melanoma was treated. TGF-alpha has also been implicated as

the growth hormone potentially responsible for the clinical features of TP and acanthosis nigricans in a patient with systemic mastocytosis [48].

It has also been suggested that the tumor secretes lytic factors that decrease the extracellular matrix viscosity and lead to the clinical findings in acanthosis nigricans [49] and the sign of LT [50].

Additionally, the cause of the cutaneous findings in those patients without an associated malignancy clearly cannot be attributed to a cancer-secreting hormone. Hormone imbalances, such as hyperinsulinemia, are associated with benign versions of acanthosis nigricans [8]. In addition, Brown and Winkelman [10] speculated that local factors, such as friction, heat, and sweating, may play a role in producing acanthosis nigricans given the pronounced distribution in flexural areas. Similarly, Breathnach and Wells [24] speculated that frictional change created by continual rubbing led, at least in part, to the palmar changes in two of their patients with tripe palms and no underlying malignancy.

There is no definite cause linked with these conditions in the literature. Ellis and Yates [5] proposed that a threshold level of growth factor and a genetic predisposition for developing seborrheic keratoses needs to be present to make one susceptible to the sign of LT. It is likely that to develop these conditions, there are both genetic and environmental factors that must be triggered.

Prognosis

The prognosis for most patients diagnosed with MAN and the sign of LT is poor as the associated tumors are usually aggressive with a high rate of mortality [4,7,10]. The average survival time is approximately 1 to 2 years after the diagnosis of cancer. Metastases were found 57% of the time in the sign of LT [4]. There is not much data available regarding survival time in patients with tripe palms, but one could speculate it is similar to MAN and the sign of LT.

Treatment

Treatment is difficult and generally aimed at the underlying tumor [5,6], as the diseases often parallel the course of the malignancies [31]. However, in up to two thirds of cases in the sign of LT, the cutaneous findings will not mimic the course of the cancer [4]. In MAN, certain palliative modalities have been beneficial for pruritus and extensive involvement, such as psoralen and UVA light treatment (PUVA) [51], radiotherapy [52], oral retinoids [53], and chemotherapy [54]. In TP, often traditional treatment with retinoids, emollients, keratolytics, and topical steroids prove ineffective [29,30,53]. In non–malignancy-associated TP, treatment with methotrexate, keratolytics, and topical steroids may be more successful [24]. Local measures, such as cryotherapy and biopsy can be employed for seborrheic keratoses that are particularly irritating [5].

Palmoplantar keratoderma

Palmoplantar keratoderma (PPK) is the thickening of the skin on the palms and soles that results from abnormal keratinization [55]. The PPKs are a diverse group of disorders that can be either acquired or hereditary. They are often categorized on the basis of histology (such as presence or absence of epidermolysis) and type of involvement (focal, diffuse, or punctate). In addition, hereditary PPKs can be associated with a number of other ectodermal abnormalities, such as changes seen in hair, nails, and teeth. Classification can often be difficult, as there is significant overlap among the categories.

A number of malignancies have been associated with various PPKs. Tripe palms (discussed in the second section of this article) is considered an

acquired PPK [55] and is almost always associated with a malignancy, usually of the stomach or lung [3]. Some hereditary PPKs, which will be the focus of this section, can also denote an increased cancer risk.

Clinical features and associated malignancies

Palmoplantar keratoderma presents as well-demarcated hyperkeratotic plaques on the palms and soles, which can be diffuse, focal, or punctate (see Table 2 for summary) [55], and it is often associated with hyperhidrosis [56]. There are some generalizations that can be made to delineate these categories. In regard to the hereditary variants, diffuse PPKs, such as epidermolytic hyperkeratosis, generally present at birth or soon thereafter and show generalized thickening of the palms and soles [57]. On the other hand, focal PPKs such as Howel-Evans syndrome, present in later childhood and show thickening only over pressure points, which may regress when the stimulation is removed. Punctate PPKs are characterized by punctate, or "cup-shaped" keratoses on acral sites, which can be accentuated over pressure points [58]. These tend to present after puberty.

The prototype of a hereditary PPK associated with a malignancy is Howel-Evans syndrome. In 1958, Howel-Evans and colleagues [56] first

Table 2
Palmoplantar keratodermas associated with malignancy

Clinical variant	Syndrome	Inheritance	Associated malignancies
Diffuse	Tripe palms	Acquired	Gastric, lung [3]
	KID syndrome	Autosomal recessive	Squamous cell carcinoma [63]
	Huriez syndrome (sclerotylosis)	Autosomal dominant	Squamous cell carcinoma in sites of PPK/atrophic skin [64]
	Diffuse PPK described in Indian family [65]	Autosomal dominant	Squamous cell carcinoma in sites of PPK [65]
	Epidermolytic PPK	Autosomal dominant	Breast and ovarian cancer reported in one family [60]
	Diffuse PPK associated with dental anomalies and hypogonadism described in one family [62]	Autosomal recessive	Squamous cell carcinoma in sites of PPK [62]
Focal	Howel-Evans syndrome	Autosomal dominant	Esophageal squamous cell carcinoma [56–58]
Punctate	Arsenic	Acquired	Basal cell carcinomas and other skin cancers, squamous cell carcinomas of the upper aerodigestive tract and urinary carcinomas [66]
	Inherited punctate PPK and malignancy described in a single four-generation family [59]	Autosomal dominant	Internal malignancies (renal, breast, colon, lung, Hodgkin's, melanoma) [59]

Abbreviations: KID, keratitis-ichthyosis-deafness syndrome; PPK, palmoplantar keratoderma.

reported an increased incidence of esophageal squamous cell carcinoma in two families in England with an autosomal dominantly inherited PPK, which they referred to as *tylosis*. There have been just a handful of families reported that are affected with this syndrome [56,57,59]. Clinically, these patients have focal hyperkeratosis, often with associated follicular lesions, such as keratosis pilaris and oral hyperkeratosis [57].

Howel-Evans and colleagues [56] found that 18 of 48 family members with tylosis developed esophageal squamous cell carcinoma, and further estimated that 96% of affected individuals would die of this cancer by age 65 if they did not die of other causes. Stevens and colleagues [57] studied a large German-American family affected with the disease and estimated a relative risk of 38 for oral or esophageal squamous cell carcinoma in affected family members with a mean age of cancer onset of 61.

Other genodermatoses with PPK may have an increased risk of malignancy as well. However, most of these reported increased cancer risks are single case reports or within one family, making a true association speculative.

A family with diffuse, epidermolytic PPK, which is caused by a keratin 9 mutation, was shown to have an increased incidence of breast and ovarian cancer [60]. However, this association was more likely the result of a BRCA1 mutation cosegregating with a keratin 9 mutation coincidentally rather than a true connection [61]. Micali and colleagues [62] found evidence in four brothers for a new, autosomal dominant syndrome characterized by a diffuse, nonepidermolytic PPK, dental anomalies, hypogenitalism, and increased incidence of squamous cell carcinomas in the affected palmoplantar sites. Others, too, have described increased incidence of squamous cell carcinomas in diffuse PPK syndromes, such as keratitis-ichthyosis-deafness (KID) syndrome [63], Huriez syndrome [64], and an Indian family with inherited tylosis [65].

Stevens and colleagues [58] reported a large, four-generation, family with an autosomal dominantly inherited punctate PPK with an increased risk of internal malignancy (23% incidence compared with 2% in unaffected individuals). The malignancies reported included Hodgkin's disease and renal, breast, pancreatic, and colon cancers.

It is worth noting that there are acquired and idiopathic forms of PPK that can also be associated with cancer. Tripe palms is a diffuse PPK associated with stomach or lung cancers [3].

Punctate keratoses can signify arsenic ingestion, which is associated with an increased incidence of basal cell carcinomas and other skin cancers, as well as internal malignancies including squamous cell carcinomas in the upper aerodigestive tract and urinary carcinomas [66].

Histopathology

Histologically, PPK is characterized by hyperkeratosis with variable acanthosis and papillomatosis [67]. The granular layer is thickened and there is generally no perivascular infiltrate. There may be epidermolytic hyperkeratosis with dyskeratotic keratinocytes in the spinous and granular layer.

Pathogenesis

Most hereditary PPKs are autosomal dominant [58]. Gene mutations in keratins have been elucidated in several of the PPKs that are unlikely to be associated with malignancy. Howel-Evans syndrome has been linked to the tylosis and esophageal cancer (TEC) locus on chromosome 17q24 distal to a keratin site. While the mechanism of action of this gene is unknown, it has been hypothesized that it may function as a tumor suppressor. Additionally, in one study, seven of the eight patients with Howel-Evans syndrome and oral/esophageal squamous cell carcinoma had a history of smoking or chewing tobacco, conferring that there may be an environmental component, in addition to the genetic one, for the development of the cancers [57]. Vitamin A has been implicated as a link between hyperkeratosis and malignancy in Howel-Evans syndrome, but the evidence is poor [68].

Treatment

Conservative management of PPKs include topical keratolytics (such as urea and salicylic acid), emollients, topical steroids and retinoids, and physical debridement, which have varied results [55]. Topical PUVA and oral retinoids can also be used in more severe disease.

Bazex syndrome

History

Acrokeratosis paraneoplastica, or Bazex syndrome, is a paraneoplastic process in which psorasiform skin lesions on the ears, nose, cheeks, and acral sites are associated with malignancy, primarily in the upper aerodigestive tract [69]. It was first described in 1922 when Gougerot and Rupp [70] reported a patient with scaly lesions on the nose, ears, and acral sites who had squamous cell carcinoma (SCC) of the tongue. However, it was not until 1965 when Bazex and colleagues [71] described a patient with SCC of the piriform fossa and a similar skin eruption that the paraneoplastic nature of the skin findings was recognized.

For clarification, "Bazex syndrome" is the name used to describe two distinct entities: (1) the paraneoplastic syndrome, as described in the preceding paragraph, and (2) a genodermatosis characterized by follicular atrophoderma, congenital hypotrichosis, and multiple basal cell malignancies. The former is the focus of this section.

Epidemiology

Like the other paraneoplastic syndromes in this article, Bazex syndrome is rare. In 2006, there were approximately 140 reported cases in the literature [72]. However, the incidence may be underestimated as the skin findings often resemble more common eczematous or papulosquamous disorders that won't encourage further workup [73]. The vast majority of reported cases occur in white males over age 40 [74,75]. In fact, Sarkar and colleagues [75] found 94% of the reported cases in men. There is no known genetic predisposition; however, HLA typing in several cases have shown HLA-A2 and/or B8 to be present, suggesting perhaps, some form of genetic susceptibility [75,76].

Clinical manifestations

The skin lesions present as symmetrical, erythematous to violaceous scaly plaques on the nose, ear helices, and distal extremities (Fig. 4) [74]. They often have a psoriatic appearance, although their distribution is not typical of psoriasis. In more advanced disease, the skin lesions can spread to the elbows and knees. Acral sites are frequently involved, including both the dorsal and palmoplantar aspects of the hands and feet. Palms and soles will often have hyperkeratotic plaques on the pressure points [77], with the central area spared [74]. In contrast to psoriasis, skin lesions in Bazex syndrome are usually ill defined with a finer, "pityrosporum" scale and often have a more bluish hue [76]. In dark-skinned individuals, the lesions may appear as hyperpigmented macules [74]. Vesicles and bullae may also be present [38,77,78]. Nails can be dystrophic with horizontal and vertical ridging and onycholysis, and there can be prominent paronychial swelling and tenderness [69,74]. Pruritus is associated with the disease 18% of the time [74].

Bazex and Griffiths [69] described three stages of the skin findings in relation to the malignancy. In the first stage, the tumor is generally "undected," although it may have already metastasized. Scaly plaques appear on the ears, nose, and digits. Paronychia and nail dystrophy may be present. Second, the malignancy becomes symptomatic and the skin findings start to spread locally and become more violaceous. Third, if the tumor remains untreated, the rash continues to expand and can

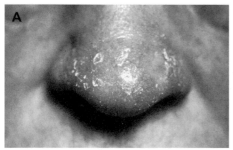
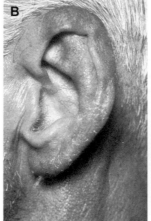
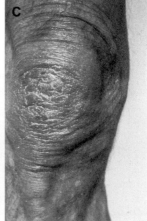

Fig. 4. Bazex syndrome on the (*A*) nose, (*B*) ear, and (*C*) knee. (*Courtesy of* Franklin Parker, MD.)

become quite extensive, involving new sites on the more proximal extremities and trunk.

Histopathology

Biopsy of skin lesions reveals varying degrees of hyperkeratosis with parakaratosis, acanthosis, and dyskeratotic keratinocytes [69,74]. There is a superficial perivascular lymphocytic infiltrate. Vacuolar change has also been reported as well as melanophages in the upper dermis. Immunofluorescence studies are generally negative. There have been reports of Bazex syndrome with positive direct immunofluorescence studies in patients with bullous skin lesions [78], bringing into question whether Bazex syndrome was occurring simultaneosly with another bullous dermatosis or manifesting itself in a different way [79].

Associated malignancies

All reported cases of Bazex syndrome have been associated with a malignancy [74]. The cutaneous findings precede the diagnosis of malignancy by an average of 11 months approximately two thirds of the time. Less often, the diagnosis occurs simultaneously, or after, the diagnosis of malignancy.

In one review, nearly 80% of the tumors arose from the acrodigestive tract (oral cavity, larynx, pharynx, lung, and esophagus) and 64% of those were SCCs [75]. Interestingly, over 50% of the reported malignancies had metastases to the cervical lymph nodes. Further, 16% of the tumors, primarily SCC, had no known primary source but were found in the cervical lymph nodes. Most of the patients (20 of 22), in whom social data were available, had a smoking and/or drinking history.

There are single cases of other malignancy associations in the literature, including ductal carcinoma of the breast [80], cholangiocarcinoma [72], adenocarcinoma of the colon [81], and Hodgkin's disease [82], among others. Bazex syndrome has also been described in conjunction with other paraneoplastic syndromes, such as acquired icthyosis. Lucker and Steijlen [82] described a patient in which symptoms of both Bazex syndrome and acquired icthyosis presented before diagnosis of Hodgkin's disease.

Pathogenesis

The etiology of Bazex syndrome is unknown, but several hypotheses have been discussed. First, there may be an immunologic mechanism in which antibodies directed against the tumor cross-react with antigens in the epidermis or basement membrane [78]. Second, the tumor may secrete a growth factor, such as TGF-alpha, that leads to epidermal growth and differentiation [82]. Third, a Vitamin A deficiency has been suggested as a mechanism, although the level has been normal in some of those tested [76]. Fourth, the occurrence of the same HLA types (A3 and B8) in several cases [75,76] raises the possibility that one must be genetically susceptible to get the disease. Last, environmental risk factors may play a role, given the specific nature of the associated malignancies (primarily SCCs of the head and neck region) and the high prevalence of risk factors for these malignancies, such as smoking and/or drinking. Likely, the etiology is a multifactorial process and requires several variables to align to manifest itself.

Treatment

The skin lesions of Bazex syndrome are notoriously resistant to therapy [69]. Treatment with keratolytics, topical steroids, and antibiotics are generally ineffective. Nevertheless, there are reports of improvement with PUVA [77] and oral retinoids [83,84]. In over 90% of cases, the cutaneous findings will parallel the course of the cancer [74]. Thus, the most efficacious therapy is to treat the underlying tumor. Interestingly, nail changes are often permanent, with a poor response to any modality of treatment [77,78].

Acquired ichthyosis

History and epidemiology

Ichthyosis orginates from the Greek word for fish, *ichthys*, and is used to describe rhomboid, or fish-like, scales on the skin [85]. Ichthyosis can be either acquired or genetic [86]. Genetic ichthyoses, such as ichthyosis vulgaris, usually present in childhood [85]. Acquired ichthyoses, on the other hand, usually present in adulthood and have been associated with a number of drugs and systemic diseases, including endocrine abnormalities, nutritional deficiencies, infection, and malignancy [85,86]. It is the latter association that will be the focus of this section.

The association of ichthyosis and malignancy was first made in 1943 by Ronchese [87] when he described a patient diagnosed with Hodgkin's disease who later developed ichthyosis. Since this first reporting, there have been a number of case reports and reviews documenting the association of acquired ichthyosis and malignancy. The incidence of the disease is unknown. Men may be more affected than women [88], and there is no reported genetic or racial predilection.

Clinical manifestations

Ichthyosis presents as small white to brown scale seen primarily on the extensor extremities and trunk [85]. There is general sparing of the flexures, palms, and soles [89]. The scale itself has been described as "rhomboid" shaped [87] or fish-like [90] with a free edge. Often, the change can be subtle. The disease tends to be worse in wintertime [85] or dry climates.

Histopathology

Histologically, the defining features of ichthyosis are hyperkeratosis with occasional parakaratosis and a decreased granular layer [85,86]. The spinous layer can be normal [86] to slightly acanthotic [89] to atrophic [91,92]. There is no dermal infiltrate [85,91,92].

Associated malignancies

The most common malignancy associated with acquired ichthyosis is Hodgkin's disease, estimated to occur nearly 70% of the time [88]. It has also been associated with other lymphoproliferative disorders, such as mycosis fungoides [93], reticulolymphosarcoma, and multiple myeloma [88]. Other nonlymphoproliferative malignancy associations have been reported, including a dysgerminoma of the ovary [94], leiomyosarcoma [95], transitional cell carcinoma of the kidney [96], and hepatocellular carcinoma [97]. Unlike other paraneoplastic syndromes in which the cutaneous manifestation often precedes the diagnosis of malignancy, ichthyotic skin changes most often occur several weeks to months after discovery of the tumor [92]. Rarely, the cutaneous findings can be the presenting sign of an internal malignancy.

Other paraneoplastic syndromes have been described to occur with acquired ichthyosis and malignancy, such as dermatomyositis [94,97], erythema gyratum repens [96], and Bazex syndrome [82].

Acquired ichthyosis has been seen with increasing frequency in AIDS patients [89], who may or may not have a tumor association, and it has been reported in patients with graft-versus-host disease following bone marrow transplantation [90]. There are many other associations, including leprosy, sarcoidosis, thyroid abnormalities, malnutrition, and cholesterol-lowering medications, such as niacin, among others, which have been summarized by Patel and colleagues [55].

Pathogenesis

Ichthyosis occurs when there is an error in cornification, a complicated process involving numerous enzymes and steps [98]. Alterations in cellular lipid content may lead to an abnormality in cornification, explaining, in part, why lipid-lowering agents can lead to the disease. Cooper and colleagues [99] applied this idea to acquired ichthyosis and malignancy and looked at epidermal and dermal lipid synthesis in patients with Hodgkin's disease and ichthyosis. They found that dermal lipid synthesis was reduced in patients with Hodgkin's disease compared with controls regardless of whether they had ichthyosis, which does not lend significant credence to this hypothesis.

Another thought is that an abnormal host immune response leads to ichthyosis [86]. This idea is based on the association of the disease with malignancies, as well as leprosy, sarcoidosis, and AIDS—all of which alter one's immune system. Additonally, Lucker and Steijlen [82] postulated that the tumor may secrete a growth factor (such as TGF-α) that leads to the skin findings, a similar mechanism to other paraneoplastic syndromes. There is little available evidence to support or refute either of these hypotheses.

Treatment

Treatment is generally aimed at the underlying tumor [89]. Other treatment modalities, such as urea, oral vitamin A, salicylic acid, and topical steroids have been tried with varied results [89,96].

References

[1] Curth HO. Skin lesions and internal carcinomas. In: Andrade R, Gumport SL, Popkin GL, Rees D, editors. Cancer of the skin: biology-diagnosis-management. Philadelphia: Saunders; 1976. p. 1308–41.

[2] Andreev VC. Malignant acanthosis nigricans. Semin Dermatol 1984;3(4):265–72.

[3] Cohen PR, Grossman ME, Silvers DN, et al. Tripe palms and cancer. Clin Dermatol 1993;11(1):165–73.

[4] Holdiness MR. On the classification of the sign of Leser-Trélat. J Am Acad Dermatol 1988;19(4):754–7.

[5] Ellis DL, Yates RA. Sign of Leser-Trélat. Clin Dermatol 1993;11(1):141–8.

[6] Schwartz RA. Acanthosis nigricans. J Am Acad Dermatol 1994;31(1):1–19.

[7] Curth HO. Cancer associated with acanthosis nigricans. Arch Surg 1943;47(6):517–52.

[8] Stuart CA, Pate CJ, Peters EJ. Prevalence of acanthosis nigricans in an unselected population. Am J Med 1989;87(3):269–72.

[9] Sedano HO, Gorlin RJ. Acanthosis nigricans. Oral Surg Oral Med Oral Pathol 1987;63(4):462–7.

[10] Brown J, Winkelmann RK. Acanthosis nigricans: a study of 90 cases. Medicine 1968;47(1):33–51.

[11] Curth HO, Hilberg AW, Machacek GF. The site and histology of the cancer associated with malignant acanthosis nigricans. Cancer 1962;15:364–82.

[12] Lee HW, Suh HS, Choi JC, et al. Hyperkeratosis of the nipple and areola as a sign of malignant acanthosis nigricans. Clin Exp Dermatol 2005;30(6):721–2.

[13] Wedge CC, Rootman DS, Hunter W, et al. Malignant acanthosis nigricans. A case report. Ophthalmology 1993;100(10):1590–2.

[14] Ramirez-Amador V, Esquivel-Pedraza L, Caballero-Mendoza E, et al. Oral manifestations as a hallmark of malignant acanthosis nigricans. J Oral Pathol Med 1999;28(6):278–81.

[15] Clarke J. Malignant acanthosis nigricans. Clin Exp Dermatol 1977;2(2):167–70.

[16] Schwartz RA, Burgess GH. Florid cutaneous papillomatosis. Arch Dermatol 1978;114(12):1803–6.

[17] Gross G, Pfister H, Hellenthal B, et al. Acanthosis nigricans maligna: clinical and virological investigations. Dermatologica 1984;168(6):265–72.

[18] McGinness J, Greer K. Malignant acanthosis nigricans and tripe palms associated with pancreatic adenocarcinoma. Cutis 2006;78(1):37–40.

[19] Mohrenschlager M, Vocks E, Wessner DB, et al. Tripe palms and malignant acanthosis nigricans: cutaneous signs of imminent metastasis in bladder cancer? J Urol 2001;165(5):1629–30.

[20] Hiranandani M, Kaur I, Singhi SC, et al. Malignant acanthosis nigricans in adrenal carcinoma. Indian Pediatr 1995;32(8):920–3.

[21] Janier M, Blanchet-Bardon C, Bonvalet D, et al. Malignant acanthosis nigricans associated with non-Hodgkin's lymphoma: report of 2 cases. Dermatologica 1988;176(3):133–7.

[22] Lam S, Stone MS, Goeken JA, et al. Paraneoplastic pemphigus, cicatricial conjunctivitis, and acanthosis nigricans with pachydermatoglyphy in a patient with bronchogenic squamous cell carcinoma. Ophthalmology 1992;99(1):108–13.

[23] Mikhail GR, Fachnie DM, Drukker BH, et al. Generalized malignant acanthosis nigricans. Arch Dermatol 1979;115(2):201–2.

[24] Breathnach SM, Wells GC. Acanthosis palmaris: tripe palms. A distinctive pattern of palmar keratoderma frequently associated with internal malignancy. Clin Exp Dermatol 1980;5(2):181–9.

[25] Razack EM, Premalatha S, Rao NR, et al. Acanthosis palmaris in a patient with bullous pemphigoid. J Am Acad Dermatol 1987;16(1 Pt 2):217–9.

[26] Millard LG, Gould DJ. Hyperkeratosis of the palms and soles associated with internal malignancy and elevated levels of immunoreactive human growth hormone. Clin Exp Dermatol 1976;1(4):363–8.

[27] Chung VQ, Moschella SL, Zembowicz A, et al. Clinical and pathologic findings of paraneoplastic dermatoses. J Am Acad Dermatol 2006;54(5):745–62; quiz 763–6.

[28] Verbov JL. Dermatoglyphics of malignant acanthosis nigricans. Clin Exp Dermatol 2005;30(3):302–3.

[29] Hazen PG, Carney JF, Walker AE, et al. Acanthosis nigricans presenting as hyperkeratosis of the palms and soles. J Am Acad Dermatol 1979;1(6):541–4.

[30] Skiljevic DS, Nikolic MM, Jakovljevic A, et al. Generalized acanthosis nigricans in early childhood. Pediatr Dermatol 2001;18(3):213–6.

[31] Dantzig PI. Sign of Leser-Trélat. Arch Dermatol 1973;108(5):700–1.

[32] De Bersaques J. Sign of Leser-Trélat [letter]. J Am Acad Dermatol 1985;12:724.

[33] Yaniv R, Servadio Y, Feinstein A, et al. The sign of Leser-Trélat associated with transitional cell carcinoma of the urinary-bladder—a case report and short review. Clin Exp Dermatol 1994;19(2):142–5.

[34] Rampen HJ, Schwengle LE. The sign of Leser-Trélat: does it exist? J Am Acad Dermatol 1989;21(1):50–5.

[35] Lindelof B, Sigurgeirsson B, Melander S. Seborrheic keratoses and cancer. J Am Acad Dermatol 1992;26(6):947–50.

[36] Grob JJ, Rava MC, Gouvernet J, et al. The relation between seborrheic keratoses and malignant solid tumours. A case-control study. Acta Derm Venereol 1991;71(2):166–9.

[37] Inamadar AC, Palit A. Eruptive seborrhoeic keratosis in human immunodeficiency virus infection: a coincidence or 'the sign of Leser-Trélat'? Br J Dermatol 2003;149(2):435–6.

[38] Hsu C, Abraham S, Campanelli A, et al. Sign of Leser-Trélat in a heart transplant recipient. Br J Dermatol 2005;153(4):861–2.

[39] Kilmer SL, Berman B, Morhenn VB. Eruptive seborrheic keratoses in a young woman with acromegaly. J Am Acad Dermatol 1990;23(5 Pt 2):991–4.

[40] Flugman SL, McClain SA, Clark RA. Transient eruptive seborrheic keratoses associated with erythrodermic psoriasis and erythrodermic drug eruption: report of two cases. J Am Acad Dermatol 2001;45 (6 Suppl):S212–4.

[41] Bruckner N, Katz RA, Hood AF. Pemphigus foliaceus resembling eruptive seborrheic keratoses. Arch Dermatol 1980;116(7):815–6.

[42] Fetil E, Ozkan S, Gurler N, et al. Recurrent Leser-Trélat sign associated with two malignancies. Dermatology 2002;204(3):254–5.

[43] Ellis DL, Kafka SP, Chow JC, et al. Melanoma, growth factors, acanthosis nigricans, the sign of Leser-Trélat, and multiple acrochordons. A possible role for alpha-transforming growth factor in

cutaneous paraneoplastic syndromes. N Engl J Med 1987;317(25):1582–7.

[44] Nanney LB, Stoscheck CM, Magid M, et al. Altered [125I] epidermal growth factor binding and receptor distribution in psoriasis. J Invest Dermatol 1986; 86(3):260–5.

[45] Douglas F, McHenry PM, Dagg JH, et al. Elevated levels of epidermal growth factor in a patient with tripe palms. Br J Dermatol 1994;130(5):686–7.

[46] Curry SS, King LE. The sign of Leser-Trélat. Report of a case with adenocarcinoma of the duodenum. Arch Dermatol 1980;116(9):1059–60.

[47] Koyama S, Ikeda K, Sato M, et al. Transforming growth factor-alpha (TGF alpha)-producing gastric carcinoma with acanthosis nigricans: an endocrine effect of TGF alpha in the pathogenesis of cutaneous paraneoplastic syndrome and epithelial hyperplasia of the esophagus. J Gastroenterol 1997;32(1):71–7.

[48] Chosidow O, Becherel PA, Piette JC, et al. Tripe palms associated with systemic mastocytosis: the role of transforming growth factor-alpha and efficacy of interferon-alfa. Br J Dermatol 1998;138(4): 698–703.

[49] Stone OJ. Acanthosis nigricans–decreased extracellular matrix viscosity: cancer, obesity, diabetes, corticosteroids, somatotrophin. Med Hypotheses 1993; 40(3):154–7.

[50] Stone OJ. The sign of Leser-Trelat: a cutaneous sign of internal malignancy: weakened subepithelial matrix from the effect of neoplasms on the extracellular matrix of the host. Med Hypotheses 1993;40(6): 360–3.

[51] Bonnekoh B, Thiele B, Merk H, et al. Systemic photochemotherapy (PUVA) in acanthosis nigricans maligna: regression of keratosis, hyperpigmentation and pruritus. Z Hautkr 1989;64(12):1059–62.

[52] Weiss E, Schmidberger H, Jany R, et al. Palliative radiotherapy of mucocutaneous lesions in malignant acanthosis nigricans. Acta Oncol 1995;34(2): 265–7.

[53] Gorisek B, Krajnc I, Rems D, et al. Malignant acanthosis nigricans and tripe palms in a patient with endometrial adenocarcinoma—a case report and review of literature. Gynecol Oncol 1997;65(3): 539–42.

[54] Anderson SH, Hudson-Peacock M, Muller AF. Malignant acanthosis nigricans: potential role of chemotherapy. Br J Dermatol 1999;141(4):714–6.

[55] Patel S, Zirwas M, English JC 3rd. Acquired palmoplantar keratoderma. Am J Clin Dermatol 2007; 8(1):1–11.

[56] Howel-Evans W, McConnell RB, Clarke CA, et al. Carcinoma of the oesophagus with keratosis palmaris et plantaris (tylosis): a study of two families. Q J Med 1958;27(107):413–29.

[57] Stevens HP, Kelsell DP, Bryant SP, et al. Linkage of an American pedigree with palmoplantar keratoderma and malignancy (palmoplantar ectodermal dysplasia type III) to 17q24. Literature

survey and proposed updated classification of the keratodermas. Arch Dermatol 1996;132(6):640–51.

[58] Stevens HP, Kelsell DP, Leigh IM, et al. Punctate palmoplantar keratoderma and malignancy in a four-generation family. Br J Dermatol 1996; 134(4):720–6.

[59] Ellis A, Field JK, Field EA, et al. Tylosis associated with carcinoma of the oesophagus and oral leukoplakia in a large Liverpool family—a review of six generations. Eur J Cancer B Oral Oncol 1994; 30B(2):102–12.

[60] Blanchet-Bardon C, Nazzaro V, Chevrant-Breton J, et al. Hereditary epidermolytic palmoplantar keratoderma associated with breast and ovarian cancer in a large kindred. Br J Dermatol 1987;117(3): 363–70.

[61] Torchard D, Blanchet-Bardon C, Serova O, et al. Epidermolytic palmoplantar keratoderma cosegregates with a keratin 9 mutation in a pedigree with breast and ovarian cancer. Nat Genet 1994;6(1): 106–10.

[62] Micali G, Nasca MR, Innocenzi D, et al. Association of palmoplantar keratoderma, cutaneous squamous cell carcinoma, dental anomalies, and hypogenitalism in four siblings with 46,XX karyotype: a new syndrome. J Am Acad Dermatol 2005; 53(5 Suppl 1):S234–9.

[63] Grob JJ, Breton A, Bonafe JL, et al. Keratitis, ichthyosis, and deafness (KID) syndrome. Vertical transmission and death from multiple squamous cell carcinomas. Arch Dermatol 1987;123(6):777–82.

[64] Delaporte E, N'guyen-Mailfer C, Janin A, et al. Keratoderma with scleroatrophy of the extremities or sclerotylosis (Huriez syndrome): a reappraisal. Br J Dermatol 1995;133(3):409–16.

[65] Yesudian P, Premalatha S, Thambiah AS. Genetic tylosis with malignancy: a study of a south Indian pedigree. Br J Dermatol 1980;102(5):597–600.

[66] Sommers SC, McManus RG. Multiple arsenical cancers of skin and internal organs. Cancer 1953; 6(2):347–59.

[67] Piepkorn MW. Alterations in the stratum corneum and epidermis. In: Barnhill RL, Crowson AN, editors. Textbook of dermatopathology. 2nd edition. New York: McGraw-Hill, Medical Pub. Division; 2004. p. 333–58.

[68] Harper PS, Harper RM, Howel-Evans AW. Carcinoma of the oesophagus with tylosis. Q J Med 1970;39(155):317–33.

[69] Bazex A, Griffiths A. Acrokeratosis paraneoplastica—a new cutaneous marker of malignancy. Br J Dermatol 1980;103(3):301–6.

[70] Gougerot H, Rupp C. Dermatose érythémato-squameuse avec hyperkératose palmo-plantaire, porectasies digitales et cancer de la langue latent. Contribution à l'étude des dermatoses monitrices de cancerParis Med 1922;43:234–7.

[71] Bazex A, Salvador R, Dupre A, et al. Syndrome paranéoplasique à type d'hyperkératose des extrèmités.

guérison après le traitement de l'épithélioma laryngé. Bull Soc Fr Dermatol Syphiligr 1965;72:182.

[72] Karabulut AA, Sahin S, Sahin M, et al. Paraneoplastic acrokeratosis of bazex (Bazex's syndrome): report of a female case associated with cholangiocarcinoma and review of the published work. J Dermatol 2006;33(12):850 4.

[73] Bolognia JL. Bazex' syndrome. Clin Dermatol 1993; 11(1):37–42.

[74] Bolognia JL, Brewer YP, Cooper DL. Bazex syndrome (acrokeratosis paraneoplastica). An analytic review. Medicine (Baltimore) 1991;70(4):269–80.

[75] Sarkar B, Knecht R, Sarkar C, et al. Bazex syndrome (acrokeratosis paraneoplastica). Eur Arch Otorhinolaryngol 1998;255(4):205–10.

[76] Jacobsen FK, Abildtrup N, Laursen SO, et al. Acrokeratosis paraneoplastica (Bazex' syndrome). Arch Dermatol 1984;120(4):502–4.

[77] Gill D, Fergin P, Kelly J. Bullous lesions in Bazex syndrome and successful treatment with oral psoralen phototherapy. Australas J Dermatol 2001;42(4):278–80.

[78] Pecora AL, Landsman L, Imgrund SP, et al. Acrokeratosis paraneoplastica (Bazex' syndrome). Report of a case and review of the literature. Arch Dermatol 1983;119(10):820–6.

[79] Mutasim DF, Meiri G. Bazex syndrome mimicking a primary autoimmune bullous disorder. J Am Acad Dermatol 1999;40(5 Pt 2):822–5.

[80] Akhyani M, Mansoori P, Taheri A, et al. Acrokeratosis paraneoplastica (Bazex syndrome) associated with breast cancer. Clin Exp Dermatol 2004;29(4):429–30.

[81] Hsu YS, Lien GS, Lai HH, et al. Acrokeratosis paraneoplastica (Bazex syndrome) with adenocarcinoma of the colon: report of a case and review of the literature. J Gastroenterol 2000;35(6):460–4.

[82] Lucker GP, Steijlen PM. Acrokeratosis paraneoplastica (Bazex syndrome) occurring with acquired ichthyosis in Hodgkin's disease. Br J Dermatol 1995;133(2):322–5.

[83] Esteve E, Serpier H, Cambie MP, et al. Bazex paraneoplastic acrokeratosis. Treatment with acitretin. Ann Dermatol Venereol 1995;122(1–2):26–9.

[84] Wishart JM. Bazex paraneoplastic acrokeratosis: a case report and response to tigason. Br J Dermatol 1986;115(5):595–9.

[85] Schwartz RA, Williams ML. Acquired ichthyosis: a marker for internal disease. Am Fam Physician 1984;29(2):181–4.

[86] Aram H. Acquired ichthyosis and related conditions. Int J Dermatol 1984;23(7):458–61.

[87] Ronchese F. Ichthyosiform atrophy of the skin in Hodgkin's disease. Archives of Dermatology and Syphilology 1943;47:778–81.

[88] Van Dijk E. Ichthyosiform atrophy of the skin associated with internal malignant diseases. Dermatologica 1963;127:413–28.

[89] Griffin LJ, Massa MC. Acquired ichthyosis and pityriasis rotunda. Clin Dermatol 1993;11(1):27–32.

[90] Dilek I, Demirer T, Ustun C, et al. Acquired ichthyosis associated with chronic graft-versus-host disease following allogeneic peripheral blood stem cell transplantation in a patient with chronic myelogenous leukemia. Bone Marrow Transplant 1998;21(11):1159–61.

[91] Sneddon IB. Acquired ichthyosis in Hodgkin's disease. Br Med J 1955;1(4916):763–4.

[92] Stevanovic DV. Hodgkin's disease of the skin. Acquired ichthyosis preceding tumoral and ulcerating lesions for seven years. Arch Dermatol 1960;82: 96–9.

[93] Eisman S, O'Toole EA, Jones A, et al. Granulomatous mycosis fungoides presenting as an acquired ichthyosis. Clin Exp Dermatol 2003;28(2):174–6.

[94] Roselino AM, Souza CS, Andrade JM, et al. Dermatomyositis and acquired ichthyosis as paraneoplastic manifestations of ovarian tumor. Int J Dermatol 1997;36(8):611–4.

[95] Farrell AM, Ross JS, Thomas JM, et al. Acquired ichthyosis, alopecia and loss of hair pigment associated with leiomyosarcoma. J Eur Acad Dermatol Venereol 1998;10(2):159–63.

[96] Ameen M, Chopra S, Darvay A, et al. Erythema gyratum repens and acquired ichthyosis associated with transitional cell carcinoma of the kidney. Clin Exp Dermatol 2001;26(6):510–2.

[97] Inuzuka M, Tomita K, Tokura Y, et al. Acquired ichthyosis associated with dermatomyositis in a patient with hepatocellular carcinoma. Br J Dermatol 2001;144(2):416–7.

[98] Patel N, Spencer LA, English JC 3rd, et al. Acquired ichthyosis. J Am Acad Dermatol 2006; 55(4):647–56.

[99] Cooper MF, Wilson PD, Hartop PJ, et al. Acquired ichthyosis and impaired dermal lipogenesis in Hodgkin's disease. Br J Dermatol 1980;102(6): 689–93.

ELSEVIER
SAUNDERS

Dermatol Clin 26 (2008) 31–43

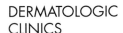

DERMATOLOGIC
CLINICS

Dermal and Pannicular Manifestations of Internal Malignancy

Roger H. Weenig, MD, MPH[a],*, Khosrow Mehrany, MD[b,c]

[a]Department of Dermatology, Dermatopathology Division, Mayo Clinic,
200 First Street SW, Rochester, MN 55905, USA
[b]Deparment of Dermatology, University of California, San Francisco, CA, USA
[c]Stanislaus Skin Cancer Clinic, 1130 Coffee Road, Suite 5B, Modesto, CA 95355, USA

The concept that noncutaneous malignances may induce paraneoplastic inflammatory reactions and neoplastic or non-neoplastic proliferations in the skin is well known. Moreover, numerous reviews, book chapters, and reports address the myriad cutaneous manifestations of internal malignancies. Previous work on this subject primarily provides lists and descriptions of dermatologic entities that are exclusively or occasionally associated with specific or varied internal cancers or precancerous states.

This review seeks to provide a different perspective to this subject by emphasizing components of the skin (the dermis and subcutis) as focal points of paraneoplastic phenomena, with the intent of broadening thinking and differential diagnoses when the findings described herein are encountered in dermatology clinics and dermatopathology laboratories.

A discussion of paraneoplastic skin disorders deserves special emphasis on the importance of correlation between clinical and pathologic findings as well as effective communication between clinicians and dermatopathologists.

Paraneoplastic skin disorders that primarily affect the epidermis (acanthosis nigricans, Bazex syndrome, dermatomyositis, necrolytic migratory erythema, and paraneoplastic pemphigus) are discussed elsewhere.

Pathophysiologic considerations

The pathogenesis of most of the malignancy-induced dermatologic disorders is complex, varied, and incompletely defined; however, recent research has provided clues into the molecular and biochemical mechanisms that drive some paraneoplastic processes. Most paraneoplastic skin disorders result directly as a cutaneous response to a tumor cell product or indirectly result from the effect of the neoplasm on another (noncutaneous) organ system. Examples of a direct cell product causing a paraneoplastic skin disorder include paraproteinemia-related skin disorders (Table 1) as well as the many hormonal and cytokine aberrations that drive malignancy-related hypercalcemia and extraskeletal calcium deposition. Indirect causes include tumors that cause secondary organ dysfunction or destruction, which then results in the skin disorder. Examples where a malignancy indirectly results in a paraneoplastic skin disorder include tumor destruction of pancreatic tissue with liberation of pancreatic enzymes followed by pancreatic panniculitis and myelofibrosis-related cutaneous extramedullary hematopoiesis.

Paraneoplastic calcium deposition of the dermis and subcutis

Hypercalcemia is a well-known paraneoplastic sign that is most prone in patients with squamous cell carcinoma of the esophagus, multiple myeloma, breast cancer, lymphoma, and osteolytic metastases. A subset of patients with paraneoplastic hypercalcemia may develop metastatic calcification, which usually occurs in the kidney or lung [1,2]. Rarely, paraneoplastic calcification may present as soft tissue calcium deposits in the dermis or subcutis (Fig. 1) or

---

* Corresponding author.
E-mail address: weenig.roger@mayo.edu
(R.H. Weenig).

0733-8635/08/$ - see front matter © 2008 Elsevier Inc. All rights reserved.
doi:10.1016/j.det.2007.08.007

Table 1
Dermal and pannicular manifestations of paraproteinemia

Finding/entities	Paraproteinemia
Calcium deposition[a]	Myeloma,
• Calcinosis cutis	various types
• *Calciphylaxis*	
Cryoglobulinemia	
• Type 1 (monoclonal)	IgG or IgM
• Type 2 (monoclonal + polyclonal)	anti-IgG IgM
Fibromucinosis	IgG-κ
• Lichen myxedematosus or scleromyxedema	
• Papular mucinosis[a]	
Hemangiomas (glomeruloid)	
• POEMS syndrome	IgA
Neutrophilic dermatoses	IgA
• Sweet syndrome	
• Pyoderma gangrenosum[a]	
• Erythema elevatum diutinum	
Xanthomatous infiltration	
• Plane xanthomas	IgG
• Necrobiotic xanthogranuloma	IgG-κ > IgG-λ
• Xanthoma disseminatum[a]	IgG
Sclerosis	
• Scleredema[a]	IgG
Urticaria	
• Schnitzler syndrome	IgM

[a] Rarely associated with paraproteinemia.

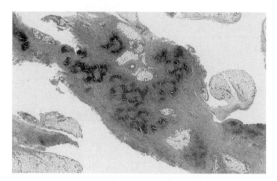

Fig. 1. Photomicrograph demonstrating septal pannicular calcium deposition in a patient with osteolytic myeloma (hematoxylin and eosin [H&E], ×10 original magnification).

[IL]-1, IL-8), and immunoglobulins (especially IgA). The latter two are of most relevance to paraneoplastic neutrophilic reactions in the skin.

Acute febrile neutrophilic dermatosis (Sweet syndrome)

Acute febrile neutrophilic dermatosis was described in 1964 by Sweet [16]. Most regard Sweet syndrome as a reactive inflammatory process that may be triggered by various stimuli. In Sweet's original series, an infectious cause was thought to be the inciting factor. Subsequently, other systemic disorders (inflammatory bowel disease, rheumatoid arthritis, sarcoidosis, drug reactions, and malignancy) were implicated in Sweet syndrome. In up to 54% of patients, a paraneoplastic association is identified [17]. A hematologic malignancy or premalignancy (paraproteinemia) is the most common paraneoplastic disorder associated with Sweet syndrome. Solid malignancies are identified in less than 10% of patients.

Patients with Sweet syndrome classically present with edematous, pseudovesicular pink-red papules and plaques, which preferentially involve the extremities but may present on any mucocutaneous site (Fig. 2). Other signs and symptoms may include arthritis, eye or conjunctival involvement, and oral lesions. Clinical variations of Sweet syndrome include bullous, atypical, and subcutaneous variants. The atypical variants include lesions that present in atypical locations and lesions that tend to develop necrotic ulceration or demonstrate significant clinical and pathologic overlap with pyoderma gangrenosum. Alternative designations (pustular vasculitis, neutrophilic dermatosis of the hands) are often

as calciphylaxis [3–6]. Malignancy-associated hypercalcemia and calcification has a variable pathogenesis, but includes tumor production of parathyroid hormone, parathyroid hormone–related peptide, vitamin D, and various cytokines, as well as up-regulation of receptor-activator of nuclear factor kappa B-Ligand (RANKL) and/or down-regulation of the RANKL-antagonist, osteoprotegerin (OPG) (Table 2) [7–15].

Paraneoplastic neutrophilic infiltration of the dermis and subcutis

A variety of stimuli may attract neutrophils to the skin, including infection, foreign material, trauma, connective tissue disease (acute and bullous lupus erythematosus, Still's disease), a variety of allergic/antigenic agents, cytokines (interleukin

Table 2
Causes and mechanisms of paraneoplastic calcium deposition of the dermis and subcutis

Tumor product	Serum Ca	Serum PO$_4$	PTH	Tumor type
PTH secreting tumors	↑	↓	↑	Parathyroid adenoma, other tumors
PTHrP secreting tumors	↑	↓	nl/↓	Breast cancer, SCC, lymphoma, myeloma
Osteolytic metastases	↑	↓	nl/↓	Tumor secretion of cytokines and PTHrP
Vitamin D secreting tumors	↑	↑	nl/↓	Lymphomas

Abbreviations: Ca, Calcium; nl, normal; PO$_4$, phosphate; PTH, parathyroid hormone; PTHrP, parathyroid hormone–related peptide; SCC, squamous cell carcinoma.

assigned to such cases, although most meet diagnostic criteria for Sweet syndrome.

Biopsy of skin involved by Sweet syndrome typically reveals a dense and diffuse dermal neutrophilic infiltrate, often associated with neutrophilic debris and marked papillary dermal edema. Histopathologic variations include a cell-poor variant, predominantly subcutaneous neutrophil infiltration in the subcutaneous variant, an infiltrate composed of histiocyte-like cells or band and stab forms in the histiocytoid variant and subepidermal separation in the bullous variant. Although Sweet syndrome is not a form of primary vasculitis, bystander neutrophilic vascular infiltration and injury may be observed occasionally and is more common in atypical cases and cases showing significant overlap with pyoderma gangrenosum. Cases with marked vascular injury also tend to be associated with cutaneous necrosis and ulceration.

Some apply a strict histologic requirement that the neutrophilic infiltrate in subcutaneous Sweet syndrome should predominantly involve the pannicular septae and that neutrophilic lobular panniculitis should be regarded as a distinct entity. However, there are no unique clinical findings, disease associations, or therapeutic differences to justify such distinction. Furthermore, most cases meet diagnostic criteria for Sweet syndrome. Subcutaneous Sweet syndrome does not appear more likely to be associated with malignancy.

Requena and colleagues [18] recently reported a series of 41 patients who presented with clinical features typical of Sweet syndrome, but with a dermal infiltrate composed of histiocyte-like cells as opposed to mature neutrophils typical of classical Sweet syndrome. The cells were demonstrated to be neutrophil precursors and the authors designated this histologic presentation as a "histiocytoid" variant of Sweet syndrome. A paraneoplastic association was not more common in their series of patients.

Rare cases of Sweet syndrome demonstrate clear morphologic features of precursor myeloid cells with band and stab forms predominating the infiltrate. These cases could be designated "histiocytoid Sweet syndrome," but "monocytoid" or "precursor myeloid" Sweet syndrome is preferred by the authors. The explanation for an immature neutrophilic infiltrate in these cases is unclear, but may be secondary to bone marrow pathology (myeloid dysplasia, myeloma, and other bone marrow–infiltrating processes) in some patients, which results in defective maturation or premature release of myeloid cells in-transit from the marrow to skin.

Treatment of paraneoplastic-associated Sweet syndrome is the same as in classical Sweet syndrome, and systemic corticosteroids remain the drug of choice. Some patients with underlying malignancy may experience chronic or recurrent eruptions of Sweet syndrome or disease flare associated with cancer relapse.

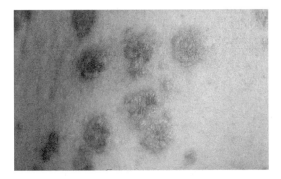

Fig. 2. Photograph of red, indurated, and edematous annular plaques typical of Sweet syndrome.

Pyoderma gangrenosum

Since the description of pyoderma gangrenosum by Brunsting, Goeckerman, and O'Leary in 1930 [19], numerous diseases (inflammatory and neoplastic) have been reported in association with this neutrophilic dermatosis. An IgA paraproteinemia is the most common neoplastic state associated with pyoderma gangrenosum. Other hematologic neoplasms reported in association with pyoderma gangrenosum include myeloma, leukemia, and polycythemia rubra vera. However, there are no reliable clinical features to predict which cases have a paraneoplastic association.

Pyoderma gangrenosum typically starts as a violaceous, tender, pustule that rapidly enlarges to a painful, necrotic supperative ulcer via a dissecting dermatitis (Fig. 3).

Histopathologic findings in pyoderma gangrenosum are NOT specific or diagnostic, but biopsy of the violaceous border of pyoderma gangrenosum demonstrates diffuse dermal neutrophilia and necrosis. Dermal edema, leukocytoclasis, and necrosis of the overlying epidermis may also be observed. Cases associated with an internal malignancy do not demonstrate unique histopathologic findings compared with other cases of pyoderma gangrenosum.

The diagnosis of pyoderma gangrenosum is one of exclusion, and many disorders may produce similar cutaneous ulceration [20]. Appropriate clinical and laboratory investigations are required to exclude alternative causes of pyoderma gangrenosum–like ulceration. Diagnostic criteria for pyoderma gangrenosum have been recommended to help guide clinical evaluation and avoid misdiagnosis [21].

Pyoderma gangrenosum is typically responsive to moderate doses of systemic corticosteroids. A variety of steroid-sparing immunosuppressive drugs, antibiotics, and biologic agents have been used to successfully manage pyoderma gangrenosum. Treatment of an associated malignancy may or may not lead to improvement of pyoderma gangrenosum.

As pyoderma gangrenosum often results in substantial loss of tissue and many of the treatments used both delay healing and increase the risk of infection, careful attention to wound care and frequent clinical reassessment are needed. During the course of treating pyoderma gangrenosum, the active inflammatory component may resolve, yet the ulceration progresses because of inadequate or inappropriate wound care, secondary infection, treatment-related delay of healing, or a combination of these. In these circumstances, the *current* cause for persistent ulceration should be addressed instead of increasing immunosuppressive therapy.

Erythema elevatum diutinum

Erythema elevatum diutinum (EED) is a chronic neutrophil-mediated vasculitis, which

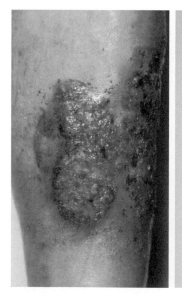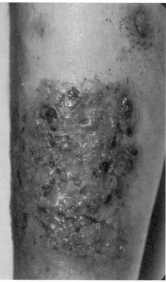

Fig. 3. Photograph of pyoderma gangrenosum demonstrating deep violaceous, boggy induration and early ulceration.

may be considered to belong to the family of neutrophilic dermatoses. A paraprotein, usually IgA, is frequently associated with EED. B-cell lymphoma, chronic lymphocytic leukemia, myelodysplastic syndrome, and myeloma have also been reported in association with EED [22–26].

Patients present with red-brown papules and nodules that tend to occur overlying boney prominences, particularly of the digits (Fig. 4). Lesions usually impart a yellowish (xanthomatous) hue.

Biopsy of involved skin reveals a spectrum of findings that depend on lesion chronicity. Early lesions reveal leukocytoclastic vasculitis (LCV) that may be indistinguishable from other causes of LCV. The histopathologic diagnosis is more apparent in older lesions that demonstrate fibrosis in addition to LCV. Foamy (xanthomatized) histiocytes and extracellular lipid or cholesterol deposits may also be observed.

EED is often responsive to dapsone as monotherapy. A combination of "anti-neutrophil" agents (eg, dapsone and colchicine) or more potent immunosuppressive therapy may be required. However, in contrast to other neutrophilic dermatoses and other forms of vasculitis, systemic steroids are often ineffective for EED.

Paraneoplastic fibrocyte disorders of the dermis and subcutis

Fibrocytes (AKA: fibroblasts) originate from bone marrow–derived CD34-positive hematopoietic precursor cells that differentiate and migrate to the skin during development and in skin remodeling/repair. The primary role of skin fibrocytes is to produce the anchoring substance (collagen, elastin, mucopolysaccharides, and proteoglycans) of the dermis and pannicular septae to which the epidermis and skin appendages attach.

A variety of disease states produce fibrocyte pathology (fibropathy) resulting in fibrocyte hyperplasia (fibrosis), excessive collagen deposition (sclerosis), mucin production (mucinosis), or a combination of these (eg, fibrosis + mucinosis in scleromyxedema; or sclerosis + mucinosis in scleredema). An IgG paraprotein is usually identified in patients with scleromyxedema and rarely in scleredema.

Scleromyxedema

Lichen myxedematosus was described by Montgomery and Underwood in 1953 and in the following year, Gottron described scleromyxedema [27,28]. Papular mucinosis is considered a localized variant of scleromyxedema with indistinguishable histopathologic findings. Monoclonal paraproteinemia (usually IgG-kappa) is identified in most patients, but is less frequent in localized disease. Progression to myeloma is rare.

The pathogenesis of scleromyxedema is not known and evidence for a direct effect of the monoclonal protein on fibroblast proliferation or mucin production is lacking [29,30]. Indirect mechanisms may be more relevant, including circulating cytokines and inflammatory mediators that stimulate dermal fibroblasts or recruit fibrocyte precursors from the bone marrow to the skin.

Several distinct clinical presentations and nosologic designations for scleromyxedema are recognized. Significant clinical overlap exists between the variants, and patients may progress from limited to widespread disease. Nonetheless, it is useful to separate limited from widespread disease and cases that present with discrete lichenoid papules compared with confluent indurated plaques, as patients with extensive disease and/or confluent plaques are more likely to have paraproteinemia and experience progressive disease. The disease tends to involve the face, trunk, and

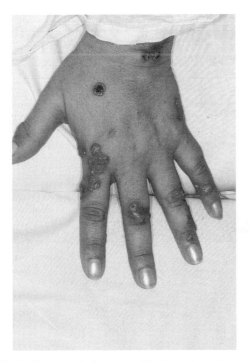

Fig. 4. Photograph showing red indurated papules and plaques overlying joints of the hand in erythema elevatum diutinum.

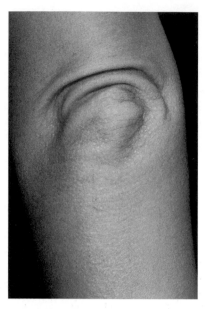

Fig. 5. Photograph of the arm and elbow of a patient with scleromyxedema showing indurated, firm skin and numerous small "lichenoid" papules.

extremities resulting in facial disfigurement and decreased flexibility of joints underlying involved skin (Fig. 5).

Muscle weakness, flexion contractors, restrictive lung disease, esophageal and upper respiratory tract involvement, pulmonary hypertension, and neurologic disorders may occur in the course of the disease. There are no tests that determine which patients will develop internal organ involvement.

Skin biopsy of involved skin reveals superficial and mid-dermal haphazard fibrosis with marked increase in dermal mucin (Fig. 6).

Treatment of scleromyxedema has been difficult historically and melphalan has been used for many years with mixed results. Recently, aggressive treatment of the paraproteinemia with bone marrow transplantation was associated with dramatic improvement of scleromyxedema [31].

Scleredema

Scleredema is a rare sclerosing disorder that Buschke [32] originally described in 1902. Three clinical variants are recognized: (1) postinfectious scleredema of youth; (2) diabetes mellitus–associated scleredema of adulthood; and (3) paraproteinemia-associated scleredema.

The etiopathogenesis of scleredema is not known, but is likely variable given the three known disease associations. Increased collagen deposition (sclerosis) with a mild increase in dermal mucin is observed in all three forms of the disease.

Patients with scleredema present with firm, waxy, indurated, nonpitting edema of the neck, shoulders, and upper back (Fig. 7). Skin of the face and arms is less commonly affected. Imperceptible blending of involved from uninvolved skin is distinct from the sharply demarcated papules and plaques of scleromyxedema. Scleredema of the esophagus, bone marrow, nerve, liver, and salivary glands has been reported, but is probably rare since most patients lack signs and symptoms of extracutaneous disease [33,34].

A punch biopsy of involved skin demonstrates a nontapered (square) appearance of the dermis at low power. The dermis is thickened relative to noninvolved skin and adnexal structures may be numerically decreased, contain less

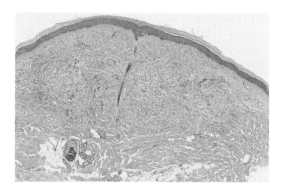

Fig. 6. Photomicrograph of scleromyxedema showing loose, haphazard fibroblast proliferation and mucin deposition in the superficial to mid-dermis (H&E, ×50 original magnification).

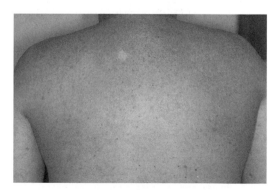

Fig. 7. Photograph of scleredema showing indurated, shiny, and waxy skin of the upper back.

periappendageal fat, and/or be located higher in the dermis. Collagen bundles are thickened and separated by subtle mucin deposits.

The course, prognosis, and response to treatment of scleredema varies by subtype and extent of disease. Postinfectious scleredema does not improve with antibiotics, but usually regresses spontaneously within 2 years of presentation. Diabetes-associated scleredema is usually chronic, but may improve with better glucose control. Paraproteinemia-associated scleredema runs a protracted course and is often unresponsive to treatment; however, extracorporeal photopheresis was reported effective in one patient [35]. Phototherapy (bath-psoralen plus ultraviolet A and ultraviolet A1) was reported effective in a few patients with scleromyxedema [36,37].

Paraneoplastic histiocytic infiltrates of the dermis and subcutis

Multicentric reticulohistiocytosis (lipoid dermatoarthritis)

Reticulohistiocytomas may present clinically as solitary or multiple lesions, or as a systemic condition (multicentric reticulohistiocytosis) associated with destructive arthritis and periodic fever. A paraneoplastic association is seen in as many as 25% of cases of multicentric reticulohistiocytosis, including leukemia and solid tumors (breast, cervix, colon, lung, pancreas, stomach, and skin [melanoma]) [38–43].

Women are affected by muticentric reticulohistiocytosis three times more frequently than males and the mean age of onset is 43 years [44]. Characteristically, the skin and mucosa of the face and hands develop reddish-brown to yellow papules and nodules (Fig. 8). Destructive arthritis of the small joints of the digits is common, but involvement of larger joints of the limbs and axial skeleton may occur. Viscera (heart, gastrointestinal tract, and lung) and the deeper soft tissues, muscle, or bone may also develop reticulohistiocytic infiltrates [45–48]. Hyperlipidemia is commonly identified in patients with multicentric reticulohistiocytosis.

Biopsy of involved skin reveals a nodular dermal to superficial pannicular infiltrate composed of numerous solitary and multinucleated histiocytes with abundant eosinophilic, "ground-glass–appearing" cytoplasm. Admixed lymphocytes are also present.

Treatment of multicentric reticulohistiocytosis has been challenging historically. Systemic immunosuppressive agents have demonstrated mixed results. Clinical improvement with bisphosphonates or tumor necrosis factor-alpha inhibitors has been reported [49,50].

Necrobiotic xanthogranuloma

Kossard and Winkelmann [51] described necrobiotic xanthogranuloma (NXG) in 1980. NXG is characterized by an infiltrative histiocytic process that results in indurated red-yellow papules, nodules, and plaques that tend to ulcerate (Fig. 9). A monoclonal protein (usually IgG-kappa) is identified in most patients. Some patients develop plasma cell dyscrasia, lymphoma, or myeloma.

Skin is the primary organ involved, but involvement other organs has been reported. The skin surrounding the eyes is preferentially

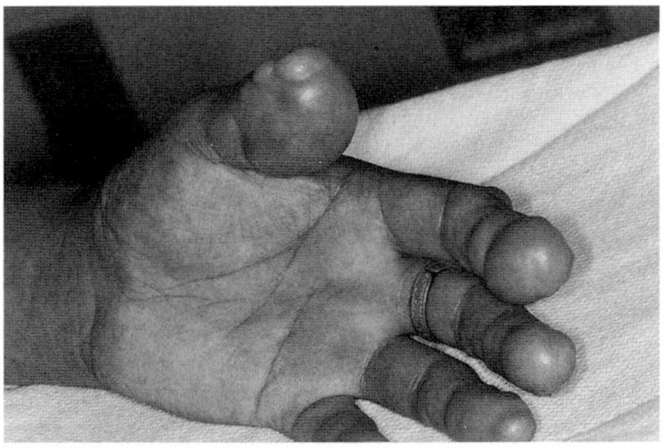

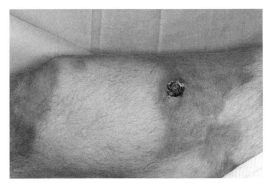

Fig. 8. Photograph of multicentric reticulohistiocytosis with indurated papules, nodules, and destructive arthritis affecting several digits of the hand.

Fig. 9. Photograph of necrobiotic xanthogranuloma showing erythematous to yellowish plaques on the thigh and knee. Note necrotic ulcer in the center of the plaque on the thigh.

involved and many patients have eye problems (ptosis, orbital mass lesions, ectropion, scleritis, episcleritis, or uveitis) [52].

Skin biopsy of NXG demonstrates aggregates of foamy "xanthomatized" histiocytes and giant cells in the dermis and/or subcutaneous tissue that surround zones of degenerated collagen. Cholesterol clefts may also be observed.

The prognosis of NXG is variable in published series, but appears to be dependent on the development of an associated lymphoproliferative disorder. However, some patients succumb to sepsis acquired from extensive nonhealing cutaneous ulceration.

No standardized treatment is established for NXG, but systemic chemotherapy (chlorambucil and melphalan), radiation, and plasmaphoresis has been helpful for some patients. A few patients have had marked improvement after bone marrow transplantation. Surgery should be avoided, as it does not appear beneficial and may actually exacerbate the disease process.

Normolipemic plane xanthoma

Plane xanthomas are characterized by variably sized yellow plaques (Fig. 10) that show regional predilection for specific disease associations (palmar crease in dysbetalipoproteinemia [53], web spaces of digits or intertriginous areas in homozygous familial hypercholesterolemia [54], and normolipemic diffuse plane xanthomas in monoclonal gammopathies, myeloma, leukemia, or lymphoma [55–57]).

As in other xanthomas, skin biopsy of plane xanthoma reveals a dermal-based proliferation of foamy, lipidized histiocytes, but these tend to be more superficial than in other xanthomas; there is

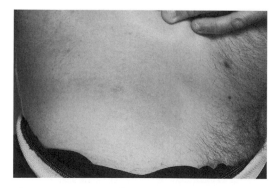

Fig. 10. Photograph of plane xanthoma in a patient with normal lipids and IgG monoclonal gammopathy.

usually no associated lymphocytic or acute inflammation.

Xanthogranuloma

Xanthogranulomas are relatively uncommon, benign, asymptomatic histiocytic proliferations that present as solitary or multiple yellow-reddish to brown dome-shaped papules or nodules in the skin (especially on the head and neck), mucosa, or eye (particularly the iris). As onset is usually early in life, the lesion is frequently referred to as "juvenile xanthogranuloma." Visceral lesions of xanthogranuloma may also occur, but are rare. When visceral lesions occur, the brain, liver, lung, and spleen are most often affected. However, numerous other organs may be involved (heart, peripheral nerves, ovaries, testes).

Lipid abnormalities are not more common in patients with xanthogranulomas.

The presence of xanthogranuloma in association with neurofibromatosis type 1 is estimated to confer a 20- to 32-fold increased risk for the development of juvenile myelomonocytic leukemia [58]. However, the absence of neurofibromatosis does not exclude leukemia risk.

Biopsy of xanthogranuloma reveals a circumscribed, dermal to subcutaneous nodular proliferation of foamy ("xanthomatized") histiocytes. Touton giant cells may be absent in early lesions, but are characteristically present in established lesions. Larger lesions may be situated entirely within the subcutis, invade skeletal muscle, or may involve deeper soft tissues.

Xanthogranulomas that present in youth often regress spontaneously within a few years of presentation, whereas adult lesions tend to persist.

Dermal and pannicular paraneoplastic proliferations

POEMS syndrome

In 1980, Bardwick and colleagues [59] coined the acronym "POEMS" to describe a multisystem, paraneoplastic syndrome with characteristic clinical features. The acronym, "POEMS," refers to symmetric, progressive, sensorimotor Polyneuropathy, Organomegally (enlarged liver, spleen, and lymph nodes), Endocrinopathy (adrenal, gonadal, pancreatic, parathyroid, pituitary, thyroid) and Edema (acsites, lower extremity edema), Monoclonal gammopathy (osteosclerotic more often than osteolytic and IgA more often than IgG or IgM), and Skin changes. "Crow-Fukase syndrome," "Takatsuki disease," "Shimpo syndrome," and PEP syndrome are other less frequently used designations for the syndrome.

Many reports of POEMS syndrome have been associated with angiofollicular lymph node hyperplasia (Castleman's disease). This led some authors to place POEMS syndrome under the rubric of multicentric Castleman's disease [60]. Although distinction between these entities is often difficult or may be arbitrary, Castleman's disease is more often associated with a polyclonal gammopathy, and is defined by distinctive lymph node histology (hyaline-vascular, plasma-cell, or mixed variants) rather than other requisite features of POEMS syndrome (such as osteosclerotic lesions and peripheral neuropathy). Still others define POEMS as a variant of osteosclerotic myeloma that is frequently accompanied by a demyelinating polyneuropathy [61–64].

The cutaneous manifestations of POEMS syndrome are manifold. Diffuse hyperpigmentation is the most sensitive skin finding (present in 71% to 93% of patients), followed by scleroderma-like skin thickening (56% to 94%), and hypertrichosis (50% to 87%) [64]. Cutaneous angiomata that present in a rapid or progressive fashion are seen less frequently (26% to 32%) [64,65], but are a more specific finding, especially if a glomeruloid histologic pattern is observed [66,67].

The pathogenesis of the angioproliferative lesions in POEMS syndrome is unknown, but an undefined angiogenic factor has been implicated. High levels of IL-1, IL-6, and tumor necrosis factor-alpha (TNF-α) have been found in the sera, lymph nodes, and skin of patients with POEMS syndrome [64,68–70]. These acute phase reactant–producing cytokines may be directly or indirectly related to the angiomata of POEMS syndrome. For example, TNF-α has been shown to stimulate polymorpholeukocytes to secrete one of the most potent angiogenic cytokines, vascular endothelial growth factor (VEGF) [71]. This is intriguing given the recent report of elevated serum VEGF in 10 patients with POEMS syndrome (15- to 30-fold greater serum VEGF than controls) [72].

Moreover, studies looking for an association of human herpes virus 8 (HHV-8) infection in POEMS syndrome have produced conflicting results. One study reported positive HHV-8 DNA sequences in 7 (54%) of 13 and positive anti-HHV-8 antibodies in 9 (50%) of 18 patients with POEMS syndrome [73]. However, rates of positivity were higher in patients who also had multicentric Castleman's disease (85% and 78% with

evidence of HHV-8 by polymerase chain reaction [PCR] and antibody detection respectively). Another study found evidence of HHV-8 in only 1 of 13 patients by PCR [74].

Paraneoplastic urticaria

Schnitzler syndrome

Schnitzler syndrome is a rare disorder characterized by urticaria, recurrent fever, bone pain, arthralgias, myalgias, and paraproteinemia. The paraprotein is composed of IgM, which is thought to form immune complexes and activate the complement cascade.

A small percentage of patients with Schnitzler syndrome will develop a lymphoproliferative disorder (lymphoplasmacytic lymphoma or Waldenstrom macroglobulinemia).

Skin biopsy of the urticarial lesions are nonspecific, but may demonstrate perivascular dermal inflammation composed of neutrophils or lymphocytes, so-called "neutrophilic" or "lymphocytic" urticaria, respectively.

Paraneoplastic vasculitis and vaso-occlusive disorders

Cryoglobulinemias

The cryoglobulinemia represent a group of disorders characterized by the presence of an immunoglobulin within the serum that precipitates in cold temperatures.

Cryoglobulinemias in which the cryoprotein is a monoclonal protein (Type I and Type II cryoglobulinemia) should be considered paraneoplastic diseases and may be associated with myeloma, lymphoma, and Waldenstrom macroglobulinemia, as well as lymphoblastic leukemias. Type III cryoglobulinemia is not associated with neoplasia per se.

The monoclonal cryoglobulin protein precipitates within the vascular lumina and frequently results in vascular occlusion and cutaneous ischemia. Acral skin (eg, ears, nose, fingers, and toes) is predisposed, but proximal regions may also be involved. Ischemic purpuric patches and acral cyanosis are typical of Type I cryoglobulinemia (Fig. 11). Histologically, skin biopsies of Type I cryoglobulinemia reveal glassy, eosinophilic deposits within dermal blood vessels. Unless there is associated ulceration, there is minimal associated inflammation. The mixed cryoglobulinemias (Type II and Type III) are more prone to immune complex formation and complement activation,

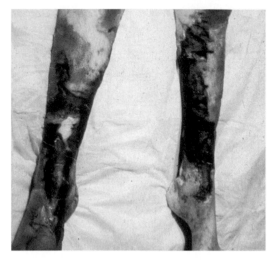

Fig. 11. Photograph of Type I cryoglobulinemia showing ischemic necrosis and ulceration of the legs.

resulting in palpable purpura clinically and leukocytoclastic vasculitis histologically.

Miscellaneous paraneoplastic disorders of the dermis and subcutis

Erythema gyratum repens

Some cases of erythema gyratum rapens–like eruptions are associated with infection (tuberculosis), connective tissue disease (lupus, Sjogren syndrome), or are idiopathic, but most cases are associated with a solid organ malignancy. The most common neoplasm associated with erythema gyratum repens is lung carcinoma. Other reported cancers include tumors of the breast, esophagus, kidney, stomach, uterus, and cervix. The eruption may proceed cancer detection by months.

Erythema gyratum repens occurs twice as frequently in men compared with women, and onset is usually in the seventh decade of life. The higher incidence of erythema gyratum repens in these groups likely reflects the higher frequency and type of malignancies in these populations.

Patients present with a distinctive patterned (gyrate "wood-grain–like") papulosquamous eruption on the extremities with tendency to generalize rapidly. Scaling is present and may be accompanied by pruritus.

Skin biopsy of erythema gyratum repens is nonspecific, but demonstrates a variably spongiotic dermatitis associated with tight ("coat-sleeve") perivascular dermal lymphocytic inflammation.

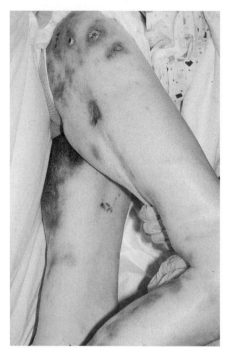

Fig. 12. Photograph of pancreatic panniculitis demonstrating numerous draining ulcers of the legs in a patient with pancreatic carcinoma.

Treatment of erythema gyratum repens usually entails treating the underlying disorder. Systemic steroids may provide symptomatic improvement for cases associated with significant pruritus, but the eruption is characteristically unresponsive to treatment.

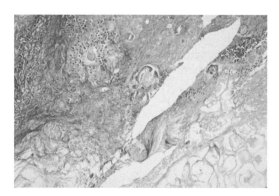

Fig. 13. Photomicrograph of pancreatic panniculitis demonstrating saponification of fat lobules, suppurative fat necrosis, and cholesterol cleft formation (H&E, ×200 original magnification).

Pancreatic panniculitis

Inflammatory or neoplastic destruction of pancreatic tissue may result in the liberation of lipase, trypsin, amylase, and phospholipase, which in turn causes enzymatic digestion (soaponification) of adipose tissue. Adipose tissue at any site (eg, subcutaneous, visceral, and mesenteric) may be involved, but the subcutaneous tissue of the lower extremities is a predisposed location.

Patients present with tender, red, subcutaneous nodules that may ulcerate and drain oily material (Fig. 12). An associated inflammatory arthritis is common, especially in cases associated with pancreatic carcinoma. The ankle joints are especially prone to arthritis in the setting of pancreatic panniculitis. Effusions of the pleura or pericardium and asities may also be observed. Peripheral blood eosinophilia is commonly seen in cases associated with pancreatic cancer and less common in cases associated with pancreatitis.

Skin biopsy of pancreatic panniculitis demonstrates acute and chronic inflammatory infiltrate of the fat lobules associated with a pathognomonic fat necrosis characterized by anucleate (ghost) fat cells that are often calcified (Fig. 13).

The overall prognosis of patients with pancreatic panniculitis is guarded, as the mortality exceeds 40% for cases associated with pancreatitis and 100% for cases associated with pancreatic carcinoma [75].

References

[1] Hall SW, Luna MA, Bedrossian C, et al. Calcinosis in nonparathyroid malignant disease: an unusual case report and clinicopathologic review of 17 cases. Med Pediatr Oncol 1978;4:49–58.

[2] Mine Y, Ito N, Tagawa M, et al. [Metastatic calcification associated with malignancy]. Gan No Rinsho 1988;34:2044–51 [in Japanese].

[3] Alvarez AJC, Saval AH, Enriquez JM, et al. Metastatic calcinosis cutis in multiple myeloma. Br J Dermatol 2000;142:820–2.

[4] Mastruserio DN, Nguyen EQ, Nielsen T, et al. Calciphylaxis associated with metastatic breast carcinoma. J Am Acad Dermatol 1999;4:295–8.

[5] Kutlu NO, Aydin NE, Aslan M, et al. Malignant melanoma of the soft parts showing calciphylaxis. Pediatr Hematol Oncol 2003;20:141–6.

[6] De Roma I, Filotico R, Cea M, et al. Calciphylaxis in a patient with POEMS syndrome without renal failure and/or hyperparathyroidism. Ann Ital Med Int 2004;19:283–7.

[7] Weiss ES, Doty J, Brock MV, et al. A case of ectopic parathyroid hormone production by a pulmonary neoplasm. J Thorac Cardiovasc Surg 2006;131: 923–4.

[8] Benit A, Allard J, Rimailho J, et al. Persistent and moderate hypercalcemia related to an ovarian clear cell adenocarcinoma: pre- and postoperative parathyroid hormone related-peptide and 1,25-dihydroxyvitamin D3 levels. J Endocrinol Invest 2006;29: 443–9.

[9] Gupta R, Neal JM. Hypercalcemia due to vitamin D-secreting Hodgkin's lymphoma exacerbated by oral calcium supplementation. Endocr Pract 2006; 12:227–9.

[10] Matsumoto T, Abe M. Bone destruction in multiple myeloma. Ann N Y Acad Sci 2006;1068:319–26.

[11] Roux S, Mariette X. The high rate of bone resorption in multiple myeloma is due to RANK (receptor activator of nuclear factor-kB) and RANK ligand expression. Leuk Lymphoma 2004;45: 1111–8.

[12] Chen G, Sircar K, Aprikian A, et al. Expression of RANKL/RANK/OPG in primary and metastatic human prostate cancer as markers of disease stage and functional regulation. Cancer 2006;107:289–98.

[13] Lau YS, Sabokbar A, Giele H, et al. Malignant melanoma and bone resorption. Br J Cancer 2006;94: 1496–503.

[14] Kitazawa S, Kitazawa R. RANK ligand is a prerequisite for cancer-associated osteolytic lesions. J Pathol 2002;198(2):228–36.

[15] Niizuma H, Fujii K, Sato A, et al. PTHrP-independent hypercalcemia with increased proinflammatory cytokines and bone resorption in two children with CD19-negative precursor B acute lymphoblastic leukemia. Pediatr Blood Cancer 2006; [Epub ahead of print].

[16] Sweet RD. An acute febrile neutrophilic dermatosis. Br J Dermatol 1964;76:349–56.

[17] Fett DL, Gibson LE, Su WP. Sweet's syndrome: systemic signs and symptoms and associated disorders. Mayo Clin Proc 1995;70:234–40.

[18] Requena L, Kutzner H, Palmedo G, et al. Histiocytoid Sweet syndrome. Arch Dermatol 2005;141: 834–42.

[19] Brunsting LA, Goeckerman WH, O'Leary PA. Pyoderma (ecthyma) gangrenosum: clinical and experimental observation in five cases occurring in adults. Arch Dermatol 1930;20:655–80.

[20] Weenig RH, Davis MDP, Dahl PR, et al. Skin ulcers misdiagnosed as pyoderma gangrenosum. N Engl J Med 2002;347:1412–8.

[21] Su WP, David MD, Weenig RH, et al. Pyoderma gangrenosum: clinicopathologic correlation and proposed diagnostic criteria. Int J Dermatol 2004; 43:790–800.

[22] Futei Y, Konohana I. A case of erythema elevatum diutinum associated with B-cell lymphoma: a rare distribution involving palms, soles, and nails. Br J Dermatol 2000;142:116–9.

[23] Delaporte E, Alfandari S, Fenaux P, et al. Erythema elevatum diutinum and chronic lymphocytic leukemia. Clin Exp Dermatol 1994;19:188.

[24] Queipo de Llano M, Yebra M, Cabrera R, et al. Myelodysplatic syndrome in association with erythema elevatum diutinum. J Rheumatol 1992;19:1005–6.

[25] Yiannias JA, el-Azhary RA, Gibson LE. Erythema elevatum diutinum: a clinical and histopathologic study of 13 patients. J Am Acad Dermatol 1992;26:38–44.

[26] Gerbig AW, Zala L, Hunziker T. [Erythema elevatum diutinum. A rare dermatosis with a broad spectrum of associated illnesses]. Hautarzt 1997;48:113–7 [in German].

[27] Montgomery H, Underwood LJ. Lichem myxedematosus; differentiation from cutaneous myxedemas or mucoid states. J Invest Dermatol 1953;20:213–36.

[28] Gottron HA. Skleromyxodem (eine eigenartige euscheinugs-form von myxothesaurodermie). Arch Klin Exp Dermatol 1954;199:71–91.

[29] Harper RA, Rispler J. Lichen myxedematosus serum stimulates skin fibroblast proliferation. Science 1978;199:545–7.

[30] Yaron M, Yaron I, Yust I, et al. Lichen myxedematosus (scleromyxedema) serum stimulates hyaluronic acid and prostaglandin E production by human fibroblasts. J Rheumatol 1985;12:171–5.

[31] Lacy MQ, Hogan WJ, Gertz MA, et al. Successful treatment of scleromyxedema with autologous peripheral blood stem cell transplantation. Arch Dermatol 2005;141:1277–82.

[32] Buschke A. Ueber Scleroedem. Berlin Klinische Wochenschrift 1902;39:955–6.

[33] Wright RA, Bernie H. Scleredema adultorum of Buschke with upper esophageal involvement. Am J Gastroenterol 1983;77:9–11.

[34] Basarab T, Burrows NP, Munn SE, et al. Systemic involvement in scleredema of Buschke associated with IgG-kappa paraproteinaemia. Br J Dermatol 1997;136:939–42.

[35] Stables GI, Taylor PC, Highet AS. Scleredema associated with paraproteinaemia treated by extracorporeal photopheresis. Br J Dermatol 2000;142:781–3.

[36] Janiga J, Ward DH, Lim HW. UVA-1 as a treatment for scleredema. Photodermatol Photoimmunol Photomed 2004;20:210–1.

[37] Hager CM, Sobhi HA, Hunzelmann N, et al. Bath-PUVA therapy in three patients with scleredema adultorum. J Am Acad Dermatol 1998;38:240–2.

[38] Bauer A, Garbe C, Detmar M, et al. [Multicentric reticulohistiocytosis and myelodysplastic syndrome]. Hautarzt 1994;45:91–6 [in German].

[39] Catterall MD, White JE. Multicentric reticulohistiocytosis and malignant disease. Br J Dermatol 1978;98:221–4.

[40] Valencia IC, Colsky A, Berman B. Multicentric reticulohistiocytosis associated with recurrent breast carcinoma. J Am Acad Dermatol 1998;39:864–6.

[41] Oliver GF, Umbert I, Winkelmann RK, et al. Reticulohistiocytoma cutis—review of 15 cases and an association with systemic vasculitis in two cases. Clin Exp Dermatol 1990;15:1–6.

[42] Snow JL, Muller SA. Malignancy-associated multicentric reticulohistiocytosis: a clinical, histological and immunophenotypic study. Br J Dermatol 1995;133:71–6.

[43] Kenik JG, Fok F, Huerter CJ, et al. Multicentric reticulohistiocytosis in a patient with malignant melanoma: a response to cyclophosphamide and a unique cutaneous feature. Arthritis Rheum 1990;33:1047–51.

[44] Barrow MV, Holubar K. Multicentric reticulohistiocytosis. A review of 33 patients. Medicine (Baltimore) 1969;48:287–305.

[45] Yee KC, Bowker CM, Tan CY, et al. Cardiac and systemic complications in multicentric reticulohistiocytosis. Clin Exp Dermatol 1993;18:555–8.

[46] Lambert CM, Nuki G. Multicentric reticulohistiocytosis with arthritis and cardiac infiltration: regression following treatment for underlying malignancy. Ann Rheum Dis 1992;51:815–7.

[47] Kamel H, Gibson G, Cassidy M. Case report: the CT demonstration of soft tissue involvement in multicentric reticulohistiocytosis. Clin Radiol 1996;51:440–1.

[48] Nakamura H, Yoshino S, Shiga H, et al. A case of spontaneous femoral neck fracture associated with multicentric reticulohistiocytosis: oversecretion of interleukin-1beta, interleukin-6, and tumor necrosis factor alpha by affected synovial cells. Arthritis Rheum 1997;40:2266–70.

[49] Goto H, Inaba M, Kobayashi K, et al. Successful treatment of multicentric reticulohistiocytosis with alendronate: evidence for a direct effect of bisphosphonate on histiocytes. Arthritis Rheum 2003;48:3538–41.

[50] Sellam J, Deslandre CJ, Dubreuil F, et al. Refractory multicentric reticulohistiocytosis treated by infliximab: two cases. Clin Exp Rheumatol 2005;23:97–9.

[51] Kossard S, Winkelmann RK. Necrobiotic xanthogranuloma with paraproteinemia. J Am Acad Dermatol 1980;3:257–70.

[52] Robertson DM, Windelmann RK. Necrobiotic xanthogranuloma. Arch Dermatol 1992;128:94–100.

[53] Alam M, Garzon MC, Salen G, et al. Tuberous xanthomas in sitosterolemia. Pediatr Dermatol 2000;17:447–9.

[54] Sethuraman G, Thappa DM, Karthikeyan K. Intertriginous xanthomas—a marker of homozygous familial hypercholesterolemia. Indian Pediatr 2000;37:338.

[55] Marcoval J, Moreno A, Bordas X, et al. Diffuse plane xanthoma: clinicopathologic study of 8 cases. J Am Acad Dermatol 1998;39:439–42.

[56] Ginarte M, Peteiro C, Toribio J, et al. Generalized plane xanthoma and idiopatic Bence-Jones proteinuria. Clin Exp Dermatol 1997;22:192–4.

[57] Wilson DE, Flowers CM, Hershgold EJ, et al. Multiple myeloma, cryoglobulinemia and xanthomatosis: distinct clinical and biochemical syndromes in two patients. Am J Med 1975;59:721–9.

[58] Zvulunov A, Barak Y, Metzker A. Juvenile xanthogranuloma, neurofibromatosis, and juvenile chronic myelogenous leukemia. World statistical analysis. Arch Dermatol 1995;131:904–8.

[59] Bardwick PA, Zvaifler NJ, Gill GN, et al. Plasma cell dyscrasia with polyneuropathy, organomegaly, endocrinopathy, M protein, and skin changes: the POEMS syndrome. Report on two cases and a review of the literature. Medicine (Baltimore) 1980; 59(4):311–22.

[60] Shahidi H, Myers JL, Kvale PA. Castleman's disease. Mayo Clin Proc 1995;70:969–77.

[61] Lacy MQ, Gertz MA, Hanson CA, et al. Multiple myeloma associated with diffuse osteosclerotic bone lesions: a clinical entity distinct from osteosclerotic myeloma (POEMS syndrome). Am J Hematol 1997;56(4):288–93.

[62] Vidakovic A, Simic P, Stojisavljevic N, et al. Polyneuropathy with osteosclerotic myeloma–POEMS syndrome. A case report. J Neurol 1992;239(1): 49–52.

[63] Brandon C, Martel W, Weatherbee L, et al. Case report 572. Osteosclerotic myeloma (POEMS) syndrome. Skeletal Radiol 1989;18(7):542–6.

[64] Soubrier MJ, Jean-Jacques D, Sauvezie BJM. POEMS syndrome: a study of 25 cases and review of the literature. Am J Med 1994;97:543–53.

[65] Zea-Mendoza A, Alonso-Ruiz A, Garcia-Vadillo A, et al. POEMS syndrome with neuroarthropathy and nodular regenerative hyperplasia of the liver. Arthritis Rheum 1984;27:1053–7.

[66] Chan JKC, Fletcher CDM, Hicklin GA, et al. Glomeruloid hemangioma. A distinctive cutaneous lesion of multicentric Castleman's disease associated with POEMS syndrome. Am J Surg Pathol 1990; 14(11):1036–46.

[67] Rongioletti F, Gambini C, Lerza R. Glomeruloid hemangioma. A cutaneous marker of POEMS syndrome. Am J Dermatopathol 1994;16(2):175–8.

[68] Rose C, Zandecki M, Copin MC, et al. POEMS syndrome: report on six patients with unusual clinical signs, elevated levels of cytokines, macrophage involvement and chromosomal aberrations of bone marrow plasma cells. Leukemia 1997;11: 1318–23.

[69] Feinberg L, Temple D, de Marchena E, et al. Soluble immune mediators in POEMS syndrome with pulmonary hypertension: case report and review of the literature. Crit Rev Oncog 1999;10:293–302.

[70] Mandler RN, Kerrigan DP, Smart J, et al. Castleman's disease in POEMS syndrome with elevated interleukin-6. Cancer 1992;69:2697–703.

[71] McCourt M, Wang JH, Sookhai S, et al. Proinflammatory mediators stimulate neutrophil-directed angiogenesis. Arch Surg 1999;134(12):1325–31 [discussion: 1331–2].

[72] Watanabe O, Maruyama I, Arimura K, et al. Overproduction of vascular endothelial growth factor/vascular permeability factor is causative in Crow-Fukase (POEMS) syndrome. Muscle Nerve 1998; 21:1390–7.

[73] Belec L, Mohamed AS, Authier FJ, et al. Human herpesvirus 8 infection in patients with POEMS syndrome-associated multicentric Castleman's disease. Blood 1999;93(11):3643–53.

[74] Papo T, Soubrier M, Marcelin AG, et al. Human herpesvirus 8 infection, Castleman's disease and POEMS syndrome. Br J Haematol 1999;104: 932–3.

[75] Heykarts B, Anseeuw M, Degreef H. Pancreatitis caused by acinous pancreatic carcinoma. Dermatology 1999;198:182–3.

ELSEVIER
SAUNDERS

Dermatol Clin 26 (2008) 45–57

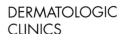
DERMATOLOGIC
CLINICS

Cutaneous Vascular Disorders Associated with Internal Malignancy

Abdel Kader El Tal, MD[a], Zeina Tannous, MD[b,c],*

[a]*Department of Dermatology, Oakwood Hospital, Cancer Center Clinic, Wayne State University, 18101 Oakwood Boulevard, Dearborn, MI 48123, USA*
[b]*Department of Dermatology, Massachusetts General Hospital, Harvard Medical School, 50 Staniford Street, 2nd Floor, Boston, MA 02114, USA*
[c]*Department of Dermatology, Boston Veterans Affairs Health Care System, Boston, MA 02130, USA*

Cutaneous vascular abnormalities can be associated with internal malignancies, and consist of a wide variety of signs and symptoms. They include flushing, telangiectasia, purpura, vasculitis, cutaneous ischemia, and thrombophlebitis. Though our current knowledge does not allow us to classify these diseases by pathophysiologic approach in all cases, the entities will be regrouped into three main categories according to etiology: (1) disorders related to vascular dilatation, (2) disorders related to vascular inflammation, and (3) disorders related to vascular occlusion (Table 1). Some of the diseases may be classified in more than one category. This article elaborates on these manifestations and presents some of the pertinent findings that may be of interest to the physician.

Disorders related to vascular dilatation

Flushing

Recurrent episodes of flushing, in the setting of an internal malignancy, may be the presenting symptom in carcinoid syndrome [1], mastocytosis [2], pheochromocytoma [3], medullary carcinoma of the thyroid [4], renal cell carcinoma [5],

* Corresponding author. Department of Dermatology, Massachusetts General Hospital, Harvard Medical School, 50 Staniford Street, 2nd Floor, Boston, MA 02114.
E-mail address: ztannous@partners.org
(Z. Tannous).

pancreatic tumors (vasoactive intestinal peptide tumor—VIPoma) [6], POEMS syndrome (polyneuropathy, organomegaly, endocrinopathy, M-protein, skin changes) [7], and harlequin syndrome [8].

Carcinoid syndrome

The incidence of carcinoid tumors is approximately 1.5 per 100,000 of the population; however, the malignant carcinoid syndrome, characterized by the cutaneous manifestations and caused by the circulating neuroendocrine mediators, occurs in fewer than 10% of the patients. Skin flushing is the most frequent clinical sign in carcinoid syndrome, appearing in 95% of patients at some time during the course of the disease [9].

A cardinal manifestation of carcinoid syndrome is paroxysms of flushing [1]. The flushing varies in color from pink-orange to bright red, violaceous, blue, and blanching white. The distribution is usually limited to the face, neck, and upper part of the trunk, and is accompanied by warmth [10]. Occasionally, the flushing can involve the entire body in severe cases [1]. Episodes are typically brief and last for a minute or two. The character of the flush is site-dependent. Tumors originating in the foregut (stomach, lung, pancreas, and biliary tract) produce a characteristic bright salmon pink to red flush [10]. Constant facial and neck erythema with a cyanotic hue characterizes midgut tumors (appendix and ileum). This characteristic flush, which is regarded as the classical carcinoid flush, develops after patients suffer from flushing attacks for several years [10]. In addition to the cyanotic hue,

Table 1
Classification of vascular abnormalities heralding an internal malignancy according to etiology

Etiology	Vascular abnormality	Associated malignancies
Vascular dilatation	Flushing	Carcinoid tumor
		Medullary thyroid carcinoma
		Systemic mastocytosis
		Pheochromocytoma
		Renal cell carcinoma
		Pancreatic tumors (VIPoma)
		Pancoast tumor (in HS)
		Superior mediastinal neurinoma (in HS)
		Myeloma (in POEMS syndrome)
	Telangiectasia	Several malignancies (in the setting of AT, BS, and RTS)
		Breast cancer
		Bronchogenic carcinoma
		Carcinoid tumor
		Adenocarcinoma of the hepatic duct
		MAE
Vascular inflammation	Vasculitis	Several malignancies, most commonly hematopoeitic
Vascular occlusion	Trousseau	Most commonly pancreas, lung, prostate, stomach, and colon
	Mondor's disease	Mostly breast carcinoma
	Deep vein thrombosis	Several malignancies, especially advanced stages
		Mucin-secreting adenocarcinomas are the most common.
	Purpura	Several malignancies, mostly hematopoeitic
		Lymphomas are most common in ITP.
		Gastric and breast carcinomas are most common in TTP.
	Cutaneous ischemia	Several malignancies, including carcinomas of pancreas, stomach, small bowel, ovary, kidney, and lymphoma and leukemia
		In the setting of cryoglobulinemia, lymphomas and multiple myeloma are the most common associated cancers.

Abbreviations: AT, ataxia-telangiectasia syndrome; BS, Bloom's syndrome; HS, harlequin syndrome; ITP, idiopathic thrombocytopenic purpura; MAE, malignant angioendotheliomatosis; POEMS syndrome, polyneuropathy, organomegaly, endocrinopathy, M-protein, skin changes; RTS, Rothmund-Thomson syndrome; TTP, thrombotic thrombocytopenic purpura; VIPoma, vasoactive intestinal peptide tumor.

features of rosacea may develop after years of flushing [10]. Flushing may be predictably induced in patients by stimuli that result in increased adrenergic activity, such as pain, anger, or embarrassment, as well as by ingestion of certain types of food (nuts and cheese) and alcohol [9]. Telangiectasias may develop on the cheeks, nose, or forehead in chronic cases. These telangiectasias may regress with the excision of the tumor [1].

The distribution of the flushing in carcinoid syndrome is similar to the distribution of flushing in physiologic conditions, and both share common triggers such as emotional stress, alcohol, and certain foods [10]. Carcinoid flushing is usually distinguishable from other types of flushing by the presence of associated systemic symptoms

such as diarrhea, shortness of breath, or wheezing. Attacks of flushing can be accompanied by hypotension. Periorbital edema, syncope, and shock were also described in severe cases [1].

Flushing attacks associated with gastric carcinoid are mediated by histamine, and can be prevented by treatment with a combination of H1 and H2 histamine antagonists [11]. The cause of the cyanotic midgut flush in carcinoid is more complex, and is likely caused by multiple mediators, including serotonin [1], tachykinins such as bradykinin [12], and prostaglandins [13].

Comparing the symptomatology of patients who have idiopathic flushing with that of patients who have carcinoid syndrome, it is noted that palpitations, syncope, and hypotension occurred more in patients who had idiopathic flushing, whereas wheezing and abdominal pain were more common in patients who had carcinoid. Diarrhea can occur in both [14].

Neuroendocrine midgut tumors are only seldom part of a familial genetic disorder such as multiple endocrine neoplasia, Type I (MEN-I) syndrome, or the von Hippel-Lindau syndrome [15].

Patients who have carcinoid disease presenting with cutaneous flushing are usually advanced in their disease, and local resection of the tumor is not feasible in these cases. Biotherapy with somatostatin analogs (octreotide and lanreotide) [15] and interferon-α are the treatment of choice for these patients [16,17]. Systemic chemotherapy and other aggressive modalities should be reserved for patients who fail other modalities of treatment [15].

Mastocytosis

Approximately 55% of mastocytosis patients develop their disease by 2 years of age [18]. The disease is equally distributed between males and females, and has been reported in all races.

Mastocytosis is classified by the World Health Organization (WHO) into five different categories: (1) cutaneous mastocytosis, (2) indolent systemic mastocytosis, (3) systemic mastocytosis with an associated clonal hematological non-mast cell lineage disease, (4) aggressive systemic mastocytosis, and (5) mast cell leukemia [2]. Patients in every category of mastocytosis can experience flushing or even vascular collapse [19]. Accordingly, cutaneous flushing in mast cell disease is not considered as an index of high burden of mast cells (B-findings) [2], nor as an indication of an impaired organ function (C-findings), but rather as an indolent finding.

Patients who have cutaneous mastocytosis, also known as urticaria pigmentosa (UP), present classically with small, yellow-tan to reddish-brown macules or slightly raised papules. These lesions become pruritic and raised with surrounding erythema when stroked firmly. Constitutional symptoms such as weight loss, fatigue, malaise, fever, gastritis, and peptic ulcer disease, in addition to liver, spleen, lymph nodes and bone marrow involvement are rather indicative of systemic involvement [2].

Mast cell granules contain histamine, heparin, and a number of acid hydrolases [8]. In addition, the stimulated mast cell can liberate arachidonic acid from its membrane phospholipids stores, metabolizing it selectively to prostaglandin (PGD2),

and leukotrienes (LTC4, LTD4, and LTE4) [20]. Mast cells are also capable of secreting cytokines such as IL-4, IL-5, IL-6, IL-8 and tumor necrosis factor (TNF)-α. Several of the clinical manifestations of mastocytosis, like vasodilation in general and flushing in particular, are based on the pathophysiologic action of these mediators.

The diagnosis of mastocytosis is suspected on clinical grounds and confirmed by histology. A first important test to perform in patients who have suspected systemic mastocytosis is measurement of serum tryptase [21]. In adults who have suspected systemic mastocytosis, a bone marrow examination should be performed [21]. In contrast, in pediatric patients, a bone marrow biopsy is not indicated unless other signs of systemic hematologic disease or aggressive type of mastocytosis are found [21].

Because no curative therapies for mastocytosis are available at present, treatment is symptomatic [22]. H1 receptor antagonists and PUVA (methoxypsoralen plus ultraviolet light) have been particularly helpful in reducing flushing as well as pruritus [23]; however, many patients continue to complain of flushing and other symptoms, mainly from the inability to block the high level of histamine with histamine antagonists and from the presence of other mast cell mediators. Patients who have mastocytosis in general should be cautioned to avoid potential mast cell degranulating agents such as ingested alcohol, anticholinergic preparations, aspirin, and other nonsteroidal anti-inflammatory agents, narcotics, and polymyxin B sulfate. In addition, heat and friction can induce systemic symptoms and should be avoided when possible [2].

Pheochromocytoma

Flushing is uncommonly associated with pheochromocytoma, and it usually occurs only after an attack, whereas pallor is present during the attack [3]. Flushing occurs as a rebound from the facial cutaneous vasoconstriction.

Medullary carcinoma of the thyroid

Cutaneous flushing in the setting of sporadic medullary thyroid carcinoma has been reported in 10% of patients [4]. These patients usually have a metastatic disease, with other systemic symptoms such as diarrhea, hoarseness, and dysphagia [24]. Medullary thyroid carcinoma may secrete many bioactive substances in addition to calcitonin, each with the potential of causing clinical symptoms such as sweating and flushing. These substances include biogenic amines, drenocortico-tropic hormone (ACTH), corticotrophin-releasing hormone, and prostaglandins [25]. Most medullary thyroid tumors present with a long-standing multinodular goiter or an asymptomatic thyroid nodule [26]. When medullary thyroid carcinoma presents with flushing, diarrhea, or bone metastasis, the prognosis is poor, and 33% of patients die within 5 years [4].

Renal cell carcinoma

Cronin and colleagues [5] and Plaksin and colleagues [27] reported on the occurrence of cutaneous flushing with renal cell carcinoma. Renal cell carcinoma may produce hormones or hormone-like substances, including parathyroid hormones, prolactin, gonadotropins, rennin, and prostaglandins, which result in downregulation of pituitary gland hormones and flushing reactions [5].

Pancreatic tumors

VIPomas are non-β islet cell neuroendocrine tumors that secrete vasoactive intestinal peptide (VIP), gastric inhibitory polypeptide (GIP), prostaglandins, and pancreatic peptides. Patients present classically with prolonged massive diarrhea associated with hypokalemia and dehydration. Though both carcinoid tumors and VIPomas present with diarrhea, flushing similar to carcinoid occurs rarely in VIPomas [6].

It is noteworthy that three of the tumors that present with flushing—pheochromocytoma, medullary thyroid carcinoma and VIPoma—can be part of MEN syndrome.

POEMS syndrome

POEMS syndrome is a variant of osteosclerotic myeloma [7]. Flushing in association with hypotension and bronchospasms in POEMS syndrome has been reported in the literature [7].

Harlequin syndrome

Harlequin syndrome is characterized by unilateral facial flushing and sweating, which are predominantly induced by heat or exercise [28]. It results from a sympathetic deficit of the third thoracic nerve [28]. The sympathetic deficit is in the nonflushing side, and the healthy side shows normal or excessive flushing or sweating [29]. The syndrome is mostly idiopathic, but has been associated with brain stem infarction, internal jugular vein catheterization [30], and high thoracic vertebral anesthesia [31]. In the setting of internal malignancies, harlequin syndrome has been associated with a contralateral lung cancer invading

the spine in a patient who had Pancoast's syndrome concomitant with Horner's syndrome [8], and in another patient who had superior mediastinal neurinoma [32].

Telangiectasia

The spectrum of occurrence of telangiectasias is wide and may range from the insignificant, as in the syndrome of hereditary benign telangiectasia, to the serious diseases such as ataxia-telangiectasia. In general, telangiectasias are classified as primary (of unknown cause) or secondary (as a result of another disease) [33]. Telangiectasias in malignancies can be either primary or secondary.

Primary telangiectasia

Ataxia-telagiectasia syndrome, Bloom's syndrome, and Rothmund-Thomson syndrome are the classic examples for the occurrence of malignancies in the setting of primary telangiectasias.

One third of patients who have ataxia-telangiectasia develop a malignancy during their lifetimes [34]. Malignancies are sometimes the presenting problem of a patient who has ataxia-telangiectasia. Roughly four fifths of all malignancies seen in ataxia telangiectasia involve the lymphoid system [35]. Leukemias constitute one fourth of malignancies, and are usually of the T-cell chronic lymphocytic type. Lymphomas, on the other hand, are mostly of the B-cell type. Nonlymphoid malignancies tend to occur in older patients, and include solid tumors of the oral cavity, breast, stomach, pancreas, ovary, and bladder, as well as others [34]. Ataxia-telangiectasia patients are prone to the development of solar keratoses and basal cell carcinomas of the face by young adulthood [36].

Heterozygote carriers of the ataxia-telangiectasia gene, though apparently healthy, still carry a 5- to 10 fold increased risk of developing neoplasms, usually of the nonlymphoid type [35]. Female carriers carry a fivefold increased risk of developing breast cancer [35]. On average, carriers of the ataxia-telangiectasia gene die 7 to 8 years earlier than noncarriers [37]. Cancer results in the increased mortality rate in these patients. Compared with noncarriers, carriers who died of cancer were on average 4 years younger than the noncarriers [37]. The gene for ataxia-telangiectasia (ATM) plays a central role in signaling DNA damage, predominantly double-stranded breaks in DNA, and in activating checkpoints to slow the progression of cells carrying the damaged DNA through the cell cycle [38]. It also overlaps with p53, and is involved directly in the regulation of the breast cancer gene product *BRCA-1* [38]. The *ATM* gene is present on chromosome 11q22.3 [39]. It is of interest that one of the most common chromosomal aberrations observed in lymphoid neoplasms is the deletion of the long arm of chromosome 11 [39]. The mechanisms for the development of cancer in these patients still remain to be fully elucidated.

Twenty percent of patients who have Bloom's syndrome develop neoplasms [40]. Half occur before the age of 20 years. Patients who have Bloom's syndrome have been estimated to have a 150- to 300 fold increased frequency of development of neoplasia. Various internal malignancies have been reported, but the most common were leukemia, lymphosarcoma, lymphoma, and carcinomas of the oral cavity, skin, breast, and digestive system [40]. The presence of increased neoplasms in Bloom's syndrome accounts for the high incidence of early mortality in these patients [41]. The defective gene in Bloom's syndrome (*BLM*) is on chromosome 15q26.1 and codes for a DNA helicase.

There are several reported instances of skin malignancies in Rothmund-Thomson syndrome patients, such as Bowen's disease [42], basal cell carcinoma [43], and malignant poroma [44]. Patients who have Rothmund-Thomson syndrome are also prone to developing squamous cell carcinoma over the poikilodermatous areas of the skin, usually by the age of 50 [45]. In addition, noncutaneous malignancies including fibrosarcoma [45], parathyroid adenoma [46], gastric carcinoma [47], and osteosarcomas [48–50] have been reported. Similar to Bloom syndrome, the defective gene in Rothmund-Thomson syndrome codes for a DNA helicase, *RECQL4*. The etiology for the development of tumors is probably related to reduced DNA repair capacity, as in Bloom's syndrome [51].

Secondary telangiectasia

Reports of secondary telangiectasias to an internal malignancy have been documented in the literature. Localized, grouped telangiectatic vessels on the anterior chest wall may be a marker for breast cancer [52]. Telangiectatic vessels may also be the first evidence of dermal or subcutaneous metastases of breast cancer, as well as of other malignant tumors [52]. A patient who has undifferentiated bronchogenic carcinoma presented with multiple telangiectasias over the palms, soles, fingers, toes, lips, and tongue [53].

Progressive telangiectases have been associated with carcinoid tumors [1] and with adenocarcinoma of the hepatic duct [52].

Generalized telangiectasia has also been a presenting manifestation of malignant angioendotheliomatosis (MAE). This is a rare entity that represents an intravascular lymphoma, hence the name intravascular lymphomatosis [54]. This multisystemic disease primarily manifests in the central nervous system and the skin [55]. In this disease, skin lesions are seen in one third of patients, usually appearing as erythematous to blue plaques or nodules on the arms, thighs, trunk, or face [55]. Telangiectasia might be prominent over lesions [56], and are typically described as painful indurated telangiectasias [57]. MAE must be differentiated from its benign counterpart, reactive angioendotheliomatosis, which can present with similar skin manifestations, but is usually limited to the skin [55]. Reactive angioendotheliomatosis occurs in the setting of hypersensitivity reactions or systemic infections, most commonly bacterial endocarditis [54].

Telangiectasia can also be a marker for the collagen-vascular disorders, including progressive systemic sclerosis, and dermatomyositis, which can be associated with an increased cancer risk. The association of collagen-vascular disorders and malignancies is discussed in the article by Pipkin and Lio, as well as in the article by Weenig and Mehrany, elsewhere in this issue.

Diseases related to vascular inflammation: vasculitis

The coexistence of a vasculitis and a neoplastic disease is rare. The types of vasculitis more often associated with neoplasia are the leukocytoclastic vasculitis (Fig. 1) and the polyarteritis nodosa (Fig. 2) [58]. The vasculitis seen in patients who have malignant neoplasms does not differ clinically from that which occurs much more commonly secondary to non-neoplastic causes. The prevalence of malignancies in patients who have vasculitis is between 3% and 8% [59].

In a review of 200 patients who had vasculitis associated with malignancy, 77.5% had a hematological malignancy, 17% had a solid tumor, and 5.5% had an unspecified malignancy [60]. In certain subtypes of vasculitis, such as in peripheral nerve and muscle vasculitis, Henoch-Schönlein purpura, and temporal arteritis, solid tumors predominate. In cutaneous leukocytoclastic vasculitis, as well as in polyarteritis nodosa, however,

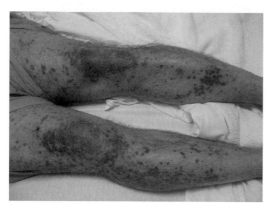

Fig. 1. Patient with acute myelogenous leukemia (AML-type 2) presenting with leukocytoclastic vasculitis (LCV) over the lower extremities. The LCV in patients with underlying malignancies does not differ from other patients with LCV clinically.

a large proportion of patients are afflicted with lymphomas or leukemias [60].

Reported hematologic malignancies associated with vasculitis include hairy cell leukemia, chronic lymphoid leukemia, myeloma, Hodgkin's disease, non-Hodgkin's lymphoma, acute myeloblastic leukemia, malignant histiocytosis, and myelodysplastic syndromes [61,62]. In solid tumors, lung cancer is the most common type (23%), followed by gastrointestinal tumors (17.5%), renal cancers (14%), cancer of the urinary bladder, prostate cancer, and breast cancer (5.3% each) [59].

Vasculitis can occur 2 to 4 years before the clinical manifestation of the tumor [60]. It can be

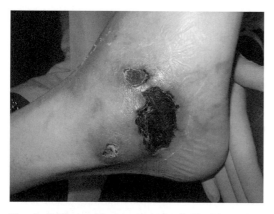

Fig. 2. Patient with cutaneous polyarteritis nodosa (PAN), presenting with necrotic skin lesions. PAN is considered among the vasculitides that are possibly associated with neoplasia.

a presenting sign in squamous cell carcinoma, particularly of the bronchus, and in renal cell carcinoma [52]. Paraneoplastic vasculitis associated with myeloproliferative and lymphoproliferative disease usually antedates the diagnosis of malignancy; however, in hairy cell leukemia, leukocytoclastic vasculitis or polyarteritis nodosa may occur after the diagnosis of the hematologic disorder [63].

A periarteritis nodosa-like syndrome has also been reported in association with hairy cell leukemia [64], acute lymphocytic leukemia [65], and multiple myeloma [66].

The pathogenetic mechanism for the occurrence of vasculitis in the setting of internal malignancy is still largely unknown. Postulated mechanisms include: (1) the formation of immune complexes of tumor-associated antigens/antibodies [67], a mechanism that may account for most leukocytoclastic paraneoplastic vasculitides; (2) a direct vascular damage by antibodies targeting endothelial cells and perhaps cross-reacting with antigens present on leukemic cells [68]; and (3) direct effect of leukemic cells (such as hairy cells) on the vascular wall [69].

When a curative treatment of the neoplasm is not possible, paraneoplastic vasculitis responds to treatment with glucocorticoids alone or in combination with immunosuppressive agents [70]. In the majority of the cases, death results from metastatic or recurrent tumor and not from vasculitis [70].

Diseases related to vascular occlusion

Thrombophlebitis and thromboembolism

Superficial thrombophlebitis of the lower limb is common, affecting 3% to 11% of the general population [71]. Isolated vein thrombophlebitis is uncommonly associated with internal malignant disease [52]. Multiple-lesion "migratory" superficial thrombophlebitis is rather more commonly associated with cancers [52]. Trousseau syndrome, defined as spontaneous, recurrent, or migratory episodes of venous thrombosis, migratory thrombophlebitis, arterial emboli secondary to nonbacterial thrombotic endocarditis, or any combination of these, was first described by Armand Trousseau as the initial sign of an underlying malignancy [72]. Interestingly, Trousseau himself subsequently presented with the syndrome he described, and died of gastric carcinoma [73]. Whereas only about 6% of patients who have deep vein thrombosis develop cancer, about 50% of patients who have migratory thrombophlebitis develop a malignant tumor [74]. Malignancies most commonly associated with Trousseau syndrome include those of the pancreas, lung, prostate, stomach, and colon, with pancreatic cancer accounting for 50% of all cases [75], as well as lymphoma and leukemia. The migratory nature of the thrombophlebitis probably relates to a generalized hypercoagulable state. Whether extensive screening for malignancy in Trousseau syndrome is warranted in asymptomatic patients is controversial; however, most authorities follow Trousseau's recommendation to search for an underlying malignancy when presented with migratory thrombophlebitis of otherwise undetermined origin [73].

Mondor's disease is a rare pathologic entity characterized by thrombophlebitis of the subcutaneous veins of the anterolateral thoraco-abdominal wall [76]. The most commonly affected vessels are the thoracoepigastric, lateral thoracic, and superior epigastric veins [77]. The condition presents as a tender or nontender palpable cord in the mammary area, radiating from the region of the areola toward the axilla, epigastrium, or subcoastal margin [76]. Rarely, the cords can assume a necklace-like appearance [78]. The palpable cord can be more appreciated upon pulling the skin or sometimes raising the limb. The condition is three times more frequent in women [78], and generally appears unilaterally [79]; it occurs bilaterally in only 3% of cases [80]. The etiology of this disease is multifactorial, and in many cases no specific etiologic factor is identified [81]. The most common etiologic factors are traumatic events, excessive physical activity, iatrogenic causes (breast surgery), inflammatory processes, infections, concomitant breast pathology (mastitis, abscess), and pendulous breast [81]. Mondor's disease has been mostly associated with breast carcinoma [76]. In a study of 63 patients who had Mondor's disease, breast cancer was reported in more than 12.7% [78]. The study authors concluded that mammography should be done in all cases [78]. The treatment of this condition is rather symptomatic and conservative, and consists of local heat application, resting of the arm, breast support, and analgesics [76].

The incidence of venous thromboembolism exhibits a fourfold increase in patients who have cancer. An underlying malignancy accounts for 10% to 20% of causes of deep vein thrombosis (DVT) [82–84]. The highest frequency of thromboembolism is noted in terminally ill cancer patients, with a 50% incidence rate reported in

postmortem studies [85]. Patients who do not have identifiable risk factors for DVT, who are older than 50 years, who present with multiple sites of venous thromboembolism, and who are resistant to therapy with oral anticoagulants appear to have a significant risk of occult cancer [86,87]. In a study reported by Adreka and colleagues [86], patients at greatest risk for cancer were of older age, had a lower hemoglobin level (<12.4 g/dL), and had an eosinophil count higher than 3%. Other studies have challenged the presence of these findings in patients who have cancer and DVT [88].

DVT of the upper limb is another complication associated with cancer, and is more frequently associated with occult malignancy as compared with the lower limb [89]. It may be a paraneoplastic phenomenon, or may result from obstruction of the venous outflow by Pancoast tumor or an axillary tumor [90].

Mucin-secreting adenocarcinomas were the most common tumors associated with DVT, and the tumors were located most commonly in the gastrointestinal tract, urogenital tract, lungs, and breasts [83]. Thrombosis is the second leading cause of death among patients who have these tumor types [91]. Thrombosis is a common complication in cancer patients undergoing surgery, radiation therapy, or chemotherapy [92].

The mechanisms of thrombosis in cancer patients are constantly being unfolded. Several recent review articles detail the known mechanisms [92]. Proposed mechanisms include: (1) change in antithrombotic and prothrombotic proteins, (2) cytokine activation and endothelial dysfunction, (3) conditions that can lead to chronic disseminated coagulation, (4) intravascular mucin secreted by tumor cells, (5) change of viscosity (such as leukemia or polycythemia vera), or (6) tumor seeding with thromboembolism [72]. Screening of coagulation parameters is not helpful, because it neither predicts the prevalence of thromboembolism events nor identifies patients who may benefit from thromboprophylaxis [93].

Treatment of thrombotic diathesis in the setting of malignancy requires treatment of the underlying tumor. As long as the tumor persists, thrombosis will be ongoing and anticoagulant therapy will be required. Anticoagulation therapy with warfarin has been disappointing in this setting [94]. Cancer patients have been included in treatment trials that compared the safety and efficacy of low-molecular weight heparin molecules (LMWH) and heparin. In six trials, there was a trend toward lesser mortality with LMWH as compared with standard heparin [92].

Purpura and ecchymoses

Only 4% to 11% of untreated patients who have malignancy have thrombocytopenia [95]. In fact, tumor cell lines that cause platelet aggregation in vitro and cause thrombocytopenia have the greatest potential for producing metastatic disease [96]. Up to 60% of patients who have IgM myeloma or Waldenstrom's macroglobulinemia have been reported as having hemorrhagic complications [97].

The von Willebrand factor (vWF) is important in the interaction between endothelium and platelets. It also stabilizes Factor VII. An acquired form of vWF has been reported with multiple myeloma, Waldenstrom's macroglobulinemia, monoclonal gammopathies, hairy cell leukemia, chronic lymphocytic leukemia, and malignant lymphomas [98]. Circulating anticoagulants to Factor VIII, abnormalities in the conversion of fibrinogen to fibrin [99], and acquired deficiencies of Factors X, IX, V, and alpha-2 subunit of plasminogen inhibitors have also been reported [100]. The presence of lupus anticoagulant was associated with cases of Hodgkin's and non-Hodgkin's lymphomas [99].

Lymphoma is the most common cause of idiopathic thrombocytopenic purpura (ITP) associated with malignant disease. Hodgkin's disease [101] and chronic lymphoid leukemia are the most recognized in this setting [102]. ITP has been also associated with solid tumors, particularly breast cancer [100]. According to de Latour and colleagues [100], an invasive ductal carcinoma of the breast, as well as a positive hormonal receptor status, appear to be more frequently associated with ITP. In general, breast cancer has a poor prognosis when associated with ITP, whereas ITP itself has a similar presentation, prognosis, and outcome as that of the nonmalignant setting [100]. Other solid tumors reported in association with ITP include ovarian cancer, cervical cancer, basal cell carcinoma, prostate cancer, poorly differentiated bronchogenic adenocarcinoma, and squamous cell carcinoma of the lung [103]. Response to conventional ITP therapy has been variable in the literature.

Disseminated intravascular coagulation (DIC) as a cause of purpura in malignant disease is associated with all hematologic malignancies, including acute lymphocytic or myelomonocytic leukemia, and particularly acute promyelocytic leukemia (APL), with an incidence of up to 100% in the latter condition [104]. Leukemias of B-cell origin, such as chronic lymphocytic leukemia and hairy cell leukemia, generally are not associated with DIC [105]. DIC has also been reported in up to 7% of solid tumors [106], and is most frequently associated with pancreatic, gastrointestinal, and prostate cancer. In cases of occult malignancy presenting with DIC, the prognosis is very poor [104]. Clinically, the oncology patient shows more commonly a chronic and subclinical compensated form of DIC with slightly altered blood coagulation parameters.

Thrombotic thrombocytopenic purpura (TTP), when associated with cancer, is usually a late sign [52]. Most cases of cancer-associated TTP have been reported in cases with adenocarcinoma, predominantly gastric and breast cancer [107]. The syndrome does not seem to be limited to patients who have advanced-stage malignant disease, but has been described as associated with tumor invasion of the bone marrow [108]. In cancer-associated TTP, the thrombotic angiopathy may be attributed to both perturbed vasculature and presence of a protease-inhibitor [108]. Results with plasma exchange in cancer-associated TTP are reported to be poor [109].

Purpura can also be associated with hyperglobulinemia seen in multiple myeloma or lymphoma. When purpura is secondary to the presence of cryoglobulins, lesions are often found in acral areas and may be associated with Raynaud's phenomenon. Benign hyperglobulinemic purpura can be associated with Sjögren's syndrome, which in turn can be associated with malignant disease.

Cutaneous ischemia

Digital gangrene, occasionally preceded by Raynaud's phenomenon, is an infrequent paraneoplastic disorder [110]. Digital ischemia may present initially as excruciating pain in the feet in the absence of physical signs.

Microvascular thrombosis of the digits may manifest as erythromelalgia. Kurzrock and Cohen [111] reviewed 60 cases of erythromelalgia with myeloproliferative disorders. The symptoms of erythromelalgia consisted of severe burning pain, erythema, and warmth of the extremities, and primarily affected the feet, and to a lesser extent, the hands. They often preceded the diagnosis of malignancy by a period of 2.5 years. Accordingly, the study authors recommended that all patients who have erythromelalgia be screened with a regular peripheral blood count.

Leukostasis is a well-known phenomenon of acute leukemia, causing infarction and hemorrhage [112,113]. This complication usually affects small vessels, and is associated with a white blood cell count of more than 150,000/mm^3.

Peripheral ischemia has been associated with many neoplasms, including carcinoma of the pancreas, stomach, small bowel, ovary, and kidney, as well as lymphoma and leukemia [52].

The peripheral cutaneous ischemia of polycythemia rubra vera appears to be secondary to the increased viscosity of the peripheral circulation associated with this disease. Similarly, some patients who have leukemia can develop leukostasis secondary to very high white blood cell concentrations.

The ischemia seen in cryoglobulinemia appears also to be secondary to increased blood viscosity. Cryoglobulinemia may be associated with multiple myeloma or with lymphoma (Fig. 3).

Arterial thrombi are less common than venous thrombi (Fig. 4). Out of 41 cancer patients who had arterial thrombi, 24 had pancreatic cancer, 10 had lung cancer, 4 had colon cancer, and 3 had adenocarcinoma of unknown origin [94]. Seventy four percent of the autopsied patients had nonbacterial thrombotic endocarditis (NBTE), with the arterial embolization being a frequent consequence of this complication [94].

In conclusion, the vascular manifestations of the skin in the setting of internal malignancies are largely nonspecific to specific kinds of tumors.

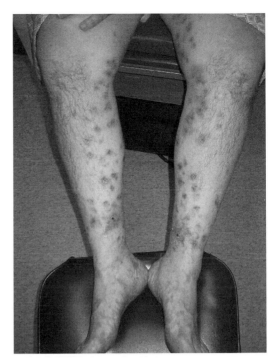

Fig. 4. Patient with thrombogenic vasculopathy with paraproteinemia presenting with arterial thrombi resulting in skin necrosis.

Nevertheless, these manifestations may be the presenting signs and symptoms of the disease. Hence, the importance of the dermatologist's role in interpreting these vascular manifestations in their appropriate setting.

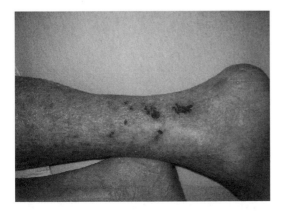

Fig. 3. Patient with cryoglobulinemia presenting with skin necrosis. Cryoglobulinemia maybe associated with myeloma or lymphoma.

References

[1] Feingold KR, Elias PM. Endocrine-skin interactions. Cutaneous manifestations of adrenal disease, pheochromocytomas, carcinoid syndrome, sex hormone excess and deficiency, polyglandular autoimmune syndromes, multiple endocrine neoplasia syndromes, and other miscellaneous disorders. J Am Acad Dermatol 1988;19(1 Pt 1):1–20.

[2] Valent P, Akin C, Sperr WR, et al. Mast cell proliferative disorders: current view on variants recognized by the World Health Organization. Hematol Oncol Clin North Am 2003;17(5):1227–41.

[3] Wilkin JK. Flushing reactions: consequences and mechanisms. Ann Intern Med 1981;95(4):468–76.

[4] Kebebew E, Ituarte PH, Siperstein AE, et al. Medullary thyroid carcinoma: clinical characteristics, treatment, prognostic factors, and a comparison of staging systems. Cancer 2000;88(5): 1139–48.

[5] Cronin RE, Kaehny WD, Miller PD, et al. Renal cell carcinoma: unusual systemic manifestations. Medicine (Baltimore) 1976;55(4):291–311.

[6] Krejs GJ. VIPoma syndrome. Am J Med 1987; 82(5B):37–48.

[7] Myers BM, Miralles GD, Taylor CA, et al. POEMS syndrome with idiopathic flushing mimicking carcinoid syndrome. Am J Med 1991;90(5): 646–8.

[8] Umeki S, Tamai H, Yagi S, et al. Harlequin syndrome (unilateral flushing and sweating attack) due to a spinal invasion of the left apical lung cancer [abstract]. Rinsho Shinkeigaku 1990;30(1): 94–9.

[9] Mohyi D, Tabassi K, Simon J. Differential diagnosis of hot flashes. Maturitas 1997;27(3):203–14.

[10] Bell HK, Poston GJ, Vora J, et al. Cutaneous manifestations of the malignant carcinoid syndrome. Br J Dermatol 2005;152(1):71–5.

[11] Roberts LJ 2nd, Marney SR Jr, Oates JA. Blockade of the flush associated with metastatic gastric carcinoid by combined histamine H1 and H2 receptor antagonists. Evidence for an important role of H2 receptors in human vasculature. N Engl J Med 1979;300(5):236–8.

[12] Zeitlin IJ, Smith AN. 5-hydroxyindoles and kinins in the carcinoid and dumping syndromes. Lancet 1966;2(7471):986–91.

[13] Smith AG, Greaves MW. Blood prostaglandin activity associated with noradrenaline-provoked flush in the carcinoid syndrome. Br J Dermatol 1974;90(5):547–51.

[14] Aldrich LB, Moattari AR, Vinik AI. Distinguishing features of idiopathic flushing and carcinoid syndrome. Arch Intern Med 1988;148(12):2614–8.

[15] De Herder WW. Tumours of the midgut (jejunum, ileum and ascending colon, including carcinoid syndrome). Best Pract Res Clin Gastroenterol 2005;19(5):705–15.

[16] Kaltsas GA, Besser GM, Grossman AB. The diagnosis and medical management of advanced neuroendocrine tumors. Endocr Rev 2004;25(3):458–511.

[17] van der Lely AJ, de Herder WW. Carcinoid syndrome: diagnosis and medical management. Arq Bras Endocrinol Metabol 2005;49(5):850–60.

[18] Tharp MD. Mastocytosis. In: Bolognia JL, Jorizzo JL, Rapini RP, editors. Dermatology, vol. 2. Philadelphia: Mosby; 2003. p. 1899–906.

[19] Travis WD, Li CY, Bergstralh EJ, et al. Systemic mast cell disease. Analysis of 58 cases and literature review. Medicine (Baltimore) 1988;67(6):345–68.

[20] Roberts LJ 2nd, Sweetman BJ, Lewis RA, et al. Increased production of prostaglandin D2 in patients with systemic mastocytosis. N Engl J Med 1980; 303(24):1400–4.

[21] Valent P, Sperr WR, Schwartz LB, et al. Diagnosis and classification of mast cell proliferative disorders: delineation from immunologic diseases and non-mast cell hematopoietic neoplasms. J Allergy Clin Immunol 2004;114(1):3–11.

[22] Escribano L, Akin C, Castells M, et al. Mastocytosis: current concepts in diagnosis and treatment. Ann Hematol 2002;81(12):677–90.

[23] Marone G, Spadaro G, Granata F, et al. Treatment of mastocytosis: pharmacologic basis and current concepts. Leuk Res 2001;25(7):583–94.

[24] Beressi N, Campos JM, Beressi JP, et al. Sporadic medullary microcarcinoma of the thyroid: a retrospective analysis of eighty cases. Thyroid 1998; 8(11):1039–44.

[25] Engelman K. Malignant carcinoid syndrome. In: DeGroot LJ, editor. 3rd edition. Textbook of endocrinology, vol. 3. Philadelphia: Saunders; 1995. p. 2649–57.

[26] Massoll N, Mazzaferri EL. Diagnosis and management of medullary thyroid carcinoma. Clin Lab Med 2004;24(1):49–83.

[27] Plaksin J, Landau Z, Coslovsky R. A carcinoid-like syndrome caused by a prostaglandin-secreting renal cell carcinoma. Arch Intern Med 1980;140(8):1095–6.

[28] Lance JW, Drummond PD, Gandevia SC, et al. Harlequin syndrome: the sudden onset of unilateral flushing and sweating. J Neurol Neurosurg Psychiatr 1988;51(5):635–42.

[29] Moon SY, Shin DI, Park SH, et al. Harlequin syndrome with crossed sympathetic deficit of the face and arm. J Korean Med Sci 2005;20(2):329–30.

[30] Coleman PJ, Goddard JM. Harlequin syndrome following internal jugular vein catheterization in an adult under general anesthetic. Anesthesiology 2002;97(4):1041.

[31] Burlacu CL, Buggy DJ. Coexisting harlequin and Horner syndromes after high thoracic paravertebral anaesthesia. Br J Anaesth 2005;95(6):822–4.

[32] Noda S. Harlequin syndrome due to superior mediastinal neurinoma. J Neurol Neurosurg Psychiatr 1991;54(8):744.

[33] Abrahamian LM, Rothe MJ, Grant-Kels JM. Primary telangiectasia of childhood. Int J Dermatol 1992;31(5):307–13.

[34] Gatti RA. Ataxia-telangiectasia. Dermatol Clin 1995;13(1):1–6.

[35] Swift M, Morrell D, Massey RB, et al. Incidence of cancer in 161 families affected by ataxia-telangiectasia. N Engl J Med 1991;325(26):1831–6.

[36] Reed WB, Epstein WL, Boder E, et al. Cutaneous manifestations of ataxia-telangiectasia. JAMA 1966;195(9):746–53.

[37] Su Y, Swift M. Mortality rates among carriers of ataxia-telangiectasia mutant alleles. Ann Intern Med 2000;133(10):770–8.

[38] Khanna KK. Cancer risk and the ATM gene: a continuing debate. J Natl Cancer Inst 2000;92(10): 795–802.

[39] Boultwood J. Ataxia telangiectasia gene mutations in leukaemia and lymphoma. J Clin Pathol 2001; 54(7):512–6.

[40] German J. Bloom's syndrome. XX. The first 100 cancers. Cancer Genet Cytogenet 1997;93(1):100–6.

[41] Gretzula JC, Hevia O, Weber PJ. Bloom's syndrome. J Am Acad Dermatol 1987;17(3):479–88.

[42] Haneke E, Gutschmidt E. Premature multiple Bowen's disease in poikiloderma congenitale with warty hyperkeratoses. Dermatologica 1979;158(5): 384–8.

[43] Berg E, Chuang TY, Cripps D. Rothmund-Thomson syndrome. A case report, phototesting, and literature review. J Am Acad Dermatol 1987;17 (2 Pt 2):332–8.

[44] Van Hees CL, Van Duinen CM, Bruijin JA, et al. Malignant eccrine poroma in a patient with Rothmund-Thomson syndrome. Br J Dermatol 1996; 134(4):813–5.

[45] Davies MG. Rothmund-Thomson syndrome and malignant disease. Clin Exp Dermatol 1982;7(4): 455.

[46] Werder EA, Murset G, Illig R, et al. Hypogonadism and parathyroid adenoma in congenital poikiloderma (Rothmund-Thomson syndrome). Clin Endocrinol (Oxf) 1975;4(1):75–82.

[47] Diem E. The Rothmund-Thomson-syndrome. A case report [abstract]. Hautarzt 1975;26(8):425–9.

[48] Dick DC, Morley WN, Watson JT. Rothmund-Thomson syndrome and osteogenic sarcoma. Clin Exp Dermatol 1982;7(1):119–23.

[49] Judge MR, Kilby A, Harper JI. Rothmund-Thomson syndrome and osteosarcoma. Br J Dermatol 1993;129(6):723–5.

[50] Drouin CA, Mongrain E, Sasseville D, et al. Rothmund-Thomson syndrome with osteosarcoma. J Am Acad Dermatol 1993;28(2 Pt 2):301–5.

[51] Smith PJ, Paterson MC. Enhanced radiosensitivity and defective DNA repair in cultured fibroblasts derived from Rothmund Thomson syndrome patients [abstract]. Mutat Res 1982;94(1):213–28.

[52] McLean DI, Haynes HA. Cutaneous manifestations of internal malignant disease: cutaneous paraneoplastic syndromes. In: Freedberg IM, Eisen AZ, Wolff K, et al, editors. Fitzpatrick's dermatology in general medicine. 6th edition. New York: McGraw-Hill; 2003. p. 1785–6.

[53] Ochshorn M, Ilie B, Blum I. Multiple telangiectases preceding the appearance of undifferentiated bronchogenic carcinoma. Dermatologica 1982;165(6): 620–3.

[54] Perniciaro C, Winkelmann RK, Daoud MS, et al. Malignant angioendotheliomatosis is an angiotropic intravascular lymphoma. Immunohistochemical, ultrastructural, and molecular genetics studies. Am J Dermatopathol 1995;17(3):242–8.

[55] Berger TG, Dawson NA. Angioendotheliomatosis. J Am Acad Dermatol 1988;18(2 Pt 2):407–12.

[56] Requena L, Sangueza OP. Cutaneous vascular proliferations. Part III. Malignant neoplasms, other cutaneous neoplasms with significant vascular component, and disorders erroneously considered as vascular neoplasms. J Am Acad Dermatol 1998;38(2 Pt 1):143–75.

[57] Wilson BB. Indurated telangiectatic plaques. Malignant angioendotheliomatosis (MAE). Arch Dermatol 1992;128(2):255–8.

[58] Diez-Porres L, Rios-Blanco JJ, Robles-Marhuenda A, et al. ANCA-associated vasculitis as paraneoplastic syndrome with colon cancer: a case report. Lupus 2005;14(8):632–4.

[59] Hayem G, Gomez MJ, Grossin M, et al. Systemic vasculitis and epithelioma. A report of three cases with a literature review. Rev Rhum Engl Ed 1997; 64(12):816–24.

[60] Kurzrock R, Cohen PR. Vasculitis and cancer. Clin Dermatol 1993;11(1):175–87.

[61] Fernandez-Miranda C, Garcia-Marcilla A, Martin M, et al. Vasculitis associated with a myelodysplastic syndrome: a report of 5 cases [abstract]. Med Clin (Barc) 1994;103(14):539–42.

[62] Hamidou MA, Boumalassa A, Larroche C, et al. Systemic medium-sized vessel vasculitis associated with chronic myelomonocytic leukemia. Semin Arthritis Rheum 2001;31(2):119–26.

[63] Gonzalez-Gay MA, Garcia-Porrua C, Salvarani C, et al. Cutaneous vasculitis and cancer: a clinical approach. Clin Exp Rheumatol 2000;18(3): 305–7.

[64] Gabriel SE, Conn DL, Phyliky RL, et al. Vasculitis in hairy cell leukemia: review of literature and consideration of possible pathogenic mechanisms. J Rheumatol 1986;13(6):1167–72.

[65] Gerber MA, Brodin A, Steinberg D, et al. Periarteritis nodosa, Australia antigen and lymphatic leukemia. N Engl J Med 1972;286(1):14–7.

[66] Hasegawa H, Ozawa T, Tada N, et al. Multiple myeloma-associated systemic vasculopathy due to crystalglobulin or polyarteritis nodosa. Arthritis Rheum 1996;39(2):330–4.

[67] Garcias VA, Herr HW. Henoch-Schonlein purpura associated with cancer of prostate. Urology 1982; 19(2):155–8.

[68] Posnett DN, Marboe CC, Knowles DM 2nd, et al. A membrane antigen (HC1) selectively present on hairy cell leukemia cells, endothelial cells, and epidermal basal cells. J Immunol 1984;132(6):2700–2.

[69] Klima M, Waddell CC. Hairy cell leukemia associated with focal vascular damage. Hum Pathol 1984; 15(7):657–9.

[70] Kurzrock R, Cohen PR, Markowitz A. Clinical manifestations of vasculitis in patients with solid tumors. A case report and review of the literature. Arch Intern Med 1994;154(3):334–40.

[71] Schonauer V, Kyrle PA, Weltermann A, et al. Superficial thrombophlebitis and risk for recurrent venous thromboembolism. J Vasc Surg 2003;37(4): 834–8.

[72] Tasi SH, Juan CJ, Dai MS, et al. Trousseau's syndrome related to adenocarcinoma of the colon

and cholangiocarcinoma. Eur J Neurol 2004;11(7):
493–6.

[73] Batsis JA, Morgenthaler TI. Trousseau syndrome
and the unknown cancer: use of positron emission to-
mographic imaging in a patient with a paraneoplastic
syndrome. Mayo Clin Proc 2005;80(4):537–40.

[74] Lesher JL Jr. Thrombophlebitis and thromboembolic problems in malignancy. Clin Dermatol
1993;11(1):159–63.

[75] Pinzon R, Drewinko B, Trujillo JM, et al. Pancreatic carcinoma and Trousseau's syndrome: experience at a large cancer center. J Clin Oncol 1986;
4(4):509–14.

[76] Mayor M, Buron I, de Mora JC, et al. Mondor's
disease. Int J Dermatol 2000;39(12):922–5.

[77] Oldfield MC. Mondor's disease. A superficial phlebitis of the breast. Lancet 1962;1:994–6.

[78] Catania S, Zurrida S, Veronesi P, et al. Mondor's disease and breast cancer. Cancer 1992;69(9):2267–70.

[79] Bartolo M, Spigone C, Antignani PL. Contribution
to the recognition of Mondor's phlebitis [abstract].
J Mal Vasc 1983;8(3):253–6.

[80] Skipworth GB, Morris JB, Goldstein N. Bilateral Mondor's disease. Arch Dermatol 1967;
95(1):95–7.

[81] Samlaska CP, James WD. Superficial thrombophlebitis. II. Secondary hypercoagulable states.
J Am Acad Dermatol 1990;23(1):1–18.

[82] Baron JA, Gridley G, Weiderpass E, et al. Venous
thromboembolism and cancer. Lancet 1998;351
(9109):1077–80. [Erratum in Lancet 2000;355
(9205):758].

[83] Lee AY, Levine MN. Venous thromboembolism
and cancer: risks and outcomes. Circulation 2003;
107(23 Suppl 1):I17–21.

[84] Prandoni P, Lensing AW, Buller HR, et al. Deep-
vein thrombosis and the incidence of subsequent
symptomatic cancer. N Engl J Med 1992;327(16):
1128–33.

[85] Ambrus JL, Ambrus CM, Mink IB, et al. Causes of
death in cancer patients. J Med 1975;6(1):61–4.

[86] Aderka D, Brown A, Zelikovski A, et al. Idiopathic
deep vein thrombosis in an apparently healthy patient as a premonitory sign of occult cancer. Cancer
1986;57(9):1846–9.

[87] Naschitz JE, Yeshurun D, Abrahamson J. Thromboembolism. Clues for the presence of occult neoplasia. Int Angiol 1989;8(4):200–5.

[88] Monreal M, Lafoz E, Casals A, et al. Occult cancer
in patients with deep venous thrombosis. A system-
atic approach. Cancer 1991;67(2):541–5.

[89] Girolami A, Prandoni P, Zanon E, et al. Venous
thromboses of upper limbs are more frequently associated with occult cancer as compared with those
of lower limbs. Blood Coagul Fibrinolysis 1999
Dec;10(8):455–7.

[90] Naschitz JE, Yeshurun D, Eldar S, et al. Diagnosis
of cancer-associated vascular disorders. Cancer
1996;77(9):1759–67.

[91] Donati MB. Cancer and thrombosis: from phleg-
masia alba dolens to transgenic mice. Thromb Haemost 1995;74(1):278–81.

[92] Walsh-McMonagle D, Green D. Low-molecular-
weight heparin in the management of Trousseau's
syndrome. Cancer 1997;80(4):649–55.

[93] Glassman AB, Jones E. Thrombosis and coagulation abnormalities associated with cancer. Ann
Clin Lab Sci 1994;24(1):1–5.

[94] Lee AY. Cancer and thromboembolic disease:
pathogenic mechanisms. Cancer Treat Rev 2002;
28(3):137–40.

[95] Sack GH Jr, Levin J, Bell WR. Trousseau's syndrome and other manifestations of chronic disseminated coagulopathy in patients with neoplasms:
clinical, pathophysiologic, and therapeutic features. Medicine (Baltimore) 1977;56(1):1–37.

[96] Sun NC, McAfee WM, Hum GJ, et al. Hemostatic
abnormalities in malignancy, a prospective study of
one hundred eight patients. Part I. Coagulation
studies. Am J Clin Pathol 1979;71(1):10–6.

[97] Gasic GJ, Gasic TB, Galanti N, et al. Platelet-
tumor-cell interactions in mice. The role of platelets
in the spread of malignant disease. Int J Cancer
1973;11(3):704–18.

[98] Fink K, Al-Mondhiry H. Idiopathic thrombocytopenic purpura in lymphoma. Cancer 1976;37(4):
1999–2004.

[99] Glaspy JA. Disturbances in hemostasis in patients
with B-cell malignancies. Semin Thromb Hemost
1992;18(4):440–8.

[100] de Latour RP, Des Guetz G, Laurence V, et al.
Breast cancer associated with idiopathic thrombo-
cytopenic purpura: a single center series of 10 cases.
Am J Clin Oncol 2004;27(4):333–6.

[101] Jakway JL. Acquired von Willebrand's disease in
malignancy. Semin Thromb Hemost 1992;18(4):
434–9.

[102] Kaden BR, Rosse WF, Hauch TW. Immune
thrombocytopenia in lymphoproliferative diseases.
Blood 1979;53(4):545–51.

[103] Porrata LF, Alberts S, Hook C, et al. Idiopathic
thrombocytopenic purpura associated with breast
cancer: a case report and review of the current literature. Am J Clin Oncol 1999;22(4):411–3.

[104] Loreto MF, De Martinis M, Corsi MP, et al. Coagulation and cancer: implications for diagnosis and
management. Pathol Oncol Res 2000;6(4):301–12.

[105] Stahl RL, Chan W, Duncan A, et al. Malignant
angioendotheliomatosis presenting as disseminated
intravascular coagulopathy. Cancer 1991;68(10):
2319–23.

[106] Sallah S, Wan JY, Nguyen NP, et al. Disseminated
intravascular coagulation in solid tumors: clinical
and pathologic study. Thromb Haemost 2001;
86(3):828–33.

[107] Antman KH, Skarin AT, Mayer RJ, et al. Micro-
angiopathic hemolytic anemia and cancer: a review.
Medicine (Baltimore) 1979;58(5):377–84.

[108] von Bubnoff N, Sandherr M, Schneller F, et al. Thrombotic thrombocytopenic purpura in metastatic carcinoma of the breast. Am J Clin Oncol 2000;23(1):74–7.

[109] Kwaan HC, Soff GA. Management of thrombotic thrombocytopenic purpura and hemolytic uremic syndrome. Semin Hematol 1997;34(2):159–66.

[110] DeCross AJ, Sahasrabudhe DM. Paraneoplastic Raynaud's phenomenon. Am J Med 1992;92(5): 571–2.

[111] Kurzrock R, Cohen PR. Erythromelalgia and myeloproliferative disorders. Arch Intern Med 1989; 149(1):105–9.

[112] McKee LC Jr, Collins RD. Intravascular leukocyte thrombi and aggregates as a cause of morbidity and mortality in leukemia. Medicine (Baltimore) 1974; 53(6):463–78.

[113] Hawley PR, Johnston AW, Rankin JT. Association between digital ischaemia and malignant disease. Br Med J 1967;3(559):208–12.

ELSEVIER
SAUNDERS

Dermatol Clin 26 (2008) 59–68

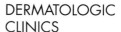

Malignancy and Cancer Treatment-Related Hair and Nail Changes

Ginette Hinds, MD, Valencia D. Thomas, MD*

Department of Dermatology, Yale Medical School, 40 Temple Street, Suite 5A, New Haven, CT 06510, USA

The relationship between a patient's overall state of health and the cutaneous adnexa is complex and dynamic. The local effects of nutrient supply, profusion, inflammation, lymphatic drainage, toxins, and physical damage may produce a myriad of abnormalities in the hair and nails. Each parameter may be affected by a systemic disease or by a remote malignancy. Through mechanisms yet to be fully understood, the hair and nails may provide important diagnostic clues to the patient's state of health.

Paraneoplastic hair and nail disorders are a set of temporally consistent, nongenetic, nonsyndromic abnormalities that are observed in association with malignancy [1]. Although some paraneoplastic hair disorders have been described, most nail changes associated with internal malignancy are nonspecific. A number of cytokine and immune-related explanations have been proposed to explain the association between cancer and paraneoplastic conditions, but no one etiologic cause has been identified. Table 1 summarizes the common hair changes associated with internal malignancies.

The treatment of cancer with chemotherapy and radiation therapy may also induce abnormalities of the hair and nails. Overall, these changes can be linked to cytotoxic affects of the drug or the effects of direct, physical radiation damage to the skin. Table 2 summarizes some of the hair changes associated with chemotherapy and radiation therapy. Establishing an understanding of the behavior of the hair and nails with respect to

systemic disease may be helpful not only in the diagnosis of occult malignancy, but can be vital in assessing a patient's overall health.

Normal hair physiology

The hair follicle is a complex structure called the pilosebaceous unit that comprises the follicle, sebaceous gland, and arrector pili muscle. It is formed by the downward growth of the epidermis and is joined by the upward growth of the dermal papillary mesenchyme in the fetal period. Follicles give rise to three different types of hairs: lanugo, terminal, and vellus hairs. Lanugo hairs can be seen in the fetal period or in early infancy. These fine hairs that are shed immediately before birth or in early infancy [2]. Vellus hairs are soft, nonpigmented hairs that can be found on the face and arms of children as well as on the face of many adult women. Terminal hairs are pigmented, longer, and more coarse than vellus hairs. These can be found on the scalp, eyebrows, and eyelashes at birth. Under the influence of androgens, vellus hairs develop into terminal hairs on the trunk, beard, axillae, and pubic area of adults [3].

Hairs cycle through three different phases: anagen, catagen, and telogen. Anagen is a growth phase that classically lasts approximately 1000 days [4]. On the scalp, approximately 80% to 90% of hairs are in anagen. This phase is followed by a short involution phase, or catagen, during which part of the lower follicle undergoes apoptosis [2]. The final phase of the hair cycle is telogen, a resting phase, lasting 3 to 4 months. After telogen, the hair is shed and the cycle begins again.

* Corresponding author.
  E-mail address: valencia.thomas@yale.edu
(V.D. Thomas).

0733-8635/08/$ - see front matter © 2008 Elsevier Inc. All rights reserved.
doi:10.1016/j.det.2007.08.003

Table 1
Common cancer-associated hair changes and their causes

Hair abnormality	Associated malignancy
Acquired hypertrichosis lanuginosa	Lung, colon, rectal, breast, renal, pancreatic, uterine, ovarian, bladder, and gallbladder cancer; lymphoma, leukemia [3]
Alopecia areata	Malignancies of the immune system, Hodgkin's lymphoma
Cicatricial alopecia	Multiple myeloma [10], plasma cell dyscrasias, plasmacytoma
Alopecia neoplastica	Metastatic breast, gastric, lung, ovarian, and colon cancers [13]; desmoplastic melanoma metastases [12], and metastatic placental trophoblastic tumors [14]

Table 2
Common chemotherapy- and radiation-associated hair changes and their causes

Hair abnormality	Associated cause
Anagen effluvium	Adriamycin, cyclophosphamide, docetaxel, daunorubicin, combination chemotherapy
Telogen effluvium	Systemic stresses: medications, surgery, pregnancy, mourning, and so on
Hair lightening or canities	Chloroquine, cyclosporine A, etretenate, interferon alpha [17,19,20]
Hair darkening	Estrogens, prostaglandin analogs, tamoxifen, electron beam radiation [19], methotrexate [21,22]
Hair texture change (curling or straightening)	Antineoplastic agents, retinoids, valproic acid indinavir, lithium [19]; interferon alpha plus ribavirin [23,24]
Follicular spicules	Multiple myeloma and cryoglobulinemia
Cicatricial alopecia	Radiation therapy, potentiated by bleomycin, chlorambucin, doxorubicin, flurouracil, cysplatin, hydroxyurea, 6-mercaptopurine, or methotrexate [27]

Paraneoplastic hair changes

Acquired hypertrichosis lanuginosa

Acquired hypertrichosis lanuginosa (AHL) is a rare paraneoplastic condition, characterized by the development of fetal-type, lanugo hair on the face. This thin, nonpigmented hair develops most commonly on the forehead, nose, and ears, but can arise on the trunk, axillae, and extremities. Fewer than 60 cases have been described in the literature [5].

AHL is most frequently associated with lung cancer and colorectal carcinomas [3]. It has also been described in association with lymphoma and leukemia, as well as with carcinomas of the breast, kidney, pancreas, uterus, ovary, bladder, and gallbladder [3]. AHL may appear from 2.5 years before the malignancy is diagnosed to 5 years after diagnosis [6]. Histologically, mantle-type lanugo hair follicles contain immature sebocytes that run parallel to the epidermal surface [3].

The differential diagnosis of AHL includes hirsutism and hypertrichosis associated with drugs or systemic diseases. Some drugs known to cause increased hair growth include cyclosporine, phenytoin, minoxidil, spirinolactone, interferon alpha, penicillin, streptomycin, zidovudine, and corticosteroids [3]. Hirsutism and hypertrichosis have also been associated with polycystic ovary syndrome, thyrotoxicosis, and porphyrias, as well as ovarian and adrenal tumors. Although

patients note an improvement in AHL with the successful treatment of their underlying malignancy, most individuals will succumb to their disease within 3 years of diagnosis [3,6,7].

Alopecia areata

Alopecia areata (AA) is usually a benign disease that presents with well-demarcated areas of nonscarring hair loss in any hair-bearing area of the body. Although the pathogenesis remains unclear, immunological investigations have shown decreased activity of T-helper and T-suppressor cells [8]. AA is commonly seen in association with autoimmune phenomena, including thyroiditis, vitiligo, and lupus erythematosus. Additionally, AA has been observed in association with malignancies of the immune system, particularly Hodgkin's lymphoma. The course of the disease tends to mirror the course of the malignancy, with total resolution reported with successful treatment of the disease [8,9]. AA presenting in a patient who have a history of a hematologic malignancy could be a sign of cancer recurrence, and should be evaluated fully with a biopsy and a referral to the patient's hematologist, if indicated.

Cicatricial alopecia

Cicatricial, or scarring, alopecia (CA) has been reported in patients who have multiple myeloma, multiple myeloma-associated amyloidosis [10], and plasma cell dyscrasias [11]. CA results when the hair follicle sustains irreversible, inflammatory damage to the follicular stem cells, preventing repair and regeneration of the follicle. Clinically, this disorder is manifested as areas of shiny, atrophic skin on the scalp without evidence of follicular ostia. This permanent hair loss can be discrete or diffuse, and may involve not only the scalp, but any hair-bearing area of the body.

CA is an inflammatory form of hair loss that must be distinguished from alopecia neoplastica (AN), a form of scarring alopecia that results from metastatic tumor invasion of the skin that results in the obliteration of hair follicles. The course of this paraneoplastic disorder has not been well-characterized; however, a report of a plasmacytoma presenting with paraneoplastic POEMS syndrome (polyneuropathy, organomegaly, endocrinopathy, M-protein, skin changes) and CA noted that the CA became quiescent after removal of the tumor [11]. The management of CA focuses on controlling inflammation in the skin through the use of topical and systemic anti-inflammatory agents. Cosmetically, full or partial hair pieces can be used with or without makeup to help minimize the appearance of the hair loss.

Alopecia neoplastica

AN is a form of cicatricial alopecia associated with primary or metastatic malignancies. Cases of AN caused by primary cutaneous malignancies, namely squamous cell carcinomas, basal cell carcinomas, cutaneous lymphomas and angiosarcoma [12], are not discussed here because they are not considered to be paraneoplastic phenomena. Cutaneous metastases resulting in AN usually present as single or multiple areas of scarring alopecia in the scalp. Cutaneous metastases occur in approximately 2% to 4% of all solid tumor cancers. The most common association is with metastatic breast carcinoma [12], but AN has been described in association with metastases from gastric, lung, colon [13], and ovarian cancers, as well as with placental trophoblastic tumors [14] and desmoplastic melanoma metastases [12]. It can present as nontender nodules, sclerodermoid plaques, or inflammatory telangiectatic lesions. AN is characterized histologically by the presence of metastatic carcinoma cells in the deep dermis or subcutis, fibrosis, miniaturization of hair follicles, and a decrease in the number of pilosebaceous units [15]. Given the variety of clinical presentations that are possible with cutaneous metastases, patches of alopecia that are treatment-resistant or patches that display atypical erythema, induration, or nodularity should be biopsied to rule out AN, particularly if the hair loss occurs in an individual who has a history of cancer. In general, cutaneous metastases are considered to be indicative of advanced tumors and poor prognosis [14].

Cancer treatment-related hair disorders

Anagen effluvium

The most common form of hair loss associated with chemotherapeutic agents is anagen effluvium. Anagen effluvium occurs after an insult to the hair follicle that impairs its mitotic or metabolic activity, and is almost exclusively seen after intake of chemotherapeutic agents such as antimetabolites, alkylating agents, and mitotic inhibitors. The inhibition of the mitotic activity in the hair matrix of actively growing anagen hair follicles leads to a narrow, weakened segment of the hair shaft, a Pohl-Pinkus constriction, that easily fractures with minimal trauma. Magnification of the hairs may show tapered fractures at the site of progressive narrowing of the hair shaft, causing tapered fractures of the hair near the follicular ostia [2].

Anagen effluvium usually begins 7 to 10 days after initiation of the chemotherapeutic agent, becomes more apparent in the subsequent 4 to 8 weeks, and persists for approximately 3 to 4 weeks [16]. Certain drugs are more likely than others to cause anagen effluvium. Examples include adriamycin, cyclophosphamide, docetaxel, and daunorubicin. Other chemotherapeutic agents, such as capecitabine, cisplatin, and carboplatin are less likely to cause hair loss [17,18]. In general, full recovery of the hair is achieved after the withdrawal of the inciting agent, though permanent, diffuse hair thinning may be observed in some.

Anagen effluvium is more frequent and severe in patients receiving combination chemotherapy than in those treated with monotherapy. Hair loss usually starts after the first or second cycle of treatment [17]. Hair shedding is usually acute and severe, and most of the scalp hair, eyebrows, and eyelashes may be temporarily lost.

Telogen effluvium

Telogen effluvium is a common form of hair loss induced by drugs or systemic stresses (such as surgery, pregnancy and extreme emotional stress [eg, mourning]) and is characterized by excessive shedding of telogen hairs 2 to 4 months after the inciting event [17]. Chemotherapeutic agents and the general stress of cancer diagnosis and treatment can induce telogen effluvium by prematurely precipitating the follicle into the resting phase.

Daily hair shedding is variable, but usually ranges between 100 and 150 hairs. Chemotherapeutic agents may induce severe shedding, however, with the loss of more than 200 to 300 hairs daily [17]. Scalp hair is most commonly affected, but loss of pubic or body hairs can occur. The duration of hair loss mirrors the duration of the stress, and full regrowth is usually achieved.

Chemotherapy-induced hair color changes

Hair color changes, either hyper- or hypopigmentation, have been anecdotally reported in association with a number of chemotherapeutic agents. In general, agents that directly influence the enzymes responsible for melanin production can affect skin and hair pigmentation, although a number of compounds may affect hair color changes through unknown mechanisms. Chemotherapeutic agents commonly associated with hypopigmentation or loss of hair color include chloroquine, cyclosporine A, etretenate, and interferon alpha [17,19,20]. The term canities is applied when all melanin pigmentation is lost from the hair. Alternatively, hair darkening has been reported with estrogens, prostaglandin analogs, tamoxifen, and electron beam radiation [19]. When patients experience the flag sign, alternating bands of color sometimes seen in various nutritional states or in association with chemotherapeutic drugs such as methotrexate, the hair appears to be darker clinically [21,22].

Chemotherapy-induced hair texture changes

Curling or straightening of the hair has been reported after the use of some antineoplastic agents, retinoids, valproic acid indinavir, and lithium [19]. Interestingly, both hair curling and hair straightening have been reported with the use of interferon alpha and ribavirin [23,24]. The amount of curl in normal hair is determined primarily by the formation of disulfide bonds between amino acid residues in the hair, with hydrogen bonding contributing additional conformational stability. Very curly hair or kinky hair has a greater number of these intermolecular bonds. Permanently straightened or curled hair has not been studied, however, and the exact mechanism of this drug-induced textural change remains unknown at this time.

Follicular spicules

Patients who have multiple myeloma and cryoglobulinemia may develop hornlike projections from hair follicles composed of the antibodies predominant in their disease [2]. Clinically, the patient may have spiny papules on the face, scalp, or neck [25]. One report noted the development of ulcerations on the trunk from this pathologic process [26].

Radiation therapy-induced hair changes

Although radiation treatment fields are designed to minimize the disruption of normal tissues, hair-bearing areas may be at risk for permanent damage. Physical treatment modalities resulting in complete destruction of hair follicles display scarring alopecia. Additionally, concomitant chemotherapeutic agents such as bleomycin, chlorambucin, doxorubicin, flurouracil, cysplatin, hydroxyurea, 6-mercaptopurine, and methotrexate may increase the radiosensitivity of target tissues [27]. In 2004, a dose-response relationship for cranial irradiation was determined for humans. The dose at which 50% of patients experienced permanent alopecia was 43 Gy [28]. Partial destruction of follicular cells may result in the hair becoming more fine, whereas melanocyte effects may result in hair color change. Topical radioprotectors, prostaglandins, keratinocyte growth factors, and many other agents that help to minimize the damage to skin are currently being investigated to help decrease cutaneous morbidity [29,30].

Paraneoplastic and cancer treatment-related nail changes

Normal nail physiology

The nail unit is composed of the nail plate, nail bed, matrix, hyponychium, and the proximal and lateral nail folds. The nail matrix is the germinal center of the nail, with the proximal matrix forming the dorsal nail plate and the distal matrix forming the ventral nail plate. The nail plate is a specialized epidermal structure formed by a process known as onycholemmal keratinization, whereby matrix cells mature, lose their nuclei and organelles, and become cemented in a thick mortar. This plate remains adherent to the nail bed to the level of the hyponychium, where there is a natural release of the nail plate (Fig. 1). The proximal and lateral nail folds have an adherent cuticle that forms a barrier to infections and external insults. In adults, transit from the proximal matrix to the hyponychium takes 6 months, whereas formation of a toenail takes 12 months [31].

Paraneoplastic nail changes

There are no nail signs pathognomonic for internal malignancy. Various systemic and local stressors, however, may result in distinct nail changes that may aid in the assessment of a patient's overall health. Chemotherapeutic agents are the most frequent cause of drug-induced nail changes [32]. The continuously dividing nail matrix cells are easily perturbed by the antimitotic activity of most chemotherapeutic agents. As with other systemic and drug-induced nail changes, most of the nails tend to be involved. Although not life-threatening, these nail changes are cosmetically distressing to many patients. Common nail changes and their definitions are summarized in Table 3.

Several chemotherapeutic have been reported in association with nail dystrophy; however, in many cases determining the exact inciting drug is difficult because most chemotherapy regimens comprise a combination of multiple agents. Docetaxel, cyclophosphamide, and doxorubicin are commonly associated with nail toxicity. Taxanes, daunorubicin, 5-fluorouracil, and vincristine have also been reported to affect the nails [33]. Please see Table 4 for a summary of nail changes and their causes.

Acquired digital clubbing

Acquired digital clubbing is an increased convex curvature of the nail plate secondary to enlargement of the soft tissue of the distal digit. The angle between the proximal nail fold and the nail plate becomes greater than 180°. Increased amounts of connective tissue and subungual edema are responsible for the thickening of the nail bed and subsequent periosteal proliferation [6].

Although the exact etiology is unknown, the pathogenesis of clubbing may be related to local tissue deoxygenation, platelet impaction of the distal digital vessels, or a humoral substance causing vasodilation in the blood vessels of the fingertips [6,34].

Clubbing has been most frequently associated with primary bronchogenic carcinoma and mesothelioma [6]. It has also been associated with gastrointestinal tumors and tumors metastatic to the lung [32,35]. Other systemic diseases commonly associated with clubbing include cardiovascular, endocrine, and gastrointestinal diseases, and congenital heart disease. Clubbing may also be

Table 3
Common nail abnormalities defined

Term	Description
Mee's lines	Nail plate parakeratosis resulting in a white, transverse nail plate band parallel to the lunula
Beau's lines	Simultaneously-appearing, transverse depressions in the nail plates of the hands, feet, or both
Onycholysis	Nail plate separation from the nail bed
Onychomadesis	Nail plate shedding
Muehrcke's lines	Blanchable, paired, white lines in the nail bed
Subungual hematoma	Nail bed hemorrhage deep to an intact nail plate
Melanonychia	Melanin pigmentation of the nail plate

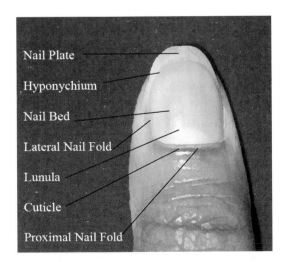

Fig. 1. Nail anatomy.

Nail Plate

Hyponychium

Nail Bed

Lateral Nail Fold

Lunula

Cuticle

Proximal Nail Fold

Table 4
Common nail changes and their causes

Nail apparatus sign	Related cause
General nail toxicity	Cyclophosphamide, doxorubicin, taxanes, daunorubicin, 5-fluorouracil, vincristine [33]
Acquired digital clubbing	Primary bronchogenic carcinoma, mesothelioma [6], gastrointestinal carcinoma, tumors metastatic to the lung [32,35]
Yellow nail syndrome	Carcinomas of the breast, endometrium, gallbladder, larynx, and lung; metastatic melanoma, metastatic sarcoma, Hodgkin's disease, and mycosis fungoides [37].
Mee's lines	Hodgkin's disease and carcinoid tumors [41]. Chemotherapeutic agents, commonly vincristine, doxorubicin, and cyclophosphamide
Melanonychia (longitudinal, transverse, or diffuse)	Breast cancer, metastatic melanoma, Peutz-Jegers syndrome, vincristine, adriamycin [44], doxorubicin [45], hydroxyurea [46], bleomycin, cyclophosphamide, daunorubicin, dacarbazine, 5- fluorouracil, methotrexate, electron beam therapy [47]
Muehrcke's lines	Hypoalbuminemia and nephrotic syndrome [41]
Hemorrhagic onycholysis	Taxane chemotherapy [48], ixabepilone [49]
Paronychia or pyogenic granulomas	Epidermal growth factor inhibitors [50,51], mitozantrone [52], taxanes [53], methotrexate [54], multiple myeloma [55], bronchogenic carcinoma [56], metastatic cancer [57]

a congenital disorder, as seen in pachydermoperiostosis [36].

Yellow nail syndrome

Yellow nail syndrome (YNS) is a rare disorder characterized by slow-growing, thickened yellow nails. In most cases, all 20 nails are involved, with transverse and longitudinal overcurvature of the nails and absent cuticles and lunulae (Fig. 2) [37]. In addition to the nail findings, YNS is characterized by lymphedema and respiratory tract involvement, including sinusitis, pleural effusions, and bronchiectasis. YNS may be inherited or acquired, with nail findings being the only manifestation of the disease in some cases. There are heterogeneous inheritance patterns, with both

autosomal dominant and recessive inheritance reported [38] in the inherited form, resulting in congenital inadequate lymphatic drainage.

Development of acquired YNS may be sporadic or associated with systemic diseases. Commonly, the disease is associated with autoimmune diseases such as systemic lupus erythematosus, rheumatoid arthritis, and thyroiditis; or infections, such as AIDS and tuberculosis. There are several case reports of paraneoplastic YNS associated with internal malignancies, including carcinomas of the breast, endometrium, gallbladder, larynx, and lung; metastatic melanoma; metastatic sarcoma; Hodgkin's disease; and mycosis fungoides [37]. Paraneoplastic YNS is thought to result from either direct tumor infiltration into already dysfunctional lymphatics, or from the release of tumor mediators that inhibit lymphatic function [39]. The differential diagnosis of YNS includes onychomycosis and pseudomonal nail infection, but involvement of all 20 nails would be highly unlikely in either of these conditions.

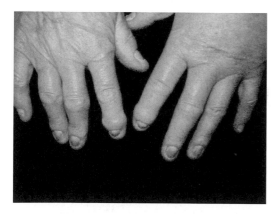

Fig. 2. Yellow nail syndrome nail changes in a patient with bronchogenic carcinoma. Note the transverse and longitudinal overcurvature of the nail plates.

Nonspecific nail changes

Chemotherapy-induced nail changes may involve the nail matrix, resulting in aberrations of nail plate growth (Mee's lines, Beau's lines, onychomadesis, or melanonychia), the nail bed (resulting in Muehrcke's lines, onycholysis, subungual hemorrhage or hematoma), or the proximal nail fold (eg, paronychia, periungual pyogenic granuloma) [33,40].

Nail plate abnormalities

Processes that interfere with nail matrix activity result in abnormalities of the nail plate. If a systemic stress or drug results in the retention of matrix keratinocyte nuclei in the nail plate (parakeratosis), a white, transverse band will appear across the nail plate (Fig. 3). This band of true leukonychia usually parallels the contour of the lunula, and is termed a Mee's line [41]. These non-blanching lines can be single or multiple on one nail plate, and usually affect multiple nails when associated with a systemic condition. Various heavy metal poisons [42] are associated with Mee's lines, as are metabolic, dermatologic, cardiopulmonary, hematologic, and renal states. Additionally, Mee's lines have been reported in association with Hodgkin's disease and carcinoid tumors [41]. Chemotherapeutic agents, commonly vincristine, doxorubicin, and cyclophosphamide, are also associated with Mee's lines.

Temporary cessation in nail growth results in plate known as Beau's lines, and complete matrix toxicity results in nail plate shedding known as onychomedesis. Beau's lines present clinically as simultaneously appearing, transverse depressions in all the nail plates (Fig. 4). The onset of this depression is usually in association with a single systemic insult such as infection, surgery, or illness. The depth of the depression is associated with the severity of matrix keratinocyte toxicity, whereas the longitudinal width corresponds with the duration of the insult [43]. If the inciting event results in full matrix toxicity, onychomedesis may

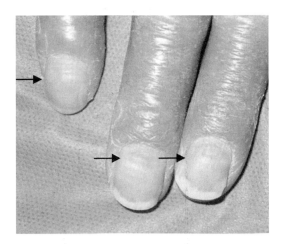

Fig. 4. Beau's lines in association with Sezary syndrome. Note the steep step-off that corresponded with the onset of erythroderma approximately 3 months before the photo.

be seen. Both Beau's lines and onychomedesis are commonly reported in association with chemotherapy.

Development of melanin pigmentation of the nail plate is termed melanonychia. Melanonychia may be normal in darkly pigmented individuals (Fig. 5), but is occasionally reported in the context of cancer and cancer treatment. Three patterns of melanonychia exist: longitudinal, transverse, and diffuse. Melanonychia are usually caused by matrix melanin deposition in the growing nail plate, and more than one pattern of melanonychia may be observed in a single nail plate. Solitary or multiple longitudinal pigmented streaks in the nail plate are usually associated with discrete pigmented lesions in the nail matrix. Longitudinal melanonychia can be common in deeply

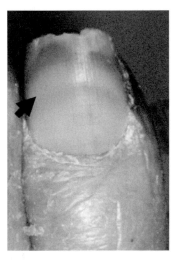

Fig. 3. Mee's line in a patient with vasculitis.

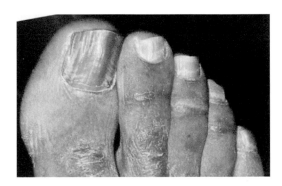

Fig. 5. Physiologic, diffuse melanonychia of the first nail plate in a darkly pigmented individual.

pigmented individuals, and can be acquired without any association to disease. These bands have been reported to arise in a number of systemic diseases and physiologic states, including Addison's disease, AIDS, hyperthyroidism, malnutrition, and pregnancy. Additionally, melanonychia striata have been reported to arise in association with breast cancer, metastatic melanoma, and Peutz-Jegers syndrome [41].

Transverse melanonychia have been reported to occur in the context of medications, including chemotherapy and electron-beam radiation therapy. Vincristine, adriamycin [44], doxorubicin [45], hydroxyurea [46], bleomycin, cyclophosphamide, daunorubicin, dacarbazine, 5-fluorouracil, methotrexate, and electron beam therapy [47] have all been reported to cause transverse melanonychia, or a mixed pattern of melanonychia. These pigmented areas tend to resolve after the completion of therapy. The band will persist in the nail plate until it eventually grows out, however.

Nail bed changes

Abnormalities in the nail bed can have many different clinical presentations; however, the overlying nail plate remains unchanged. Vascular congestion in the nail bed can result in the formation of blanchable, paired, white lines termed Muehrcke's lines. These apparent leukonychia are most commonly seen in association with hypoalbuminemia and nephrotic syndrome [41]. If nail bed hemorrhage occurs, a subungual hematoma may occur. If the hematoma is severe, the nail plate may become completely detached from the nail bed with a loss of the nail. Taxane chemotherapy agents such as docetaxel and paclitaxel are common inducers of hemorrhagic onycholysis, resulting in suppuration and hemorrhage of the nail bed with subsequent nail plate loss [48]. Ixabepilone [49] has also been noted to result in this form of nail loss.

Proximal nail fold changes

The proximal nail fold can be affected by a number of nonspecific systemic conditions. Paronychia, inflammation of the nail folds, may be observed in the context of a number of drugs, or pyogenic granulomas, lobular tumors of capillaries, may be seen in a variety of conditions. Epidermal growth factor inhibitors [50,51], mitozantrone [52], taxanes [53], and methotrexate [54] have been associated with paronychia, pyo-

genic granulomas, or both. Chronic paronychia has also been reported in association with multiple myeloma [55], bronchogenic carcinoma [56], and metastatic cancer [57].

Summary

The hair and nails may be affected by malignancy, systemic diseases, medications, or physical factors. Although hair and nail abnormalities are usually of great cosmetic concern to the patient, they may indicate even greater medical concerns that should not be overlooked. Early identification and management of internal disease is paramount to early intervention, and may be vital in improving overall morbidity and mortality.

References

[1] Curth HO. Skin lesions and internal carcinoma. In: Andrade R, editor. Cancer of the skin: biology, diagnosis, management. Philadelphia: Saunders; 1976.

[2] Weedon D. Diseases of cutaneous appendages. In: Weedon D, editor. Skin pathology. 2nd Edition. London: Elsevier Science Limited; 2002. p. 456–501.

[3] Farina MC, Tarin N, Grilli R, et al. Acquired hypertrichosis lanuginosa: case report and review of the literature. J Surg Oncol 1998;68(3):199–203.

[4] Whiting DA. Structural abnormalities of the hair shaft. J Am Acad Dermatol 1987;16:1–25.

[5] Vulink AJ, ten Bokkel Huinink D. Acquired hypertrichosis lanuginosa: a rare cutaneous paraneoplastic syndrome. J Clin Oncol 2007;25(12):1625–6.

[6] Kurzrock R, Cohen PR. Cutaneous paraneoplastic syndromes in solid tumors. Am J Med 1995;99: 662–71.

[7] Perez-Losada E, Pujol RM, Domingo P, et al. Hypertrichosis lanuginosa acquisita preceding extraskeletal Ewing's sarcoma. Clin Exp Dermatol 2001;26:182–3.

[8] Mlczoch L, Attarbaschi A, Dworzak M, et al. Alopecia areata and multifocal bone involvement in a young adult with Hodgkin's disease. Leuk Lymphoma 2005;46(4):623–7.

[9] Chan PD, Berk MA, Kucuk O, et al. Simultaneously occurring alopecia areata and Hodgkin's lymphoma: complete remission of both diseases with MOPP/ABV chemotherapy. Med Pediatr Oncol 1992;20:345–8.

[10] Bayer-Garner IB, Smoller BR. The spectrum of cutaneous disease in multiple myeloma. J Am Acad Dermatol 2003;48(4):497–507.

[11] Weichenthal M, Stemm AV, Ramsauer J, et al. POEMS syndrome: cicatricial alopecia as an unusual cutaneous manifestation associated with an

underlying plasmacytoma. J Am Acad Dermatol 1999;40(5 Pt 2):808–12.

[12] Crotty K, McCarthy W, Quinn M, et al. Alopecia neoplastica caused by desmoplastic melanoma. Aust J Dermatol 2003;44(4):295–8.

[13] Gül U, Kılıç A, Akbaş A, et al. Alopecia neoplastica due to metastatic colon adenocarcinoma. Acta Derm Venereol 2007;87:93–4.

[14] Chung JJ, Namiki T, Johnson DW. Cervical cancer metastasis to the scalp presenting as alopecia neoplastica. Int J Dermatol 2007;46(2):188–9.

[15] Kim HJ, Min HG, Lee ES. Alopecia neoplastica in a patient with gastric carcinoma. Br J Dermatol 1999;141(6):1122–4.

[16] Hussein AM. Chemotherapy-induced alopecia: new developments. South Med J 1993;86:489–96.

[17] Tosti A, Pazzaglia M. Drug reactions affecting hair: diagnosis. Dermatol Clin 2007;25(2):223–31.

[18] Yun SJ, Kim SJ. Hair loss pattern due to chemotherapy-induced anagen effluvium: a cross-sectional observation. Dermatology 2007;215(1):36–40.

[19] Routhouska S, Gilliam AC, Mirmirani P. Hair depigmentation during chemotherapy with a class III/V receptor tyrosine kinase inhibitor. ArchDermatol 2006;142:1477–9.

[20] Rebora A, Delmonte S, Parodi A. Cyclosporin A-induced hair darkening. Int J Dermatol 1999;38(3):229–30.

[21] Cline DJ. Changes in hair color. Dermatol Clin 1988;6(2):295–303.

[22] Wheeland RG, Burgdorf WH, Humphrey GB. The flag sign of chemotherapy. Cancer 1983;51(8):1356–8.

[23] Bessis D, Luong SM, Blanc P, et al. Straight hair associated with interferon-alfa plus ribavirin in hepatitis C infection. Br J Dermatol 2002;147:392.

[24] Tinio P, Hadi S, Al-Ghaithi K, et al. Segmental vitiligo and hair curling after interferon alpha and ribavirin treatment for hepatitis C. Skinmed 2006;5(1):50–1.

[25] Braun RP, Skaria AM, Saurat JH, et al. Multiple hyperkeratotic spicules and myeloma. Dermatology 2002;205(2):210–2.

[26] Satta R, Casu G, Dore F, et al. Follicular spicules and multiple ulcers: cutaneous manifestations of multiple myeloma. J Am Acad Dermatol 2003; 49(4):736–40.

[27] Susser WS, Whitaker-Worth DL, Grant-Kels JM. Mucocutaneous reactions to chemotherapy. J Am Acad Dermatol 1999;40:367–400.

[28] Lawenda BD, Gagne HM, Gierga DP, et al. Permanent alopecia after cranial irradiation: dose-response relationship. Int J Radiat Oncol Biol Phys 2004; 60(3):879–87.

[29] Metz JM, Smith D, Mick R, et al. A phase I study of topical tempol for the prevention of alopecia induced by whole brain radiotherapy. Clin Cancer Res 2004;10(19):6411–7.

[30] Cuscela D, Coffin D, Lupton GP, et al. Protection from radiation-induced alopecia with topical

application of nitroxides: fractionated studies. Cancer J Sci Am 1996;2(5):273–8.

[31] Fleckman P. Structure and function of the nail unit. In: Scher RK, Daniel CR, editors. Nails: diagnosis, therapy, surgery. 3rd edition. Philadelphia: Elsevier Saunders; 2005. p. 13–25.

[32] Paus R, Peker S. Biology of hair and nails. In: Bolognia JL, Jorizzo JL, Rapini RP, editors. Dermatology. 1st edition. Philadelphia: Mosby; 2003. p. 1007–32.

[33] Chen W, Yu YS, Liu YH, et al. Nail changes association with chemotherapy in children. J Eur Acad Dermatol Venereol 2007;21:186–90.

[34] Dickinson CJ. The aetiology of clubbing and hypertrophic osteoarthropathy. Eur J Clin Invest 1993;23: 330–8.

[35] Benedeck TG. Paraneoplastic digital clubbing and hypertrophic osteoarthropathy. Clin Dermatol 1993;11:53–9.

[36] Tosti A, Piraccini BM. Nail disorders. In: Bolognia JL, Jorizzo JL, Rapini RP, editors. Dermatology. 1st edition. Philadelphia: Mosby; 2003. p. 1061–78.

[37] Iqbal M, Rossoff LJ, Marzouk KA, et al. Resolution of yellow nails after successful treatment of breast cancer. Chest 2000;117(5):1516–8.

[38] Lambert EM, Dziura J, Kauls L, et al. Yellow nail syndrome in three siblings: a randomized double-blind trial of topical vitamin E. Pediatr Dermatol 2006;23(4):390–5.

[39] Thomas PS, Sidhu B. Yellow nail syndrome and bronchial carcinoma [letter]. Chest 1987;92:191.

[40] Daniel CR III, Scher RK. Nail changes secondary to systemic drugs or ingestants. J Am Acad Dermatol 1984;10:250–8.

[41] Lawry M, Daniel CR. Nails in systemic disease. In: Scher RK, Daniel CR, editors. Nails: diagnosis, therapy, surgery. 3rd edition. Philadelphia: Elsevier Saunders; 2005. p. 147–76.

[42] Piraccini BM, Iorizzo M. Drug reactions affecting the nail unit: diagnosis and management. Dermatol Clin 2007;25(2):215–21, vii.

[43] Piraccini BM, Iorizzo M, Starace M, et al. Drug-induced nail diseases. Dermatol Clin 2006;24(3): 387–91.

[44] Dasanu CA, Vaillant JG, Alexandrescu DT. Distinct patterns of chromonychia, Beau's lines, and melanoderma seen with vincristine, adriamycin, dexamethasone therapy for multiple myeloma. Dermatol Online J 2006;12(6):10.

[45] M I, Khairkar PH. Doxorubicin induced melanonychia. Indian Pediatr 2003;40(11):1094–5.

[46] Oh ST, Lee DW, Lee JY, et al. Hydroxyurea-induced melanonychia concomitant with a dermatomyositis-like eruption. J Am Acad Dermatol 2003; 49(2):339–41.

[47] Quinlan KE, Janiga JJ, Baran R, et al. Transverse melanonychia secondary to total skin electron

beam therapy: a report of 3 cases. J Am Acad Dermatol 2005;53(2 Suppl 1):S112–4.

[48] Roh MR, Cho JY, Lew W. Docetaxel-induced onycholysis: the role of subungual hemorrhage and suppuration. Yonsei Med J 2007;48(1):124–6.

[49] Alimonti A, Nardoni C, Papaldo P, et al. Nail disorders in a woman treated with ixabepilone for metastatic breast cancer. Anticancer Res 2005;25(5): 3531–2.

[50] Segaert S, Van Cutsem E. Clinical signs, pathophysiology and management of skin toxicity during therapy with epidermal growth factor receptor inhibitors. Ann Oncol 2005;16(9):1425–33 [epub 2005, Jul 12].

[51] Chang GC, Yang TY, Chen KC, et al. Complications of therapy in cancer patients: case 1. Paronychia and skin hyperpigmentation induced by gefitinib in advanced non-small-cell lung cancer. J Clin Oncol 2004;22(22):4646–8.

[52] Freiman A, Bouganim N, O'Brien EA. Case reports: mitozantrone-induced onycholysis associated with subungual abscesses, paronychia, and pyogenic granuloma. J Drugs Dermatol 2005;4(4):490–2.

[53] Nicolopoulos J, Howard A. Docetaxel-induced nail dystrophy. Australas J Dermatol 2002;43(4):293–6.

[54] Wantzin GL, Thomsen K. Acute paronychia after high-dose methotrexate therapy. Arch Dermatol 1983;119(7):623–4.

[55] Ahmed I, Cronk JS, Crutchfield CE 3rd, et al. Myeloma-associated systemic amyloidosis presenting as chronic paronychia and palmodigital erythematous swelling and induration of the hands. J Am Acad Dermatol 2000;42(2 Pt 2):339–42.

[56] Shepherd DM, Dzikowski CM, Chussid F. Bronchogenic carcinoma mimicking paronychia and osteomyelitis in the great toe. J Foot Ankle Surg 1997;36(2):115–9.

[57] Henderson JJ. Metastatic carcinoma in the hand presenting as an acute paronychia. Br J Clin Pract 1987;41(6):805–6.

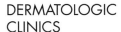

DERMATOLOGIC
CLINICS

ELSEVIER
SAUNDERS

Dermatol Clin 26 (2008) 69–87

Genodermatoses with Cutaneous Tumors and Internal Malignancies

Brian Somoano, MD[a], Hensin Tsao, MD, PhD[b],*

[a]Department of Dermatology, Stanford University Medical Center, 900 Blake Wilbur Drive, Stanford, CA 94305, USA
[b]Department of Dermatology, Massachusetts General Hospital, 622 Bartlett Hall,
48 Blossom Street, Boston, MA 02114, USA

Dermatologists have long appreciated the clustering of specific skin findings in kindreds in frequencies above those in the general population. The term genodermatoses has come to define this large group of heterogeneous disorders whose etiology results from a known or suspected underlying genetic abnormality. A subset of these inherited diseases has been shown to be associated with the development of skin and internal tumors. Although the constellation of anomalies in these familial syndromes are presumed to be pathogenically related, it is also recognized that confounding environmental factors can lead to the collection of sporadic malignancies within families. For example, related individuals who have similar lifelong exposure to excess ultraviolet radiation may all be prone to developing skin cancer, potentially simulating a true inherited susceptibility such as that seen in hereditary melanoma.

Despite these challenges, several clinical clues suggest a true inherited predisposition to skin and internal malignancies. One or several specific tumor types are usually noted in numerous relatives, often in multiple generations on one side of the family. These neoplasms also tend to develop at a significantly younger age than normal, and multiple primary tumors in a given individual are not uncommon.

Furthermore, powerful new genetic tools are also continuously adding to our understanding of the molecular events underlying these genodermatoses, and a continuing medical education (CME) report recently reviewed many of these enabling technologies in detail [1]. These advances have in turn resulted in an ever-growing number of available genetic tests for their associated mutations. A good understanding of the clinical features and molecular studies available for these genodermatoses is especially prudent for dermatologists, because the often subtle cutaneous findings can be among the first stigmata of these disorders, and function as early indicators of an underlying predisposition to potentially grave malignancies.

Once suspected, a multidisciplinary approach is recommended, because genetic counselors and geneticists can help to ensure that an informed decision can be made about testing. Many factors must be considered, including the potential psychosocial consequences of this information on the patient and relatives, which test to offer, any associated costs, and the potential risks for genetic discrimination. Furthermore, genetic analysis may not always be available, or may be of only limited utility, and diagnoses are often made on the basis of clinical findings alone. Additional information about the availability of genetic counseling can be found at the National Society of Genetic Counselors' Web site (www.nsgc.org). The authors have previously reviewed the predictive value of many of the genetic tests available for these disorders, as well as the specific laboratories in the United States and abroad offering these services [2]. Given the rapidly changing nature of genetic testing availability, the regularly updated Web site www.genetests.org is an especially practical resource for this information.

---

* Corresponding author.

E-mail address: tsao.hensin@mgh.harvard.edu
(H. Tsao).

Genodermatoses with cutaneous tumors and internal malignancies

It is possible to divide this group of disorders into two general categories based on the malignant potential of the most characteristic cutaneous tumors (Box 1). Group I is composed of disorders that feature prominent cutaneous malignancies and occasional visceral neoplasms (eg, basal cell carcinomas in nevoid basal cell carcinoma syndrome). In comparison, disorders in Group II manifest chiefly benign cutaneous neoplasms, or rare cutaneous malignancies, and internal tumors (eg, hamartomas in Cowden disease). Although multiple endocrine neoplasia Type IIb could belong among the syndromes in Group II, its characteristic dermatologic features are mainly limited to oral mucosa, and it has not been included in this article.

This article focuses on our current understanding of the clinical manifestations and underlying genetic anomalies of those genodermatoses that manifest cutaneous and internal tumors, whether benign or malignant. Because a comprehensive discussion is not feasible given the limitations of this article, exceedingly rare disorders have not been included, and the corresponding Online Mendelian Inheritance in Man (OMIM) reference number is provided for each disorder as an additional resource.

Box 1. Genodermatoses with cutaneous and internal tumors and abbreviations used

Group I: prominent cutaneous malignancies
Nevoid basal cell carcinoma syndrome (NBCCS)
Familial melanoma (FM)
Xeroderma pigmentosum (XP)

Group II: chiefly benign tumors of the skin
Cowden syndrome (CS)
Muir-Torre syndrome (MTS)
Gardner syndrome (GS)
Tuberous sclerosis (TS)
Neurofibromatosis 1 (NF1)
Neurofibromatosis 2 (NF2)
Birt-Hogg-Dube (BHD)
Hereditary leiomyomatosis and renal cell cancer (HLRCC)

Group I

Nevoid basal cell carcinoma syndrome

Nevoid basal cell carcinoma syndrome (NBCCS) (Gorlin syndrome, basal cell nevus syndrome; OMIM 109,400) is an autosomal dominant (AD) genodermatosis characterized by basal cell carcinomas (BCCs), odontogenic keratocysts, and a wide spectrum of developmental anomalies and extracutaneous neoplasms. Prevalence ranges from 1 in 56,000 to 1 in 164,000 [3,4].

Cutaneous features

Affected individuals are predisposed to the development of numerous premature BCCs, occurring in over 80% of Caucasian patients who have NBCCS. A mean age of 20 years at first diagnosis has been reported [4], and although thousands can develop during one's lifetime, an average of eight lesions has been suggested. Clinically, the BCCs can resemble acrochordons or vascular lesions, and a large number of tan pedunculated papules at an unusually early age should raise suspicion for this disorder [5]. Although they can occur at any site, the face, neck, and trunk are most common [3]. As a result, noninvasive treatment options have been considered, such as topical 5-fluorouracil [6] or photodynamic therapy [7], to avoid significant surgical scarring and possibly even prevent new lesions. Possible immunoprevention of BCCs with recombinant hedgehog-interacting protein has also been proposed [8].

Acral pitting is another characteristic feature of NBCCS, occurring in about 80% of patients [4]. These present as persistent tiny, asymptomatic depressions, and are often subtle and overlooked. Immersion of hands in water can make them more pronounced, and characteristic red globules on dermoscopy may facilitate their identification [9]. Up to one half of patients may also manifest epidermal cysts or facial milia [4,10], and discrete patches of long pigmented hair have recently been reported on several patients [11].

Extracutaneous tumors and features

Odontogenic keratocysts of the jaw develop in nearly 75% of affected patients [12] at a mean age of 15 years [4], and are considered a major criteria in establishing a clinical diagnosis of NBCCS (Box 2) [12]. These cystic lesions usually result in swelling or pain, though they can be asymptomatic, and appear as radiolucencies on imaging. About 4% of patients develop medulloblastomas,

Box 2. Diagnostic criteria: nevoid basal cell carcinoma syndrome

Major criteria
Multiple (>2) BCCs, or one before the age of 30 years
Odontogenic keratocysts of the jaw (proven by histology)
Multiple (>2) palmar or plantar pits
Bilamellar calcification of the falx cerebri
Bifid, fused, or markedly splayed ribs
First-degree relative who has NBCCS

Minor criteria
Macrocephaly determined after adjustment for height
Congenital malformations: cleft lip or palate, frontal bossing, "coarse face," or moderate or severe hypertelorism
Other skeletal abnormalities: Sprengel's deformity, marked pectus deformity, or marked syndactyly of the digits
Radiological abnormalities: bridging of the sella turcica; vertebral anomalies such as hemivertebrae, fusion or elongation of the vertebral bodies; modeling defects of the hands and feet; or flame-shaped lucencies of the hands or feet
Ovarian fibroma
Medulloblastoma

Diagnosis requires one of the following
Two major criteria, or
One major and two minor criteria

Data from Kimonis VE, Goldstein AM, Pastakia B, et al. Clinical manifestations in 105 persons with nevoid basal cell carcinoma syndrome. Am J Hum Genet 1997;69:299–308.

Molecular genetics (PTCH gene on chromosome 9q22.3)

Soon after linkage analysis mapped the NBCCS gene to chromosome 9q22.3-q31, germ-line mutations in the *patched (PTCH)* gene were identified in affected patients, as well as in somatic DNA in sporadic BCCs [15]. Clinical genetic testing is available at several laboratories, and recent data by Klein and colleagues [16] show that *PTCH* mutations can be identified in about 60% of pedigrees meeting the clinical diagnostic criteria for NBCCS. A relatively high number of NBCCS cases, about half, are thought to be caused by de novo mutation [16].

Familial melanoma

Familial melanoma (FM) (familial atypical multiple-mole and melanoma [FAMMM] syndrome, dysplastic nevus syndrome [DNS]; OMIM 155,600) represents a group of heterogeneous disorders of likely polygenic etiology characterized by a predisposition to cutaneous melanoma. A subset of patients also exhibit an inherited susceptibility to numerous atypical nevi, in which case the term FAMMM syndrome or DNS has been used. Ten percent of melanoma occurs in patients who have a family history of this disease [17]. Nevertheless, given that shared environmental exposures in families can lead to the clustering of sporadic melanomas mimicking an inherited susceptibility, an accurate estimate of FM can be difficult. The true prevalence of FAMMM syndrome is especially challenging, given that unlike many classic genodermatoses in which a well-defined set of anomalies is characteristic of the disorder, nevus phenotype varies broadly along a continuous spectrum, and no well-quantified number of lesions or degree of atypia is widely recognized as diagnostic.

Cutaneous features

The predisposition toward multiple and early-onset tumors seen in other hereditary cancer syndromes is also evident in FM. In a study by Puig and colleagues [18], germline mutations in the main locus associated with FM (*CDKN2A*) were more frequent in those who had multiple primary melanomas (MPM), and lower age at diagnosis (33 versus 46 years) was noted among carriers of these mutations. In addition, FAMMM patients also manifest numerous melanocytic nevi, often numbering more than 100. Many of these display clinically atypical features including large size (6 mm or greater in diameter),

and about 1% to 2% of all of these brain tumors occur in the setting of NBCCS [12,13]. Numerous other neoplasms have been reported, including meningiomas, cardiac and ovarian fibromas, ovarian desmoids, and sarcomas [4,10,12–14]. Other anomalies include ectopic intracranial calcification of the falx cerebri (in about 65% of patients) [12], macrocephaly and frontal bossing, and other skeletal abnormalities.

irregular or poorly defined borders, or significant color variegation.

Extracutaneous tumors and features

Patients who have FM and associated *CDKN2A* mutations impairing p16 function may be predisposed to developing pancreatic cancer [19,20], with one study estimating a 22 fold increased risk for this malignancy [19]. It has also recently been suggested that a specific common *CDKN2A* variant (A148T) may also be associated with multiple internal malignancies in Poland, including breast cancer [21,22], although other studies suggest it may not segregate with melanoma [23].

Molecular genetics (CDKN2A gene on chromosomes 9p21)

Work by Cannon-Albright and colleagues [24] with melanoma kindreds supported linkage to an area within chromosome 9p21 believed to represent a melanoma-susceptibility locus, with subsequent studies using positional cloning to provide strong evidence for a candidate gene in this region [25,26]. Germline mutations in *CDKN2A*, as this gene has since been designated, have been identified in numerous FM kindreds, confirming its role in a subset of families [27]. *CDKN2A* is now known to be comprised of four exons (1a, 1b, 2, and 3) that encode the proteins p16 and p14ARF that help regulate cell cycle progression, and significant progress is being made in understanding their role in the pathogenesis of melanoma [28]. The study of melanoma-prone families who had no identifiable *CDKN2A* mutations has led to the discovery of less common susceptibility loci. The seventh FM kindred with germline mutation in the cyclin-dependent protein kinase (*CDK4*) gene on chromosome 12q14 was recently reported [29], and a susceptibility locus on chromosomes 1p22 has also been proposed [30].

The incidence of melanoma among carriers of deleterious *CDKN2A* mutations varies based on several factors. Bishop and colleagues [31] showed that mutation penetrance at age 80 years among multiple case families was 58% in Europe, 76% in the United States, and 91% in Australia, suggesting that environmental factors might be at play. More recently, analysis of buccal smears from 3626 patients who had melanoma in the general population estimated *CDKN2A* penetrance at 28% by age 80 years [32]; likely lower than previous reports, given that these patients were not selected for family history. Other factors modifying *CDKN2A* penetrance include number of nevi, dysplastic nevi, and sunburns [33], as well as melanocortin-1 receptor gene variants [34], all of which increase lifetime risk of melanoma in mutation carriers. Genetic testing is available through several clinical laboratories. Although *CDKN2A* mutations occur in fewer than 1% to 2% of all melanoma patients [18,35], it is estimated that these can be identified in 10% to 25% of those who have FM [36], depending on personal and family history. For example, mutations occur in 20% to 40% of those who have three or more affected relatives [35,37], whereas patients who have a personal history of two or three primary melanomas have a 10% or 40% chance of carrying a mutation, respectively [18]. Despite its commercial availability, testing is still controversial, because additional studies are needed to clarify what role this genetic information will play in patient care.

Xeroderma pigmentosum

Xeroderma pigmentosum (XP) (OMIM 194,400, 133,510, 278,700-278,800) is an autosomal recessive (AR) genodermatosis characterized by extreme photosensitivity and cutaneous malignancies as a result of defective DNA repair. Disease frequency in the United States is about 1:250,000, though it occurs more commonly in Japan [38].

Cutaneous features

The cutaneous manifestations of XP first present at a median age of 1 to 2 years, though an abnormally prominent sunburn response or photo-distributed freckling can be noted as early as infancy [39]. Marked xerosis and classic signs of photoaging, including actinic lentigenes and poikiloderma (atrophy, mottled hyper and hypopigmentation, and telangiectasias), become increasingly evident throughout childhood. Multiple early-onset cutaneous malignancies, primarily in sun-exposed regions, is another hallmark feature of XP, first presenting at a median age of 8 years [39,40]. Affected patients have a 2000 fold increased risk for BCCs, squamous cell carcinomas (SCCs), and melanoma [41] (>95% of which develop on the head and neck) [39], and are 10,000 times more likely to develop SCC on the tip of the tongue than unaffected individuals of comparable age [41]. The associated morbidity and mortality of these malignancies can be great, illustrated by an estimated 70% survival rate at 40 years of age [39].

Extracutaneous tumors and features

Ocular pathology is also common in XP, and involves the more photoexposed structures such as the lids, cornea, and conjunctiva [39]. Photophobia is most commonly reported, but conjunctivitis, ectropion, and corneal opacification are also often seen [42]. Ocular neoplasms develop in 10% to 20% of XP patients, usually SCCs, BCCs, or melanoma, although a case of conjunctival atypical fibroxanthoma was recently reported [42]. Neurologic anomalies also occur in about 30% of affected patients, especially in groups XPA and XPD, with slowly progressive neurological degeneration contributing to intellectual impairment, sensorineural deafness, and hyporeflexia [39,43]. Aspiration from dysphagia and rarely vocal cord paralysis may also be seen [43,44]. A 10 to 20 fold increased risk of internal malignancies has also been described in affected patients, and leukemia and cancers of the lung, breast, pancreas, stomach, brain, and testicles have all been reported in association with XP [39–41,45].

Molecular genetics (8 XP genes on various chromosomes)

About 80% of XP results from a defect in any one of seven genes encoding proteins critical in the nucleotide excision repair (NER) pathway, which consequently results in uncorrected ultraviolet (UV)-induced DNA lesions that can be propagated and tumorogenic [41]. Each of these NER genes corresponds to one of seven unique XP complementation subgroups (designated XPA–XPG) that differ in frequency and clinical characteristics. For example, although groups XPA and XPC both represent about 25% of cases and affected patients have similar skin findings, a broad spectrum of neurologic abnormalities is common in the former, but rarely seen in the latter. An estimated 20% of patients are designated XP variants, because the causative gene (XPV) is not directly involved in NER, but rather encodes a polymerase likely involved in postreplication repair. Alterations in XPD occur in 15% of cases, and XPB, XPE, XPF, and XPG occur less frequently. Genetic testing for mutations in XPA and XPC via sequence analysis is now clinically available, although some suggest that it should be used primarily to confirm a diagnosis among those previously screened for abnormalities in DNA repair by one of several functional assays available at research laboratories.

Several areas of active investigation have stemmed directly from our understanding of the molecular basis of XP. Numerous reports have documented a possible association between polymorphisms in the XP DNA repair genes (especially XPC and XPD) and risk for different internal tumors, especially lung cancer [46], and work with XPC deficient mice is helping to shed light on melanoma photocarcinogenesis [47].

Group II

Cowden syndrome

Cowden syndrome (CS) (Cowden Disease, multiple hamartoma syndrome; OMIM 158,350) is an AD familial cancer syndrome characterized by mucocutaneous hamartomas and a predisposition for various benign and malignant extracutaneous tumors, especially of the breast, thyroid, and endometrium. Although disease prevalence has been estimated at 1 in 200,000 [48], it has been suggested that many cases go undiagnosed as a result of the diverse, often subtle, clinical stigmata among affected patients that may be overlooked [49].

Cutaneous features

The benign mucocutaneous findings in CS are hallmark features of this disorder, and are among the "pathognomonic criteria" in establishing a clinical diagnosis (Box 3). Facial trichilemmomas usually present as asymptomatic, skin-colored to yellow-tan papules, and multiple oral papillomas, fibromas on histology, produce the characteristic "cobblestone" appearance often seen on the lips or buccal mucosa. Acral keratoses, and less commonly lipomas and angiomas, can also be seen. Although various skin cancers have also been reported in CS patients, including BCC, SCC, melanoma, Merkel cell carcinoma, and trichilemmomal carcinoma, a true hereditary predisposition has not been established [15].

Extracutaneous tumors and features

Internal malignancies represent the bulk of the "major" diagnostic criteria of CS, and are a source of significant morbidity and mortality in affected kindreds. Affected women have a lifetime risk of breast cancer ranging from 25% to 50%, and nearly two thirds of women can develop benign breast disease [50,51]. Thyroid abnormalities are estimated to affect 62% of CS patients [50], including thyroid cancer in 10% of cases [52]. The true risk for other reported malignancies are less well-established, and endometrial cancer may also affect 5% to 10% of affected women [53].

Box 3. Diagnostic criteria: Cowden syndrome

Pathognomonic criteria
- Adult Lhermitte-Duclos disease (LDD)
- Mucocutaneous lesions
  Facial trichilemmomas
  Acral keratoses
  Papillomatous papules

Major criteria
- Breast cancer
- Thyroid cancer, especially follicular thyroid carcinoma
- Macrocephaly ($\geq$97th percentile)
- Endometrial cancer

Minor criteria
- Other thyroid lesions (eg, adenoma or multinodular goiter)
- Mental retardation (IQ$\leq$75)
- Gastrointestinal hamartomas
- Fibrocystic disease of the breast
- Lipomas
- Fibromas
- Genitourinary tumors (especially renal cell carcinoma)
- Genitourinary structural manifestations
- Uterine fibroids

Operational diagnosis of CS requires any single pathognomonic criterion, but
- Mucocutaneous lesions alone if
  $\geq$6 facial papules with $\geq$3 trichilemmomas, or
  Cutaneous facial papules and oral mucosal papillomatosis, or
  Oral mucosal papillomatosis and acral keratoses, or
  $\geq$6 palmar/plantar keratoses
- $\geq$2 major criteria
- One major and $\geq$3 minor criteria
- $\geq$4 minor criteria

Operational diagnosis for individual in a family where one relative is diagnostic for CS requires >one of the following
- A pathognomonic criterion
- Any one major criterion
- Two minor criteria
- History of Bannayan-Riley-Ruvalcaba syndrome

Data from the National Comprehensive Cancer Network Clinical Practice Guidelines in Oncology, version 1. 2007. Available at: http://www.nccn.org/professionals/physician_gls/PDF/genetics_screening.pdf. Accessed June 23, 2007.

Furthermore, although up to 60% of patients may develop gastrointestinal polyps [50], with a recent report documenting the possibility of malignant transformation [54], increased risk for colorectal cancer has not been proven. Other important features include macrocephaly and Lhermitte-Duclos disease, a hamartoma of the cerebellum now considered pathognomonic for CS if onset is in adulthood [55].

Molecular genetics (PTEN/MMAC1 gene on chromosome 10q23)

Around the time Nelen and colleagues [56] revealed evidence of linkage to markers on chromosome 10q22-23 in CS, a tumor suppressor gene designated *PTEN/MMAC1* was identified in this locus from work with sporadic breast and brain tumors [57,58]. The role of *PTEN* in the etiology of CS was subsequently confirmed when inactivating mutations were demonstrated in germline DNA of affected patients [59]. Clinical genetic testing is available, and among patients meeting diagnostic criteria for CS, sequence analysis has identified *PTEN* germline mutations in about 80% of cases [60]. *PTEN* promoter analysis may also reveal mutations in another 10% of patients [60].

In addition to CS, *PTEN/MMAC1* has been associated with other disorders, often referred to collectively as the *PTEN* hamartoma tumor syndrome (PHTS). *PTEN/MMAC1* germline mutations have been identified in about 50% to 60% of patients who have Bannayan-Riley-Ruvalcaba syndrome (BRRS), 20% of patients who have Proteus syndrome, and 50% of those who have a Proteus-like syndrome [53]. It has recently been suggested that modulation of *PTEN/MMAC1* inactivation at the transcription level may be an important influential factor in determining the ultimate phenotype in the PHTS [61].

Muir-Torre syndrome

Muir-Torre syndrome (MTS) (OMIM 158,320) is a genodermatosis considered a phenotypic variant of hereditary non-polyposis colon cancer (HNPCC), with both disorders sharing an AD transmission, causative mutations in mismatch-repair genes, and an inherited susceptibility to internal tumors, especially gastrointestinal adenocarcinomas. The additional finding of cutaneous sebaceous tumors or keratoacanthomas (KAs) is unique to MTS. Although only 5 of the 538 HNPCC patients recently screened by Ponti and colleagues [62] (1%) had the characteristic tumors diagnostic of MTS, it has been suggested that limited skin examinations and underreporting of sebaceous tumors and KAs likely underestimate the true frequency of this disorder [62,63].

Cutaneous features

Sebaceous tumors usually present in the sixth decade of life as solitary or multiple, skin-colored to pink-yellow firm papules or nodules, arising primarily on the face or scalp. Among the 143 sebaceous tumors in MTS reviewed by Cohen and colleagues [64], benign lesions predominated (68% adenomas and 27% epitheliomas). Nevertheless, sebaceous carcinomas were identified in 30% of

patients, with more than half of these originating in meibomian glands [64]. Keratoacanthomas occur in about a quarter of probands [65], although multiple lesions, early onset, or sebaceous differentiation more reliably establish a diagnosis of MTS.

Extracutaneous tumors and features

Colorectal carcinomas represent about one half of the internal tumors in MTS, and age at diagnosis tends to precede sporadic lesions in the general population by about 10 years [64]. Whereas genitourinary carcinomas are also common, composing about one quarter of these tumors, various other malignancies, including those of the breast, head and neck, small bowel, and blood, represent fewer than 7% of cases.

Molecular genetics (MSH2 gene on chromosome 2p22)

By working with two large families manifesting the MTS phenotype, Hall and colleagues [66] were able to map the disease locus to a region of chromosome 2p that had previously been shown to be linked to HNPCC. Subsequently, germline mutations in the mismatch-repair (MMR) genes *MLH1* and *MSH2* were identified in 13 patients [67], establishing the role of these known HNPCC disease-causing genes in the etiology of MTS. The microsatellite instability (MSI) that has served as the genetic signature of HNPCC tumors has indeed also been observed in many MTS associated sebaceous tumors and KAs [15].

Numerous tests are available in the workup of MTS. The 2004 revised Bethesda guidelines for HNPCC suggest either immunohistochemical (IHC) testing for loss of gene expression or MSI analysis initially, and if positive, proceeding with germline analysis [68]. Although sebaceous adenomas and KAs are now included among tumors in MTS eligible for MSI testing, some propose that solitary sebaceous carcinomas are rare enough to also warrant analysis [62]. Although detection rates vary, MSI was recently identified in 71% of the cutaneous and visceral neoplasms of MTS patients [69]. Furthermore, Mangold and colleagues [70] showed that among 41 patients preselected for MMR deficiency via MSI or IHC evaluation, germline mutations were detected in 66% (27 of 41 cases), more than 90% of which were located in *MSH2*.

Gardner syndrome

Gardner syndrome (GS) (familial adenomatous polyposis [FAP]; OMIM 175,100) is an AD disorder currently recognized as a phenotypic variant of FAP, distinguished by the additional findings of skin cysts and osseous and soft tissue tumors in addition to colonic adenomatous polyposis. Because many FAP patients can manifest these lesions, the term GS is used primarily when these extraintestinal findings are especially prominent.

Cutaneous features

Subcutaneous nodules are common in GS, representing a combination of follicular cysts, lipomas, and fibromas. Among these, epidermoid cysts predominate [71], and are commonly noted on the head, neck, or extremities. They often precede detection of colonic polyps and, although multiple lesions are common and can be of cosmetic concern, significant disfigurement is rare [71]. Osteomas, benign tumors of bone tissue, were among the earliest described features of GS and often present as slowly enlarging growths of the skull, especially the mandible [72].

Extracutaneous tumors and features

As in FAP, GS is characterized by intestinal polyposis and, if untreated, inevitable progression to colorectal adenocarcinoma by a mean age of 39 years [73]. Affected females may also be prone to thyroid cancer, especially papillary carcinoma, with reports suggesting nearly a 100 fold incidence over the general public [74,75]. Other extracolonic malignancies disproportionately affecting these patients include duodenal and pancreatic adenocarcinomas and hepatoblastomas, and the association of FAP and CNS tumors, usually medulloblastomas, has been termed Turcot syndrome [73].

Desmoid tumors are significantly more common in FAP (relative risk of 852) [76] than in the general population, and can be found in 12% to 18% of patients who have GS [15]. Most arise in the abdomen or abdominal wall, and although benign, are locally invasive [76]. Gardner fibromas, the suspected desmoid precursor lesion, is now also being recognized as a common finding in GS, and 69% (16 of 23) of these benign soft tissue lesions were recently shown to occur in individuals who have a family history of APC [77]. Multiple pigmented ocular fundus lesions (termed congenital hypertrophy of the retinal pigment epithelium) are also characteristic of GS, found in about 90% of affected patients and bilaterally in nearly 80% [78]. Supernumerary teeth and other dental anomalies are also often appreciated [79].

Molecular genetics (APC gene on chromosome 5q21-q22)

Soon after karyotypic analysis of a suspected GS patient revealed deletion of chromosome 5q, Leppert and colleagues [15] refined the disease locus by demonstrating linkage to the 5q22 region. Mutations in the germline of families who have FAP were subsequently identified in a gene called adenomatous polyposis coli (APC) [80], and its role in the etiology of both FAP and GS has since been established. About 25% of APC mutations in FAP are thought to be de novo, and gene penetrance is nearly 100% [81]. Clinical genetic testing for APC-associated disorders is now broadly available, with disease-causing alterations identified in 85% to 90% of standard cases when both allele-specific expression analysis and protein truncation testing is used [82]. Because large deletions are not detected by some conventional methods, but may be responsible for 10% to 50% of apparently mutation negative families who have typical FAP, some argue that deletion screening (such as by multiplex ligation-dependent probe amplification) should be considered [83,84].

Efforts have been made to establish genotype-phenotype correlations, with work by Wallis and colleagues [85] suggesting that more distal APC mutations (codons 1395–1493) may predispose to the prominent extraintestinal findings of GS. Speake and colleagues [86] recently reported that 22 FAP patients who carried a specific FAP mutations (3' to codon 1399) had a 65% risk of postoperative mesenteric desmoids. Given that desmoid-related complications, including death, were numerous, the question of mutation-directed management strategies such as endoscopic management of polyps or delay of prophylactic colectomy was raised.

Tuberous sclerosis

Tuberous sclerosis (TS) (Bourneville disease, epiloia, tuberous sclerosis complex; OMIM 191,100-TSC1; 191,092-TSC2) is an AD disorder characterized by a constellation of chiefly benign tumors of the brain, skin, heart, kidneys, and lungs. Incidence can range from 1 in 5800 to 1 in 10,000 [87]. Most diagnoses are made during the first few years of life, but variable expressivity can make early detection difficult. In addition, a high percentage of cases (about 66%) are thought to be sporadic.

Cutaneous features

The cutaneous manifestations of TS compose 4 of the 11 major features of the clinical diagnostic criteria (Box 4) [88] and, cosmetic issues aside, do not pose a serious threat to one's health. These occur in almost all affected patients, though age of onset can vary by lesion [89,90]. Oval hypomelanotic macules, often called ash-leaf spots, are among the earliest skin findings in TS, detected in about 90% of affected children by 2 years of age [91]. Numerous tiny hypopigmented (confetti) macules can also be seen, especially in the pretibial region [91]. Shagreen patches are collagenomas that develop in about half of TS

Box 4. Diagnostic criteria: tuberous sclerosis

Major features
- Facial angiofibromas or forehead plaque
- Nontraumatic ungula or periungual fibroma
- Hypomelanotic macules ($\geq$3)
- Shagreen patch (connective tissue nevus)
- Multiple retinal nodular hamartomas
- Cortical tuber[a]
- Subependymal nodule
- Subependymal giant cell astrocytoma
- Cardiac rhabdomyoma, single or multiple
- Lymphangiomyomatosis[b]
- Renal angiomyolipoma[b]

Minor features
- Multiple randomly distributed pits in dental enamel
- Hamartomatous rectal polyps[c]
- Bone cysts[d]
- Cerebral white matter radial migration lines[a,d,e]
- Gingival fibromas
- Nonrenal hamartoma[c]
- Retinal achromic patch
- "Confetti" skin lesions
- Multiple renal cysts[c]

Definite TS complex
- Two major features, or
- One major feature with two minor features

Probable TS complex
- One major feature and one minor feature

Possible TS complex
- One major feature, or
- Two or more minor features

---

[a] When cerebral cortical dysplasia and cerebral white matter migration tracts occur together, they should be counted as one feature of TSC, not two.

[b] When both lymphangiomyomatosis and renal angiomyolipomas are present, other features of TS must be present before the diagnosis of TSC is made.

[c] Histologic confirmation is suggested.

[d] Radiographic confirmation is sufficient.

[e] Some feel $\geq$3 radial migration lines should constitute a major sign.

Data from Roach ES, Gomez MR, Northrup H. Tuberous sclerosis complex consensus conference: revised clinical diagnostic criteria. J Child Neurol 1998;13(12):624–8.

patients, usually presenting in early childhood as skin-colored to yellow plaques favoring the lumbosacral area [89,91]. In comparison, facial angiofibromas are most common in late childhood through adolescence, occurring in about 75% of patients. Previously referred to by the misnomer "adenoma sebaceum," these small, firm, skin-colored to red, dome-shaped papules favor the cheeks and perinasal regions, and although asymptomatic, can be fairly disfiguring. Up to 20% of TS patients will develop periungual fibromas, small firm papules arising from the nail folds or below the nail plate, and tan fibrous plaques of the face have also been described [89,91].

A recent review of 58 adults who had TS suggests that oral findings may be more common than previously thought, with multiple dental enamel pitting observed in nearly all patients (97%) [92]. Oral fibromas were identified in 69% of patients, most commonly on the gingiva, and several cases of gingival overgrowth were also documented.

Extracutaneous tumors and features

Although various types of CNS abnormalities can be seen in TS, including subependymal glial nodules and giant cell astrocytomas, it is the cortical and subcortical tubers (occurring in over 80% of patients) that are most correlated with the often debilitating cerebral dysfunction that affects patients [90]. Nearly 80% will experience seizures [93], often pharmacoresistant and requiring surgery [94]. Furthermore, some degree of learning or behavioral impairment is common, and it has been suggested that 25% to 50% have features of autism spectrum disorder [95]. Renal cysts and tumors are also estimated to affect 80% of patients by the end of childhood, of which the majority (75%) are benign angiomyolipomas [96]. Over time, these can be complicated by renal failure or life-threatening bleeding, making renal disease an important cause of death in TS, second to only central nervous system (CNS) pathology [97].

Cardiac rhabdomyomas occur in over 50% of newborns who have TS [98,99]. Although associated heart failure and arrhythmias have been reported, serious complications are relatively uncommon, and many lesions resolve spontaneously [99,100]. Lymphangiomyomatosis, an abnormal smooth-muscle proliferation in the lungs, disproportionately affects women who have TS, among which an estimated incidence of 26% to 39% has been reported [90].

Molecular genetics (TSC1 and TSC2 genes on chromosomes 9q34 and 16p13.3 respectively)

Evidence of TS linkage to chromosome 9q34 (TSC1) arose as early as 1987 [101], but it was not until 1994 that significant support for a second locus at 16p31 (TSC2) was reported [102]. Subsequent studies have shown that disease causing mutations are much more common in the TSC2 gene, accounting for 70% to 90% of TS kindreds [90]. Clinical genetic testing for deleterious mutations in both of these genes is now widely available, and a mutation detection rate of 85% has been reported among those who have a definite clinical diagnosis of TS [103]. Recent studies suggest that mutations in TSC2 predispose to a more severe phenotype than their TSC1 counterparts, and patients who have TSC2 mutations specifically of de novo origin may have an even more aggressive clinical course [103].

Neurofibromatosis type 1

Neurofibromatosis type 1 (NF1) (von Recklinghausen's disease, peripheral neurofibromatosis; OMIM 162,200) is an AD neurocutaneous disorder characterized by peripheral neurofibromas, café au lait spots (CALS) and visceral tumors. Prevalence is estimated at 1 in 3000 [104], making NF1 among the more common genodermatoses, and about 50% of these represent new mutations [105]. Although penetrance is nearly 100%, clinical expressivity is extremely variable, making it difficult to predict the ultimate phenotype.

Cutaneous features

CALS, presenting as well-circumscribed hyperpigmented macules, are usually the first manifestation of this disorder, occasionally present at birth, and are noted in over 99% of patients by 5 years of age [106]. Because about 2% of all newborns in the general population have CALS [107], as do 10% of adults [108], more than six (each ≥1.5 cm if postpubertal, ≥0.5 cm if prepubertal) are required to meet clinical diagnostic criteria (Box 5) [109]. Axillary or inguinal freckling (Crowe's sign) frequently develops in childhood, and affects nearly 90% of affected patients [110,111]. Multiple melanomas have also been reported in a few NF1 patients [112], though no clear association has yet been established.

Multiple cutaneous neurofibromas, dermal proliferations of neural tissue, are a hallmark of NF1. These tend to arise in later childhood as

Box 5. Diagnostic criteria: neurofibromatosis 1

- Six or more café au lait macules
  >1.5 cm in postpubertal individuals
  >0.5 cm in prepubertal individuals
- Two or more neurofibromas of any type, or one or more plexiform neurofibromas
- Freckling of axillae or inguinal area
- Optic glioma
- Two or more Lisch nodules
- A distinctive bony lesion
  Sphenoid bone dysplasia, or
  Thinning of the long bone cortex
    (with or without pseudoarthrosis)
- First-degree relative who has NF1 by these criteria

Diagnosis of NF1 requires: two or more of the above features
Data from Neurofibromatosis—conference statement. Arch Neurol 1988;45:575–8.

soft, skin-colored, dome-shaped or pedunculated papules or nodules, and affect nearly 60% of patients by 10 years of age [106]. Though benign, disfigurement from hundreds of lesions can be of real concern. Plexiform neurofibromas are less common, affecting about one quarter of patients [111], but represent an important source of morbidity because up to one half can be symptomatic. They often also increase in size, and may encroach on surrounding tissues, with a recent study reporting only a 33% rate of complete tumor resection in a pediatric population [106].

Extracutaneous tumors and features

Patients who have NF1 also have a greater than 2.5 fold risk for malignancy than the general population, with a cumulative risk of 20% by 50 years of age [113]. Malignant peripheral nerve sheath tumors (MPNST) are highly aggressive neoplasms that may occur in up to 8% to 13% of patients [114], capable of originating from malignant transformation of plexiform neurofibromas. Although some studies have described higher mortality rates in NF1-related tumors versus sporadic lesions (5-year survival of 21% versus 42%) [114], recent reports suggest that these may actually be equivalent [115]. CNS tumors are also common, and up to 15% of children who have NF1 develop optic pathway gliomas [106], and another 2.5% have astrocytomas [116]. Other studies suggest increased incidence of hematologic malignancies, especially juvenile myelomonocytic leukemia, in affected children (221 fold risk) [117], and a possible predisposition to breast cancer among females less than 50 years of age who have NF1 [113].

Asymptomatic pigmented hamartomas of the iris (Lisch nodules) are relatively specific for NF1, and thus can aid in diagnosis. These increase in frequency with age, noted in about one quarter of affected patients less than 6 years of age but in greater than 80% to 90% of those over age 10 [106,118], and are best detected by ophthalmologic slit lamp examination. Other endocrinologic (pheochromocytomas, carcinoids) musculoskeletal (pseudoarthrosis, scoliosis) cardiovascular (hypertension) and neurologic (learning disabilities, seizures) abnormalities may also occur more frequently than in the general population [111].

Molecular genetics (NF1 gene on chromosome 17q11.2)

Although linkage of NF1 families to chromosome 17 had been reported by 1987 [15], it was not until 3 years later that the disease-causing gene (designated *NF1*) was identified in the germline of affected patients [119,120]. This large gene encodes a type of GTPase-activating protein (designated neurofibromin), therefore accelerating the inactivation of the proto-oncogene p21 ras and regulating cellular proliferation [121]. Clinical genetic testing is available, and about 95% of causative mutations can be identified via a multistep protocol using a protein truncation test, followed by either pertinent sequencing analysis or one of several additional studies (eg, fluorescence in situ hybridization [FISH], Long-range RT-PCR, Southern blot analysis) [122]. Mattocks and colleagues [123] have suggested that automated comparative sequence analysis may be a preferable option, capable of identifying mutations in 89% of NF1 patients with a single method. Nevertheless, because the diagnosis is made based on clinical presentation, genetic testing is infrequently indicated.

Genotype-phenotype correlation in NF1 also continues to be an area of active investigation, and studies suggest that patients who have causative microdeletions may be prone to a more severe clinical presentation, with a greater burden of neurofibromas, worse cognitive deficits, and dysmorphic features [124]. More recently, 21 unrelated NF1 probands with a milder phenotype (few or no neurofibromas) were all found to harbor the same 3-bp deletion in exon 17 of *NF1* [125].

Neurofibromatosis type 2

Neurofibromatosis type 2 (NF2) (central neurofibromatosis, bilateral acoustic neurofibromatosis; OMIM 101,000) is an AD disorder characterized by bilateral vestibular schwannomas (VS) and some of the cutaneous features of NF1. With an incidence of 1 in 25,000 [126], it occurs about one tenth as often as NF1. Although NF2 is classically recognized as an adult disease (average age of onset of 21 years) [127,128], reports have suggested that symptoms can present much earlier (at 5.5 to 7 years of age) [129], and a recent series of 24 affected children showed a mean age at diagnosis of 8.8 years [129]. A more recently recognized disease entity (designated schwannomatosis) shares features with NF2, characterized by numerous schwannomas but lacking vestibular involvement [130].

Cutaneous features

Cutaneous tumors, primarily schwannomas but occasionally neurofibromas, are the initial presenting feature in 10% to 30% of cases, and can eventually be found in up to 70% of affected patients [127,131]. Clinical presentation can be variable and often subtle, ranging from skin-colored or pigmented subcutaneous nodules to well-circumscribed dermal plaques, and associated hair may be noted [128]. Multiple lesions have also been associated with a more severe phenotype, with earlier onset of disease and increased morbidity [129,131]. CALS are identified in nearly one half of patients, but rarely as six or more lesions [127,128,131].

Extracutaneous tumors and features

Bilateral VS (acoustic neuromas), benign tumors of the eighth cranial nerve, are a diagnostic criterion (Box 6) [132] and the hallmark feature of NF2. A rare occurrence in the general population, these neoplasms develop in nearly 100% of probands by the fourth decade of life [127] and slow, steady growth is often seen, estimated at just over 1 mm per year in one series [133]. Subsequent progressive hearing loss is common (the initial symptom in 60% of adults who have NF2), and tinnitus and loss of balance are also reported [127,128,131]. Malignant transformation is rare,

---

Box 6. Diagnostic criteria: neurofibromatosis 2

- Bilateral vestibular schwannomas, or
- A first-degree relative who has NF2 and any one of the following:
  Unilateral vestibular schwannoma
  Meningioma
  Neurofibroma
  Glioma
  Schwannoma
  Juvenile posterior subcapsular lens opacity

Data from National Institutes of Health Consensus Development Conference statement on acoustic neuroma, December 11–13, 1991. The Consensus Development Panel. Arch Neurol 1994;51:201–7.

---

but half of these reported cases have occurred in NF2 patients undergoing treatment with radiation therapy, even though more than 90% of irradiated VS do not occur in the setting of NF2 [134]. Thus, many still argue caution with use of this treatment modality.

In comparison, children are more likely to present with ocular complaints or neurologic deficits from other CNS tumors [129]. Seventy percent to 90% of all NF2 patients develop spinal tumors, predominantly schwannomas but also intramedullary astrocytomas and ependymomas [127,135,136]. About one half of patients develop meningiomas [127] and when this tumor is identified in any child, an underlying *NF2* mutation is usually involved [137]. Cataract, especially of the posterior subcapsular type, is noted in at least one third of pediatric patients [129], and these lens opacities occur in about 80% of all NF2 patients [138].

Molecular genetics (NF2 gene on chromosome 22q12.2)

Evidence of disease linkage to chromosome 22q12.2 surfaced in 1986 as a result of NF2 tumor analysis [139]. Rouleau and colleagues [140] substantiated these findings by mapping NF2 kindreds to this chromosomal region. The causative gene (designated *NF2*) was later identified after alterations in the germline of affected families and characteristic NF2 tumors were demonstrated

[141]. *NF2* encodes for a product designated "merlin" (moezin, ezrin, radixin-like protein), which some have proposed may direct growth-factor receptor signaling or cell adhesion, although the exact role of these mechanisms in its tumor suppressor function is not yet clear [142].

About 50% of all NF2 cases result from de novo mutations, and a very high rate of mosaicism has been identified in this group (about 25% of patients) [143]. As a result, recent genetic testing strategies that employ both mutation scanning and testing for deletions and duplications have resulted in detection rates around 90% among familial NF2, but only 60% to 70% for sporadic cases [144,145].

Birt-Hogg-Dube syndrome

Birt-Hogg-Dube syndrome (BHD) (OMIM 135,150) is a rare AD genodermatosis predisposing to a combination of benign cutaneous tumors, pulmonary cysts/spontaneous pneumothoraces, and renal neoplasia.

Cutaneous features

Patients who have BHD usually develop multiple firm, asymptomatic, skin-colored papules on the face, neck, or upper torso, often noted in the third or fourth decade [146]. These lesions represent a combination of fibrofolliculomas, a hamartoma of the hair follicle that is among the most specific findings in this syndrome, as well as trichodiscomas and acrochordons [146].

Extracutaneous tumors and features

Nearly 90% of BHD patients have numerous, bilateral lung cysts on chest CT, and about one quarter have a history of spontaneous pneumothorax, occurring at a median age of 38 years [147]. Studies also show a sevenfold increased risk for benign or malignant renal tumors in BHD [148], occurring in about 25% of affected patients at a median age of 48 years at diagnosis [149,150]. The predominant histologic tumor type is the oncocytic hybrid (combination of oncocytes and chromophobe cells) [149]. Bilateral and multifocal tumors are common, and death from metastatic disease has been reported [149]. Multiple other findings have been reported in the setting of BHD (colonic polyps/carcinoma, parotid oncocytomas, parathyroid adenomas, as well as lipomas and angiolipomas) [150], although it is not clear that affected patients are actually predisposed to developing these lesions.

Molecular genetics (BHD on chromosome 17p11.2)

Genetic linkage analysis studies in 2001 allowed the BHD locus to be mapped to chromosome 17p11.2 [151,152], and germline mutations were subsequently detected in a gene *BHD* (also called *FLCN*) in affected kindreds [153]. It is estimated that *BHD* mutations are identified in about 85% of affected families by direct sequencing analysis [147,150].

Hereditary leiomyomatosis and renal cell cancer

Hereditary leiomyomatosis and renal cell cancer (HLRCC) (multiple cutaneous and uterine leiomyomatosis, Reed's syndrome, multiple leiomyomatosis, familial leiomyomatosis cutis et uteri; OMIM 150,800) is an AD disorder characterized by cutaneous and uterine leiomyomata and renal cancer.

Cutaneous features

Cutaneous leiomyomas, benign smooth muscle tumors of the skin, occur in about three quarters of affected patients [154], developing at a mean age of 24 years [155]. These present as smooth, firm, skin-colored to red-tan papules or nodules, in most cases on the torso or extremities [154], and up to 90% of patients may report some degree of sensitivity or pain with trauma or extremes in temperature [155].

Extracutaneous tumors and features

Nearly all women who have HLRCC (75%–100%) develop uterine leiomyomas, commonly known as fibroids [156]. Lesions tend to be of greater size and number than usual, and also develop earlier (mean age of 31 years) than in the general population, although patients often struggle with menorrhagia, pain, or difficulty conceiving for years before diagnosis [155]. Patients are also predisposed to renal cancers, and these have been identified in 18 of the 56 HLRCC families (32%) followed by Wei and colleagues [154], with a median age of 39 years at diagnosis [156]. Tumors are usually solitary, but behave aggressively, and nearly 50% may have metastatic disease on initial presentation [156].

Molecular genetics (FH gene at chromosome 1q42.3-43)

Shortly after genome-wide linkage analysis mapped the HLRCC disease locus to chromosome 1q42.3 [157], Tomlinson and colleagues [158] established that germline mutations in the fumarate hydrates gene (*FH*) predisposed to this disorder. Clinical genetic testing is available at a few laboratories, and recent reports suggest that direct sequencing analysis may be able to detect disease causing mutations in over 90% of HLRCC families [154]. When *FH* mutations cannot be identified despite high clinical suspicion, FH enzyme activity testing may help confirm a diagnosis [159].

Summary

Progress in molecular biology continues to shed light on the genetic mutations at play in these and other genodermatoses. Furthermore, these technologies have also contributed to the advent of genetic tests capable of identifying not only deleterious mutations at rates higher than even just a few years back, but also many of the common polymorphisms that may someday have a far-reaching impact on the health of the general population as well. Despite these advances, a keen appreciation for the dermatologic features in these disorders remains crucial to facilitate early diagnosis and minimize the significant morbidity that can result from their susceptibility to the various cutaneous and internal malignancies described above.

References

[1] Tsai KY, Tsao H. Primer on the human genome. J Am Acad Dermatol 2007;56(5):719–35.

[2] Somoano B, Niendorf KB, Tsao H. Hereditary cancer syndromes of the skin. Clin Dermatol 2005;23(1):85–106.

[3] Evans DG, Ladusans EJ, Rimmer S, et al. Complications of the naevoid basal cell carcinoma syndrome: results of a population based study. J Med Genet 1993;30(6):460–4.

[4] Shanley S, Ratcliffe J, Hockey A, et al. Nevoid basal cell carcinoma syndrome: review of 118 affected individuals. Am J Hum Genet 1994;50: 282–90.

[5] Chiritescu E, Maloney ME. Acrochordons as a presenting sign of nevoid basal cell carcinoma syndrome. J Am Acad Dermatol 2001;44(5):789–94.

[6] van Ruth S, Jansman FG, Sanders CJ. Total body topical 5-fluorouracil for extensive non-melanoma skin cancer. Pharm World Sci 2006;28(3):159–62.

[7] Chapas AM, Gilchrest BA. Broad area photodynamic therapy for treatment of multiple basal cell carcinomas in a patient with nevoid basal cell carcinoma syndrome. J Drugs Dermatol 2006; 5(2 Suppl):3–5.

[8] Vogt A, Chuang PT, Hebert J, et al. Immunoprevention of basal cell carcinomas with recombinant

hedgehog-interacting protein. J Exp Med 2004; 199(6):753–61.

[9] Kolm I, Puig S, Iranzo P, et al. Dermoscopy in Gorlin-Goltz syndrome. Dermatol Surg 2006; 32(6):847–51.

[10] Gorlin RJ. Nevoid basal cell carcinoma syndrome. Medicine 1987;66:98–110.

[11] Wilson LC, Ajayi-Obe E, Bernhard B, et al. Patched mutations and hairy skin patches: a new sign in Gorlin syndrome. Am J Med Genet A 2006;140(23):2625–30.

[12] Kimonis VE, Goldstein AM, Pastakia B, et al. Clinical manifestations in 105 persons with nevoid basal cell carcinoma syndrome. Am J Hum Genet 1997;69:299–308.

[13] Evans DG, Farndon PA, Burnell LD, et al. The incidence of Gorlin syndrome in 173 consecutive cases of medulloblastoma. Br J Cancer 1991;64: 959–61.

[14] Thrum K, Gajda M, Settmacher U. Large mediastinal sarcoma in a patient with Gorlin-Goltz syndrome. Thorac Cardiovasc Surg 2006;54(6): 437–9.

[15] Tsao H. Update on familial cancer syndromes and the skin. J Am Acad Dermatol 2000;42(6):939–69 [quiz 970–932].

[16] Klein RD, Dykas DJ, Bale AE. Clinical testing for the nevoid basal cell carcinoma syndrome in a DNA diagnostic laboratory. Genet Med 2005; 7(9):611–9.

[17] Rivers JK. Melanoma. Lancet 1996;347(9004): 803–6.

[18] Puig S, Malvehy J, Badenas C, et al. Role of the CDKN2A locus in patients with multiple primary melanomas. J Clin Oncol 2005;23(13):3043–51.

[19] Goldstein AM, Fraser MC, Struewing JP, et al. Increased risk of pancreatic cancer in melanomaprone kindreds with p16INK4 mutations. N Engl J Med 1995;333:970–4.

[20] Hille ETM, van Duijn E, Gruis NA, et al. Excess cancer mortality in six Dutch pedigrees with the familial atypical multiple mole-melanoma syndrome from 1830 to 1994. J Invest Dermatol 1998;110: 788–92.

[21] Debniak T, Gorski B, Huzarski T, et al. A common variant of CDKN2A (p16) predisposes to breast cancer. J Med Genet 2005;42(10):763–5.

[22] Debniak T, Scott RJ, Huzarski T, et al. CDKN2A common variant and multi-organ cancer risk— a population-based study. Int J Cancer 2006; 118(12):3180–2.

[23] Orlow I, Begg CB, Cotignola J, et al. CDKN2A germline mutations in individuals with cutaneous malignant melanoma. J Invest Dermatol 2007; 127(5):1234–43.

[24] Cannon-Albright LA, Goldgar DE, Meyer LJ, et al. Assignment of a locus for familial melanoma, MLM, to chromosome 9p13-p22. Science 1992; 258:1148–52.

[25] Kamb A. A cell cycle regulator potentially involved in genesis of many tumor types. Science 1994;264: 436–9.

[26] Nobori T, Miura K, Wu DJ, et al. Deletions of the cyclin-dependent kinase-4 inhibitor gene in multiple human cancers. Nature 1994;368:753–6.

[27] Hussussian CJ, Struewing JP, Goldstein AM, et al. Germline p16 mutations in familial melanoma. Nat Genet 1994;8:15–21.

[28] Miller AJ, Mihm MC Jr. Melanoma. N Engl J Med 2006;355(1):51–65.

[29] Pjanova D, Engele L, Randerson-Moor JA, et al. CDKN2A and CDK4 variants in Latvian melanoma patients: analysis of a clinic-based population. Melanoma Res 2007;17(3):185–91.

[30] Gillanders E, Hank Juo SH, Holland EA, et al. Localization of a novel melanoma susceptibility locus to 1p22. Am J Hum Genet 2003;73(2):301–13.

[31] Bishop DT, Demenais F, Goldstein AM, et al. Geographical variation in the penetrance of CDKN2A mutations for melanoma. J Natl Cancer Inst 2002; 94(12):894–903.

[32] Begg CB, Orlow I, Hummer AJ, et al. Lifetime risk of melanoma in CDKN2A mutation carriers in a population-based sample. J Natl Cancer Inst 2005;97(20):1507–15.

[33] Chaudru V, Chompret A, Bressac-de Paillerets B, et al. Influence of genes, nevi, and sun sensitivity on melanoma risk in a family sample unselected by family history and in melanoma-prone families. J Natl Cancer Inst 2004;96(10):785–95.

[34] Box NF, Duffy DL, Chen W, et al. MC1R genotype modifies risk of melanoma in families segregating cdkn2a mutations. Am J Hum Genet 2001;69(4). 765–73.

[35] Kefford RF, Newton Bishop JA, Bergman W, et al. Counseling and DNA testing for individuals perceived to be genetically predisposed to melanoma: a consensus statement of the Melanoma Genetics Consortium. J Clin Oncol 1999;17(10):3245–51.

[36] Goldstein AM, Struewing JP, Chidambaram A, et al. Genotype-phenotype relationships in U.S. melanoma-prone families with CDKN2A and CDK4 mutations. J Natl Cancer Inst 2000;92(12): 1006–10.

[37] Goldstein AM, Tucker MA. Screening for CDKN2A mutations in hereditary melanoma. J Natl Cancer Inst 1997;89:676–7.

[38] Cleaver JE, Kraemer KH. Xeroderma pigmentosum and cockayne syndrome. In: Scriver CR, Beaudet AL, Sly WS, et al, editors. The metabolic and molecular bases of inherited disease. vol. 3. New York: McGraw-Hill; 1995. p. 4393–419.

[39] Kraemer KH, Lee MM, Scotto J. Xeroderma pigmentosum. Cutaneous, ocular, and neurologic abnormalities in 830 published cases. Arch Dermatol 1987;123(2):241–50.

[40] Kraemer KH, Lee MM, Andrews AD, et al. The role of sunlight and DNA repair in melanoma and nonmelanoma skin cancer. The xeroderma pigmentosum paradigm. Arch Dermatol 1994;130(8): 1018–21.

[41] Bootsma D, Kraemer KH, Cleaver JE, et al. Nucleotide excision repair syndromes: xeroderma pigmentosum, Cockayne syndrome, and trichothiodystrophy. In: Vogelstein BV, Kinzler K, editors. The genetic basis of human cancer. New York: McGraw Hill; 1998. p. 245–74.

[42] Shao L, Newell B, Quintanilla N. Atypical fibroxanthoma and squamous cell carcinoma of the conjunctiva in xeroderma pigmentosum. Pediatr Dev Pathol 2007;10(2):149–52.

[43] Kraemer KH, Patronas NJ, Schiffmann R, et al. Xeroderma pigmentosum, trichothiodystrophy and Cockayne syndrome: a complex genotype-phenotype relationship. Neuroscience 2007;145(4): 1388–96.

[44] Ohto T, Iwasaki N, Okubo H, et al. Life-threatening vocal cord paralysis in a patient with group A xeroderma pigmentosum. Pediatr Neurol 2004; 30(3):222–4.

[45] Kraemer KH, Lee MM, Scotto J. DNA repair protects against cutaneous and internal neoplasia: evidence from xeroderma pigmentosum. Carcinogenesis 1984;5(4):511–4.

[46] Kiyohara C, Yoshimasu K. Genetic polymorphisms in the nucleotide excision repair pathway and lung cancer risk: a meta-analysis. Int J Med Sci 2007;4(2):59–71.

[47] Yang G, Curley D, Bosenberg MW, et al. Loss of xeroderma pigmentosum C (Xpc) enhances melanoma photocarcinogenesis in ink4a-arf-deficient mice. Cancer Res 2007;67(12):5649–57.

[48] Nelen MR, Kremer H, Konings IB, et al. Novel PTEN mutations in patients with Cowden disease: absence of clear genotype-phenotype correlations. Eur J Hum Genet 1999;7(3):267–73.

[49] Schrager CA, Schneider D, Gruener AC, et al. Clinical and pathological features of breast disease in Cowden's syndrome: an underrecognized syndrome with an increased risk of breast cancer. Hum Pathol 1998;29(1):47–53.

[50] Starink TM, van der Veen JP, Arwert F, et al. The Cowden syndrome: a clinical and genetic study in 21 patients. Clin Genet 1986;29:222–33.

[51] Brownstein MH, Wolf M, Bikowski JB. Cowden's disease: a cutaneous marker of breast cancer. Cancer 1978;41(6):2393–8.

[52] Eng C, Parsons R. Cowden syndrome. In: Vogelstein B, Kinzler KW, editors. The genetic basis of human cancer. New York: McGraw Hill; 1998. p. 519–25.

[53] Pilarski R, Eng C. Will the real Cowden syndrome please stand up (again)? Expanding mutational and clinical spectra of the PTEN hamartoma tumour syndrome. J Med Genet 2004;41(5):323–6.

[54] Bosserhoff AK, Grussendorf-Conen EI, Rubben A, et al. Multiple colon carcinomas in a patient with

Cowden syndrome. Int J Mol Med 2006;18(4): 643–7.

[55] Robinson S, Cohen AR. Cowden disease and Lhermitte-Duclos disease: an update. Case report and review of the literature. Neurosurg Focus 2006; 20(1):E6.

[56] Nelen MR, Padberg GW, Peeters EA, et al. Localization of the gene for Cowden disease to chromosome 10q22-23. Nat Genet 1996;13:114–6.

[57] Li J, Yen C, Liaw D, et al. PTEN, a putative tyrosine phosphatase gene mutated in human brain, breast and prostate cancer. Science 1997;275: 1943–7.

[58] Steck PA, Pershouse MA, Jasser SA, et al. Identification of a candidate tumour suppressor gene, MMAC1, at chromosome 10q23.3 that is mutated in multiple advanced cancers. Nat Genet 1997;15: 356–62.

[59] Liaw D, Marsh DJ, Li J, et al. Germline mutations of the PTEN gene in Cowden disease, an inherited breast and thyroid cancer syndrome. Nat Genet 1997;16:64–7.

[60] Zhou XP, Waite KA, Pilarski R, et al. Germline PTEN promoter mutations and deletions in Cowden/Bannayan-Riley-Ruvalcaba syndrome result in aberrant PTEN protein and dysregulation of the phosphoinositol-3-kinase/Akt pathway. Am J Hum Genet 2003;73(2):404–11.

[61] Sarquis MS, Agrawal S, Shen L, et al. Distinct expression profiles for PTEN transcript and its splice variants in Cowden syndrome and Bannayan-Riley-Ruvalcaba syndrome. Am J Hum Genet 2006;79(1):23–30.

[62] Ponti G, Losi L, Pedroni M, et al. Value of MLH1 and MSH2 mutations in the appearance of Muir-Torre syndrome phenotype in HNPCC patients presenting sebaceous gland tumors or keratoacanthomas. J Invest Dermatol 2006; 126(10):2302–7.

[63] Lynch HT, Fusaro RM, Lynch PM. Sebaceous skin lesions as clues to hereditary non-polyposis colorectal cancer. J Invest Dermatol 2006;126(10): 2158–9.

[64] Cohen PR, Kohn SR, Kurzrock R. Association of sebaceous gland tumors and internal malignancy: the Muir-Torre syndrome. Am J Med 1991;90: 606–13.

[65] Akhtar S, Oza KK, Khan SA, et al. Muir-Torre syndrome: case report of a patient with concurrent jejunal and ureteral cancer and a review of the literature. J Am Acad Dermatol 1999; 41(5 Pt 1):681–6.

[66] Hall NR, Murday VA, Chapman P, et al. Genetic linkage in Muir-Torre syndrome to the same chromosomal region as cancer family syndrome. Eur J Cancer 1994;30A:180–2.

[67] Kruse R, Rutten A, Lamberti C, et al. Muir-Torre phenotype has a frequency of DNA mismatch-repair-gene mutations similar to that in hereditary nonpolyposis colorectal cancer families defined by the Amsterdam criteria [published erratum appears in Am J Hum Genet 1998 Oct;63(4):1252]. Am J Hum Genet 1998;63(1):63–70.

[68] Umar A, Boland CR, Terdiman JP, et al. Revised Bethesda Guidelines for hereditary nonpolyposis colorectal cancer (Lynch syndrome) and microsatellite instability. J Natl Cancer Inst 2004;96(4): 261–8.

[69] Ponti G, Losi L, Di Gregorio C, et al. Identification of Muir-Torre syndrome among patients with sebaceous tumors and keratoacanthomas: role of clinical features, microsatellite instability, and immunohistochemistry. Cancer 2005;103(5): 1018–25.

[70] Mangold E, Pagenstecher C, Leister M, et al. A genotype-phenotype correlation in HNPCC: strong predominance of MSH2 mutations in 41 patients with Muir-Torre syndrome. J Med Genet 2004; 41(7):567–72.

[71] Leppard B, Bussey HJ. Epidermoid cysts, polyposis coli and Gardner's syndrome. Br J Surg 1975;62: 387–93.

[72] Bilkay U, Erdem O, Ozek C, et al. Benign osteoma with Gardner syndrome: review of the literature and report of a case. J Craniofac Surg 2004;15(3): 506–9.

[73] Burt RW. Colon cancer screening. Gastroenterology 2000;119(3):837–53.

[74] Bell B, Mazzaferri EL. Familial adenomatous polyposis (Gardner's syndrome) and thyroid carcinoma. A case report and review of the literature. Dig Dis Sci 1993;38(1):185–90.

[75] Herve R, Farret O, Mayaudon H, et al. [Association of Gardner syndrome and thyroid carcinoma]. Presse Med 1995;24(8):415 [in French].

[76] Lynch HT, Fitzgibbons R Jr. Surgery, desmoid tumors, and familial adenomatous polyposis: case report and literature review. Am J Gastroenterol 1996;91(12):2598–601.

[77] Coffin CM, Hornick JL, Zhou H, et al. Gardner fibroma: a clinicopathologic and immunohistochemical analysis of 45 patients with 57 fibromas. Am J Surg Pathol 2007;31(3):410–6.

[78] Traboulsi EI, Krush AJ, Gardner EJ, et al. Prevalence and importance of pigmented ocular fundus lesions in Gardner's syndrome. N Engl J Med 1987;316:661–7.

[79] Carl W, Herrera L. Dental and bone abnormalities in patients with familial polyposis coli. Semin Surg Oncol 1987;3(2):77–83.

[80] Groden J, Thliveris A, Samowitz W, et al. Identification and characterization of the familial adenomatous polyposis coli gene. Cell 1991;66: 589–600.

[81] Bisgaard ML, Fenger K, Bulow S, et al. Familial adenomatous polyposis (FAP): frequency, penetrance, and mutation rate. Hum Mutat 1994;3(2): 121–5.

[82] Powell SM, Petersen GM, Krush AJ, et al. Molecular diagnosis of familial adenomatous polyposis. N Engl J Med 1993;329(27):1982–7.

[83] Michils G, Tejpar S, Thoelen R, et al. Large deletions of the APC gene in 15% of mutation-negative patients with classical polyposis (FAP): a Belgian study. Hum Mutat 2005;25(2):125–34.

[84] Aretz S, Stienen D, Uhlhaas S, et al. Large submicroscopic genomic APC deletions are a common cause of typical familial adenomatous polyposis. J Med Genet 2005;42(2):185–92.

[85] Wallis YL, Morton DG, McKeown CM, et al. Molecular analysis of the APC gene in 205 families: extended genotype-phenotype correlations in FAP and evidence for the role of APC amino acid changes in colorectal cancer predisposition. J Med Genet 1999;36(1):14–20.

[86] Speake D, Evans DG, Lalloo F, et al. Desmoid tumours in patients with familial adenomatous polyposis and desmoid region adenomatous polyposis coli mutations. Br J Surg 2007; [epub ahead of print].

[87] Osborne JP, Fryer A, Webb D. Epidemiology of tuberous sclerosis. Ann N Y Acad Sci 1991;615:125–7.

[88] Roach ES, Gomez MR, Northrup H. Tuberous Sclerosis Complex Consensus Conference: revised clinical diagnostic criteria. J Child Neurol 1998;13(12):624–8.

[89] Webb DW, Clarke A, Fryer A, et al. The cutaneous features of tuberous sclerosis: a population study. Br J Dermatol 1996;135(1):1–5.

[90] Crino PB, Nathanson KL, Henske EP. The tuberous sclerosis complex. N Engl J Med 2006;355(13):1345–56.

[91] Jozwiak S, Schwartz RA, Janniger CK, et al. Skin lesions in children with tuberous sclerosis complex: their prevalence, natural course, and diagnostic significance. Int J Dermatol 1998;37(12):911–7.

[92] Sparling JD, Hong CH, Brahim JS, et al. Oral findings in 58 adults with tuberous sclerosis complex. J Am Acad Dermatol 2007;56(5):786–90.

[93] Webb DW, Fryer AE, Osborne JP. Morbidity associated with tuberous sclerosis: a population study. Dev Med Child Neurol 1996;38(2):146–55.

[94] Thiele EA. Managing epilepsy in tuberous sclerosis complex. J Child Neurol 2004;19(9):680–6.

[95] Wiznitzer M. Autism and tuberous sclerosis. J Child Neurol 2004;19(9):675–9.

[96] Ewalt DH, Sheffield E, Sparagana SP, et al. Renal lesion growth in children with tuberous sclerosis complex. J Urol 1998;160(1):141–5.

[97] Shepherd CW, Gomez MR, Lie JT, et al. Causes of death in patients with tuberous sclerosis. Mayo Clin Proc 1991;66(8):792–6.

[98] Gibbs JL. The heart and tuberous sclerosis. An echocardiographic and electrocardiographic study. Br Heart J 1985;54(6):596–9.

[99] Smith HC, Watson GH, Patel RG, et al. Cardiac rhabdomyomata in tuberous sclerosis: their course and diagnostic value. Arch Dis Child 1989;64(2):196–200.

[100] Jozwiak S, Kawalec W, Dluzewska J, et al. Cardiac tumours in tuberous sclerosis: their incidence and course. Eur J Pediatr 1994;153(3):155–7.

[101] Fryer AE, Chalmers A, Connor JM, et al. Evidence that the gene for tuberous sclerosis is on chromosome 9. Lancet 1987;1:659–61.

[102] Povey S, Burley MW, Attwood J, et al. Two loci for tuberous sclerosis: one on 9q34 and one on 16p13. Ann Hum Genet 1994;58(Pt 2):107–27.

[103] Sancak O, Nellist M, Goedbloed M, et al. Mutational analysis of the TSC1 and TSC2 genes in a diagnostic setting: genotype—phenotype correlations and comparison of diagnostic DNA techniques in tuberous sclerosis complex. Eur J Hum Genet 2005;13(6):731–41.

[104] Lammert M, Friedman JM, Kluwe L, et al. Prevalence of neurofibromatosis 1 in German children at elementary school enrollment. Arch Dermatol 2005;141(1):71–4.

[105] Gutmann DH, Aylsworth A, Carey JC, et al. The diagnostic evaluation and multidisciplinary management of neurofibromatosis 1 and neurofibromatosis 2. JAMA 1997;278(1):51–7.

[106] Boulanger JM, Larbrisseau A. Neurofibromatosis type 1 in a pediatric population: Ste-Justine's experience. Can J Neurol Sci 2005;32(2):225–31.

[107] Alper JC, Holmes LB. The incidence and significance of birthmarks in a cohort of 4641 newborns. Pediatr Dermatol 1983;1(1):58–68.

[108] Kopf AW, Levine LJ, Rigel DS, et al. Congenital-nevus-like nevi, nevi spili, and cafe-au-lait spots in patients with malignant melanoma. J Dermatol Surg Oncol 1985;11(3):275–80.

[109] Neurofibromatosis—conference statement. Arch Neurol 1988;45:575–8.

[110] Huson SM, Harper PS, Compston DA. Von Recklinghausen neurofibromatosis. A clinical and population study in south-east Wales. Brain 1988;111(Pt 6):1355–81.

[111] Friedman JM, Birch PH. Type 1 neurofibromatosis: a descriptive analysis of the disorder in 1728 patients. Am J Med Genet 1997;70(2):138–43.

[112] Barringer CB, Gorse SJ, Rigby HS, et al. Multiple malignant melanomas in association with neurofibromatosis type 1. J Plast Reconstr Aesthet Surg 2006;59(12):1359–62.

[113] Walker L, Thompson D, Easton D, et al. A prospective study of neurofibromatosis type 1 cancer incidence in the UK. Br J Cancer 2006;95(2):233–8.

[114] Evans DG, Baser ME, McGaughran J, et al. Malignant peripheral nerve sheath tumours in neurofibromatosis 1. J Med Genet 2002;39(5):311–4.

[115] Anghileri M, Miceli R, Fiore M, et al. Malignant peripheral nerve sheath tumors: prognostic factors and survival in a series of patients

treated at a single institution. Cancer 2006; 107(5):1065–74.

[116] Blatt J, Jaffe R, Deutsch M, et al. Neurofibromatosis and childhood tumors. Cancer 1986;57(6):1225–9.

[117] Stiller CA, Chessells JM, Fitchett M. Neurofibromatosis and childhood leukaemia/lymphoma: a population-based UKCCSG study. Br J Cancer 1994;70:969–72.

[118] Lewis RA, Riccardi VM. Von Recklinghausen neurofibromatosis. Incidence of iris hamartomata. Ophthalmology 1981;88(4):348–54.

[119] Wallace MR, Marchuk DA, Anderson LB, et al. Type 1 neurofibromatosis gene: identification of a large transcript disrupted in three NF 1 patients. Science 1990;249:181–6.

[120] Cawthon RM, Weiss R, Xu G, et al. A major segment of the neurofibromatosis type 1 gene: cDNA sequence, genomic structure, and point mutations. Cell 1990;62:193–201.

[121] Lee MJ, Stephenson DA. Recent developments in neurofibromatosis type 1. Curr Opin Neurol 2007;20(2):135–41.

[122] Messiaen LM, Callens T, Mortier G, et al. Exhaustive mutation analysis of the NF1 gene allows identification of 95% of mutations and reveals a high frequency of unusual splicing defects. Hum Mutat 2000;15(6):541–55.

[123] Mattocks C, Baralle D, Tarpey P, et al. Automated comparative sequence analysis identifies mutations in 89% of NF1 patients and confirms a mutation cluster in exons 11-17 distinct from the GAP related domain. J Med Genet 2004; 41(4):E48.

[124] Mensink KA, Ketterling RP, Flynn HC, et al. Connective tissue dysplasia in five new patients with NF1 microdeletions: further expansion of phenotype and review of the literature. J Med Genet 2006;43(2):E8.

[125] Upadhyaya M, Huson SM, Davies M, et al. An absence of cutaneous neurofibromas associated with a 3-bp inframe deletion in exon 17 of the NF1 gene (c.2970-2972 delAAT): evidence of a clinically significant NF1 genotype-phenotype correlation. Am J Hum Genet 2007;80(1):140–51.

[126] Evans DG, Moran A, King A, et al. Incidence of vestibular schwannoma and neurofibromatosis 2 in the North West of England over a 10-year period: higher incidence than previously thought. Otol Neurotol 2005;26(1):93–7.

[127] Parry DM, Eldridge R, Kaiser-Kupfer MI, et al. Neurofibromatosis 2 (NF2): clinical characteristics of 63 affected individuals and clinical evidence for heterogeneity. Am J Med Genet 1994;52:450–61.

[128] Evans DG, Huson SM, Donnai D, et al. A genetic study of type 2 neurofibromatosis in the United Kingdom. II. Guidelines for genetic counselling. J Med Genet 1992;29(12):847–52.

[129] Ruggieri M, Iannetti P, Polizzi A, et al. Earliest clinical manifestations and natural history of neurofibromatosis type 2 (NF2) in childhood: a study of 24 patients. Neuropediatrics 2005;36(1):21–34.

[130] MacCollin M, Chiocca EA, Evans DG, et al. Diagnostic criteria for schwannomatosis. Neurology 2005;64(11):1838–45.

[131] Mautner VF, Lindenau M, Baser ME, et al. Skin abnormalities in neurofibromatosis 2. Arch Dermatol 1997;133(12):1539–43.

[132] National Institutes of Health Consensus Development Conference statement on acoustic neuroma, December 11–13, 1991. The Consensus Development Panel. Arch Neurol 1994;51:201–7.

[133] Slattery WH 3rd, Fisher LM, Iqbal Z, et al. Vestibular schwannoma growth rates in neurofibromatosis type 2 natural history consortium subjects. Otol Neurotol 2004;25(5):811–7.

[134] Evans DG, Birch JM, Ramsden RT, et al. Malignant transformation and new primary tumours after therapeutic radiation for benign disease: substantial risks in certain tumour prone syndromes. J Med Genet 2006;43(4):289–94.

[135] Mautner VF, Tatagiba M, Lindenau M, et al. Spinal tumors in patients with neurofibromatosis type 2: MR imaging study of frequency, multiplicity, and variety. AJR Am J Roentgenol 1995;165:951–5.

[136] Evans DG, Huson SM, Donnai D, et al. A clinical study of type 2 neurofibromatosis. Q J Med 1992; 84:603–18.

[137] Evans DG, Watson C, King A, et al. Multiple meningiomas: differential involvement of the NF2 gene in children and adults. J Med Genet 2005; 42(1):45–8.

[138] Bouzas EA, Freidlin V, Parry DM, et al. Lens opacities in neurofibromatosis 2: further significant correlations. Br J Ophthalmol 1993;77:354–7.

[139] Seizinger BR, Martuza RL, Gusella JF. Loss of genes on chromosome 22 in tumorigenesis of human acoustic neuroma. Nature 1986;322:644–7.

[140] Rouleau GA, Wertelecki W, Haines JL, et al. Genetic linkage of bilateral acoustic neurofibromatosis to a DNA marker on chromosome 22. Nature 1987;329:246–8.

[141] Rouleau GA, Mere P, Lutchman M, et al. Alteration in a new gene encoding a putative membrane-organizing protein causes neuro-fibromatosis type 2. Nature 1993;363:515–21.

[142] McClatchey AI, Giovannini M. Membrane organization and tumorigenesis—the NF2 tumor suppressor, merlin. Genes Dev 2005;19(19):2265–77.

[143] Kluwe L, Mautner V, Heinrich B, et al. Molecular study of frequency of mosaicism in neurofibromatosis 2 patients with bilateral vestibular schwannomas. J Med Genet 2003;40(2):109–14.

[144] Wallace AJ, Watson CJ, Oward E, et al. Mutation scanning of the NF2 gene: an improved service based on meta-PCR/sequencing, dosage analysis,

and loss of heterozygosity analysis. Genet Test 2004;8(4):368–80.

[145] Kluwe L, Nygren AO, Errami A, et al. Screening for large mutations of the NF2 gene. Genes Chromosomes Cancer 2005;42(4):384–91.

[146] Birt AR, Hogg GR, Dube WJ. Hereditary multiple fibrofolliculomas with trichodiscomas and acrochordons. Arch Dermatol 1977;113(12):1674–7.

[147] Toro JR, Pautler SE, Stewart L, et al. Lung cysts, spontaneous pneumothorax, and genetic associations in 89 families with Birt-Hogg-Dube syndrome. Am J Respir Crit Care Med 2007;175(10):1044–53.

[148] Zbar B, Alvord WG, Glenn G, et al. Risk of renal and colonic neoplasms and spontaneous pneumothorax in the Birt-Hogg-Dube syndrome. Cancer Epidemiol Biomarkers Prev 2002;11(4):393–400.

[149] Pavlovich CP, Grubb RL 3rd, Hurley K, et al. Evaluation and management of renal tumors in the Birt-Hogg-Dube syndrome. J Urol 2005; 173(5):1482–6.

[150] Schmidt LS, Nickerson ML, Warren MB, et al. Germline BHD-mutation spectrum and phenotype analysis of a large cohort of families with Birt-Hogg-Dube syndrome. Am J Hum Genet 2005; 76(6):1023–33.

[151] Schmidt LS, Warren MB, Nickerson ML, et al. Birt-Hogg-Dube syndrome, a genodermatosis associated with spontaneous pneumothorax and kidney neoplasia, maps to chromosome 17p11.2. Am J Hum Genet 2001;69(4):876–82.

[152] Khoo SK, Bradley M, Wong FK, et al. Birt-Hogg-Dube syndrome: mapping of a novel hereditary neoplasia gene to chromosome 17p12-q11.2. Oncogene 2001;20(37):5239–42.

[153] Nickerson ML, Warren MB, Toro JR, et al. Mutations in a novel gene lead to kidney tumors, lung wall defects, and benign tumors of the hair follicle in patients with the Birt-Hogg-Dube syndrome. Cancer Cell 2002;2(2):157–64.

[154] Wei MH, Toure O, Glenn GM, et al. Novel mutations in FH and expansion of the spectrum of phenotypes expressed in families with hereditary leiomyomatosis and renal cell cancer. J Med Genet 2006;43(1):18–27.

[155] Alam NA, Barclay E, Rowan AJ, et al. Clinical features of multiple cutaneous and uterine leiomyomatosis: an underdiagnosed tumor syndrome. Arch Dermatol 2005;141(2):199–206.

[156] Grubb RL 3rd, Franks ME, Toro J, et al. Hereditary leiomyomatosis and renal cell cancer: a syndrome associated with an aggressive form of inherited renal cancer. J Urol 2007;177(6):2074–9 [discussion 2079–80].

[157] Launonen V, Vierimaa O, Kiuru M, et al. Inherited susceptibility to uterine leiomyomas and renal cell cancer. Proc Natl Acad Sci U S A 2001;98(6): 3387–92.

[158] Tomlinson IP, Alam NA, Rowan AJ, et al. Germline mutations in FH predispose to dominantly inherited uterine fibroids, skin leiomyomata and papillary renal cell cancer. Nat Genet 2002;30(4): 406–10.

[159] Pithukpakorn M, Wei MH, Toure O, et al. Fumarate hydratase enzyme activity in lymphoblastoid cells and fibroblasts of individuals in families with hereditary leiomyomatosis and renal cell cancer. J Med Genet 2006;43(9): 755–62.

ELSEVIER
SAUNDERS

Dermatol Clin 26 (2008) 89–102

DERMATOLOGIC
CLINICS

Tumor Invasion of the Skin

Gabriela Rolz-Cruz, MD[a], Caroline C. Kim, MD[b],*

[a]*Clinical Unit for Research Trials in Skin, Department of Dermatology, Brigham and Women's Hospital,
221 Longwood Avenue, Boston, MA 02115, USA*
[b]*Pigmented Lesion Clinic, Department of Dermatology, Beth Israel Deaconess Medical Center,
330 Brookline Avenue, Shapiro 2nd Floor, Boston, MA 02215, USA*

Internal malignancies can invade the skin through hematogenous spread, lymphatic spread, or by direct extension from a primary tumor. Clinicians must keep a high level of awareness to detect metastatic skin disease, because it is sometimes overlooked and difficult to diagnose. The recognition of skin lesions associated with an underlying systemic malignancy is of great importance for prompt diagnosis and for the initiation of proper treatment. In addition, skin lesions characteristic of previously diagnosed or disseminated malignancies may help the clinician restage a disease for a more accurate prognosis.

This article discusses several solid organ and hematologic neoplasms that can metastasize to the skin. Special emphasis is placed on the most frequent solid and hematological malignancies that have cutaneous metastases, including breast cancer, melanoma, lung cancer, colon cancer, and leukemia. In addition, mammary and extramammary Paget's disease are further discussed as examples of direct extension of primary tumors to the skin.

Metastasis

The most accepted definition of metastasis in the literature is "a neoplastic lesion arising from another neoplasm with which it is no longer in contiguity" [1,2]. Lambert and Schwartz [3] suggested that in the context of dermatology,

the following definition is more appropriate: "a neoplastic lesion arising form another neoplasm with which it is no longer in contiguity or in close proximity within the same tissue." Their rationale is that in certain cutaneous neoplasms regression may have occurred, or satellite lesions may be present, and these are not considered metastases.

Metastases of internal malignancies to the skin are not uncommon, but occur less often when compared with metastases to other organs of the body [1,4–11]. Cutaneous metastases account for 0.7% to 9.0% of all metastases [1,4,12,13]. They may represent the first sign of an internal malignancy and can be difficult to diagnose [4,14]. Cutaneous metastases may also be the first manifestation of extranodal disease, which may require alteration in therapy. The prognosis of most patients who have internal malignancies has improved over the last several decades, however, the presence of skin metastases still represent a grave prognostic sign. This is especially true for metastatic disease arising from cancer of the lung, ovary, cervix, upper digestive tract, and upper respiratory tract [6,9,14].

Mechanisms of metastasis

Cutaneous metastases from internal malignancies are not random, but follow definite patterns of distribution [13]. The mechanism by which metastases occur is complex and is accomplished only by few cells in a given neoplasm [2,14]. Cancer metastasis is a dynamic process consisting of a series of interrelated mechanisms that must occur to successfully accomplish the end result.

* Corresponding author.
E-mail address: ckim3@bidmc.harvard.edu
(C.C. Kim).

0733-8635/08/$ - see front matter. Published by Elsevier Inc.
doi:10.1016/j.det.2007.08.004

The outcome of the disseminating tumor cells depends both on intrinsic properties of the tumor cells and their interactions with host factors [15]. The details of the intricate process of tumor metastasis are beyond the scope of this article, but are discussed briefly below.

After an initial transforming event, neoplastic cells start growing and expanding. The mass of cells growing up to 1 mm in diameter is supplied nutrients by simple diffusion. Subsequently, the tumor secretes pro-angiogenic factors, establishing a new capillary network from the host's tissues. There is local tumor cell invasion of the host stroma that includes the basement membrane, which occurs via a number of adhesion molecules and proteolytic enzymes [15]. Tumor cells are then able to penetrate thin-walled lymphatic and blood vessels, which are interconnected, entering the circulation. The survival of tumor cells within the vessel is limited by mechanical trauma and clearance by the immune system [2,6,15]. Once the tumor cells have survived in the circulation, they settle into organ capillary beds. This process may be random or it may be site-specific, in which case tumor cells select a specific organ vessel wall, bypassing other organs. After tumor cell emboli reach a tissue bed, extravasation must occur. The final step for a successful metastatic process is the proliferation of the tumor cell in the new tissue bed [2,9,15]. The final distribution of metastatic cells is determined by three distinct patterns:

1. Mechanical tumor stasis is the most common pattern encountered, accounting for 50% to 60% of the distribution of metastases. The tumor cells distribute in the first capillary bed they encounter, and their distribution is determined by anatomic proximity and lymphatic drainage patterns in relation to the primary tumor. Head and neck tumors usually metastasize on a mechanical or anatomic basis. Therefore, their metastases remain confined to the head and neck [2].
2. Site-specific attachment of tumor cells to a specific organ occurs when regional organs are bypassed and there is a selectivity to metastasize to specific distant organs. There are factors that favor this specificity, such as organ-specific adhesion molecules located in the vessel wall. Two examples of site-specific metastasis include prostate cancer metastasizing to bone, and melanoma metastasizing to the brain [2].

3. The nonspecific pattern of metastases refers to some highly aggressive tumors that have the ability to adhere to vessel walls of many organs and establish metastatic colonies in various sites. This is probably because of the production of autocrine growth factors that allow cells to proliferate in various environments [2].

Anatomic distribution of metastasis

The trunk is the most common site for a cutaneous metastasis, with breast cancer and lung cancer being the most frequently seen [1]. Colorectal carcinoma, which is the second most common primary carcinoma in both men and women, can also metastasize to the abdominal wall or perineal area late in the disease.

The scalp is another common site for skin metastases, and should be carefully examined in all cancer patients [4,7]. It provides a vascular, immobile environment, suitable for the proliferation of tumor cells [7]. On the scalp, metastases can take the form of single or multiple firm nodules, sometimes resembling turban tumors, but it can also present as alopecia, as can be seen in metastatic breast cancer in the form of alopecia neoplastica [7,9,16]. The recognition of scalp metastases from renal cell carcinoma is important, primarily because of its relative frequency and early presentation [1,11,14]. In men, scalp metastases often originate from primary cancers of the lung or kidney. In women, the primary cancer commonly originates in the breast, and it usually metastasizes to the scalp late in the disease [1,11].

Local metastases may also develop in the cutaneous surface of scars of surgical incisions from any prior primary tumor resection [1,14]. In one series, "iatrogenic metastases" were the most common manifestation of local metastases, with nodules appearing in pre-existing surgical scars approximately 1 year after the first surgery [1,4,9,11]. New nodules in or near an old scar should always be examined histologically [1].

Solid organ malignancies that metastasize to the skin

Cutaneous metastases from solid primary tumors are uncommon, accounting for only 0.7% to 9% of all metastases. The relative incidence and site of origin of metastatic skin disease correlates with the most common types of primary cancer in each gender (Table 1). Melanoma has recently been reported to be the most common cancer that metastasizes to skin in men (32% of all cases), whereas breast cancer is the most common type of skin metastasis in women (69% of all cases) [14]. Other common primary malignancies that metastasize to the skin include lung, gastrointestinal and genitourinary, head and neck, endocrine, and oral cavity cancers [14,17]. Because cutaneous metastasis often present as asymptomatic, painless, firm or doughy skin-colored nodules with a broad clinical differential, it is imperative to biopsy any new suspicious growth for histologic examination and confirmation of disease. Diagnosis of cutaneous metastasis can reveal an otherwise undiagnosed occult malignancy, can help restage a known disease, and may dramatically alter treatment course [1,9].

Breast cancer

Breast cancer is the most common cancer in women, and it is the most frequently encountered type of cutaneous metastasis in dermatology [1,9]. Two large studies investigating cutaneous

Table 1
Most common internal malignancies and location of cutaneous metastasis

	Internal malignancy (% skin metastasis)	Location of cutaneous metastasis
Women	Breast (69%–70%)	Chest, abdomen most common; scalp, neck, upper extremities, back less common
	Melanoma (5%–12%)	Lower extremities
	Colon cancer (9%)	Abdomen, pelvis
	Lung cancer (4%)	Chest wall, back, scalp
	Ovarian cancer (4%)	Abdomen, back
Men	Melanoma (32%)	Chest, back, extremities
	Lung cancer (24%–29%)	Chest wall, back, scalp
	Colon cancer (11%–19%)	Abdomen, pelvis
	Squamous cell cancer of oral cavity (11.5%)	Head, neck
	Renal cell carcinoma (4%)	Scalp

metastases have reported that breast cancer was the source of 69% to 70% of the cases [14,18]. It is the most common cancer in women that metastasizes to the skin [1,4,16]. Cutaneous metastases usually occur after the discovery of the primary tumor and present at a later stage of disease compared with other cancers that metastasize to the skin [13].

There are eight well-described clinicopathologic types of skin involvement from breast cancer. These patterns are not restricted to breast cancer, but are seen more often in this patient population because of the high frequency of this type of malignancy Table 2 [1,12].

En cuirasse metastatic carcinoma

En cuirasse metastatic carcinoma was described in 1838 by Velpeau as "cancer en cuirasse" because it resembles the encasement in armor of a cuirassier, a cavalry solider [14,19,20]. Years later, in 1922, Hanley saw a resemblance to the skin in chronic lymphatic obstruction, so he named it pachydermia [20]. It is a fibrotic metastatic process characterized by a diffuse morphea-like induration of the skin, and it is synonymous with the term "acarcine eburnee" [1,14]. Carcinoma en cuirasse has been reported in a few cases to be the presenting sign of breast cancer, consisting of extensive skin involvement. It more commonly presents as a local recurrence following therapy for an underlying breast cancer, usually following mastectomy, chemotherapy, or radiotherapy [19]. En cuirasse metastatic carcinoma is not specific to the breast; it may be seen in lung, gastrointestinal tract, kidney, and other metastasizing malignancies [1,19,20]. There is one reported case of carcinoma en cuirasse presenting in the scrotum [21].

There are two stages described as part of the development for carcinoma en cuirasse: an early stage of swelling with pitting edema, followed by a later stage characterized by thickened and leather-type skin [19]. It begins as scattered, firm, papules and nodules that overlie an erythematous or red-blue smooth cutaneous surface. It evolves into a sclerodermoid plaque with no inflammatory changes associated with it [1,12,20]. Mullinax and Cohen [20] described a case of carcinoma en cuirasse presenting as keloid-like nodules. Some symptoms associated with carcinoma en cuirasse are pruritus, pain, edema, bleeding, and foul-smelling discharge [19].

Table 2
Skin involvement in breast cancer: clinicopathological types

Type	Clinical presentation	Histology	Differential diagnosis
En cuirasse metastastic carcinoma	Fibrotic diffuse morphea-like induration	Densely fibrotic tissue. Tumor cells in "Indian file" pattern, which are tumor cells forming small lines between collagen bundles	Scleroderma, morphea
Inflammatory metastatic carcinoma	Erythematous patch or plaque with active spreading border	Tumor cells within the dilated lymphatics in the upper and lower dermis with no acute inflammatory infiltrate.	Erysipelas or cellulitis
Telangiectatic metastatic breast carcinoma (TMBC)	Red to yellow violaceous papulovesicles	Adenomatous tumor cells in congested blood vessels in the upper dermis	Stewart-Treves syndrome and lymphangioma
Nodular metastatic carcinoma	Resembles intertriginous dermatitis; fissures may be present	Grouped tumor cells in dermal stroma	If pigmented, it may look like a melanoma or pigmented basal cell carcinoma. One case appeared like a keratoacanthoma.
Alopecia neoplastica	Single or multiple areas of scarring alopecia on the scalp	Metastatic carcinoma cells in a dense, collagenous stroma with loss of pilosebaceous units	Discoid lupus erythematosus, lichen planopilaris, pseudopelade, morpheaform basal cell carcinoma
Breast carcinoma of the inframammary crease	Resembles intertriginous dermatitis; fissures may be present	Tumor masses infiltrate a fibrous sroma, forming acini. Malignant cells are present in lymphatics of middle and deep dermis	Basal cell carcinoma, squamous cell carcinoma, a callus, epidermal cyst, fissure or intertrigo
Metastatic mammary carcinoma of the eyelid with histiocytoid histology	Painless eyelid swelling with induration and nodularity	Prominent histiocytoid features	Basal cell carcinoma
Paget's disease	Sharply demarcated plaque or patch, or erythema and scaling on the nipple or areola	Large pale cells lying singly or in nests along the basement membrane of the epidermis. May replace the epidermis focally or full thickness	Eczematous dermatitis, dermatophyte infection, psoriasis, contact dermatitis, and erosive adenomatosis of the nipple

Histologically, the tissue shows fibrosis, with a few tumor cells in an "Indian file" pattern, representing tumor cells lining up between collagen bundles. The matrix is densely fibrotic with decreased vascularity, which makes these tumors highly resistant to chemotherapy [19,20]. Multiple treatments modalities have been tried, including intralesional chemotherapy, radiotherapy, hormonal antagonists, and some snake venoms such as crotoxin and dardiotoxin (VRCTC-310) [20].

Inflammatory metastatic carcinoma

Inflammatory metastatic carcinoma was described in 1924 by Lee and Tannenbaum when they reported breast cancer in association with overlying inflammatory skin changes. In 1931, Rasch termed it as carcinoma erysipelatoides [10,13]. This type of skin metastases accounts for 1% to 4% of all metastases in the United States, and it is most frequently associated with intraductal breast cancer [5,13]. Clinically, it presents as an erythematous patch or plaque with an active spreading border resembling erysipelas or cellulitis, and it is frequently misdiagnosed. The classic toxic symptoms associated with erysipelas are not seen [1,10–13].

Histologically, tumor cells lie within the dilated lymphatics with no acute inflammatory infiltrate [1,11,14]. The obstruction induces lymphedema and may be the cause of the erythema [11]. The differential diagnosis of inflammatory metastatic carcinoma includes erythema annulare centrifugum [1]. Metastases of this type are more common in breast cancer, but may also be seen from primary cancers of the parotid, tonsils, colon, pancreas, stomach, rectum, melanoma, lung, and pelvic organs such as ovary, uterus, and prostate [1,5,14,22].

Telangiectatic metastatic breast carcinoma

Telangiectatic metastatic breast carcinoma (TMBC) was first described by Newcomb in 1924 [23]. It represents metastatic breast cancer presenting clinically as pinpoint telangiectasia caused by dilated capillaries [1]. TMBC can also present clinically as red to yellow to violaceous papulovesicles resembling lymphangioma circumscriptum, ipsilateral to the side affected by breast cancer [24]. A violaceous hue can be seen with blood in dilated vascular channels. Papules may appear on a background resembling inflammatory metastatic carcinoma [1]. There is a rare variant described as purpuric plaques clinically resembling cutaneous vasculitis [12]. There are also cases in the literature where TMBC has been described as mimicking angiosarcoma, as well as pigmented metastatic melanoma [1,24].

Histologically, there are adenomatous tumor cells found in congested small vessels, mainly in the upper dermis. The tumor nests usually lie free in vascular lumen, and central necrosis of tumor masses can be seen. TMBC preferentially affects the congested blood capillaries of the upper dermis, whereas carcinoma erysipelatoides affects the lymphatics of both upper and lower dermis [24]. The differential diagnosis of TMBC includes Stewart-Treves syndrome (STS), lymphangioma, and metastatic melanoma. Distinction between STS and TMBC may be difficult when the tumor growth is poorly differentiated. In such cases the use of monoclonal antikeratin and antidesmosome antibodies can be helpful [24].

Nodular metastatic carcinoma

Nodular metastatic carcinoma presents clinically as multiple noninflammatory papules or nodules. Histologically they represent grouped tumor cells in dermal stroma [5]. Occasionally, nodular metastatic carcinoma may be solitary, bullous, or ulcerated [1]. Some cases have presented as a pigmented nodule with irregular borders, which may be suggestive of melanoma or pigmented basal cell carcinoma [1,12]. It may also present as a dome-shaped nodule with a central core, similar to a keratoacanthoma [1].

Alopecia neoplastica

Alopecia neoplastica refers to a rare presentation of metastatic breast cancer on the scalp [7,14]. It presents as circular plaques of scarring alopecia that can occur in a single or multiple areas [7]. These metastatic plaques are painless, nonpruritic, and well-demarcated, often with a red-pink color and a smooth surface that changes into an uneven surface as the lesion evolves [1,16]. The consistency of the lesions has been described as hard, and the skin is not easily wrinkled in the affected areas [16]. The lesions can resemble discoid lupus erythematosus, lichen planopilaris, pseudopelade, or morpheaform basal cell carcinoma [1].

Histological examination of the scalp tissue reveals cells in a dense collagenous stroma with loss of pilosebaceous units, which correlates clinically with a reduced number of hair follicles [7,16]. The mechanism behind the loss of the pilosebaceous unit is not completely understood, but some authors attribute it to the fibrosis [16]. A skin biopsy and breast examination should be considered in an adult woman who has new-onset alopecia [1].

Breast carcinoma of the inframammary crease

Breast carcinoma of the inframammary crease is a very rare, slow-growing entity accounting for fewer than 2% of breast cancers [24]. It occurs in women who have pendulous breasts and resembles intertriginous dermatitis. It begins as a lesion that may look like a callus, and then it can slowly become fissured, first invading the skin, then the deeper breast tissue, until it reaches the fascia

[25]. These lesions appear as exophytic nodules that clinically may resemble basal cell carcinoma, squamous cell carcinoma, a callus, epidermal cyst, fissure, or intertrigo [1,12,25]. The histological diagnosis is difficult to make. Therefore, some authors recommend taking a large, deep biopsy specimen if suspecting this entity, because most of these lesions are initially reported as basal cell epithelioma. Deeper sectioning of the specimen allows the diagnosis to be established. Histologically, there are masses of cells with hyperchromatic nuclei. Most tumor masses infiltrate a fibrous stroma forming acini containing eosinophilic material. Malignant cells are present in the lymphatics of the middle and deep dermis [25].

Metastatic mammary carcinoma of the eyelid with histiocytoid histology

Metastatic mammary carcinoma of the eyelid with histiocytoid histology has been described in 13 patients. It presents as painless eyelid swelling with induration or nodularity. Histologically it shows prominent histiocytoid features [1].

Paget's disease

Paget's disease was first described in 1874 by Sir James Paget as persistent breast eczema in association with breast cancer [1]. It is a cutaneous infiltration from breast cancer and clinically appears as a sharply demarcated plaque or patch or erythema and scaling that occurs on the nipple or areola associated with an underlying breast cancer. It can be unilateral or bilateral, and may develop from ectopic breast tissue as well as from a supernumerary nipple. The prognosis is better when there is no palpable tumor and no adenopathy. It may occur together with other cutaneous breast metastases like nodular or en cuirasse [1]. Paget's disease is further discussed later in this article.

Other described clinical presentations of cutaneous metastasis of breast cancer include locoregional metastasis of the anterior chest wall in or near areas that have been previously treated by surgery or radiotherapy [12,13], a herpes zoster-like unilateral vesicular eruption [12], and skin lesions mimicking malignant melanoma [26].

Melanoma

Although melanoma is a primary skin cancer, it also frequently metastasizes to other parts of the skin [1]. This can occur in in-transit metastasis, with tumor spread via the lymphatics in between the primary tumor and draining lymph node basin, and in distant metastatic spread. Lookingbill found that it was the cancer that most frequently metastasized to the skin overall [12]. Melanoma was reported to be the most common cancer that metastasizes to skin in men, representing up to 32% of all cases, whereas it represented 5% to 12% of the cases in women [14]. Clinically, metastatic lesions can present as skin-colored pink or dark blue–black papules and nodules on the skin. In-transit metastases are found in the vicinity of the primary tumor, whereas hematogenously spread metastases can be found anywhere on the skin surface.

Lung cancer

Lung cancer is the leading cause of cancer deaths in both men and women in the United States and throughout the world. Metastatic lung cancer to the skin is more common in men than in women. The incidence of lung cancer metastasizing to the skin in men has been reported to be 24% to 29%, versus 4% in women [17,18]. Cutaneous metastases most commonly appear on the chest wall and back, and they may also appear on the scalp; however, they may appear on any surface, including the scrotum. Metastatic lesions have been described as occurring as single or multiple firm or doughy skin-colored nodules. In addition, there have been reports of oat cell carcinoma having a vascular appearance, zosteriform pattern, as well as arising at the site of a burn scar [1,4,27]. Pulmonary mesothelioma has been reported to metastasize to the skin by direct extension along needle biopsy tracts or surgical scars [27].

Colorectal carcinoma

Colorectal carcinoma is the second most common primary carcinoma in both men and women. The incidence with which it metastasizes to the skin is 11% to 19% in men, and 9% in women [14,18]. Cutaneous metastases appear on the abdomen and perineal regions, usually after the colorectal tumor has been diagnosed [1]. Most primary tumors with skin metastases originate in the rectum [1]. A variety of cutaneous metastatic presentations of colorectal carcinoma have been described, including: (1) metastatic inflammatory carcinoma of the inguinal region, supraclavicular area, or face and neck [1,4]; (2) pedunculated nodules on buttocks, scrotum, chest wall, abdomen, and back [1,4]; (3) grouped vascular nodules (botryoid) on skin of the groin and scrotum [1]; (4) facial tumor; and (5) scalp cyst resembling a pilar cyst [1].

Squamous cell carcinoma of the oral cavity

Cutaneous metastases from oral cavity squamous cell carcinoma usually occur in men who have a history of a primary tumor. It represented 11.5% of the cutaneous skin metastases in one series [14]. Morphologically, cutaneous metastasis of this malignancy can appear as multiple nodules or as ulcers on the head and neck [1,14]. The metastases are most often located in actinically damaged skin of the head and neck. Their clinical and histologic appearance is almost indistinguishable from primary cutaneous squamous cell carcinoma [1].

Renal cell carcinoma

Renal cell carcinoma (RCC) has a 4% to 6% incidence of metastasizing to the skin [14,28,29]. Cutaneous RCC metastases are important for the clinician to recognize because they can be the first sign of underlying disease. The metastases have a unique appearance, usually presenting as a vascular nodule on the scalp that may bleed. Renal cell carcinoma is highly vascular, and often metastasizes to distant sites through hematogenous spread. Cutaneous metastases typically can appear erythematous or violaceous to brown or black in color. Skin lesions are usually well-circumscribed cutaneous nodules. They have also been reported to present as a cutaneous horn [1]. The scalp is a common location for skin metastasis from RCC [11,14,28]. Cutaneous lesions from RCC may resemble Kaposi's sarcoma, hemangioma, or pyogenic granuloma.

Histologically, cutaneous metastases predominantly involve the dermis, with occasional extension into the subcutis. There is usually a narrow zone of superficial dermis separating the lesion form the epidermis, also called a grenz zone. Metastatic lesions often preserve histologic similarities to the primary tumor [29].

The prognosis for patients who have cutaneous metastases from RCC is poor. Most patients die within several months of diagnosis. The treatment options are therefore limited and palliative [29].

Carcinoma of the ovary

The incidence of carcinoma of the ovary found to metastasize to the skin is approximately 4% [14,28]. Metastases from carcinoma of the ovary are most commonly located in the trunk. It may present as a nodule involving the umbilicus, representing a contiguous extension from the peritoneum. Morphologically, cutaneous metastases have also been reported as having an inflammatory appearance, as well as a zosteriform pattern [1].

Esophageal cancer

Metastatic esophageal cancer represents from 3% to 8.6% of all cutaneous metastases [1,14]. The metastases may appear as scalp tumors or as widespread cutaneous nodules. The most common histologic types are adenocarcinoma, squamous cell carcinoma, mucoepidermoid carcinoma, and small cell carcinoma [1].

Gastric adenocarcinoma

Gastric adenocarcinoma is an uncommon source of cutaneous metastases, accounting for approximately 2% of all cutaneous metastases [14]. The most common locations for cutaneous metastasis include the head, eyebrow, neck, axilla, chest, and fingers [1]. Clinically, cutaneous metastases can appear as nonspecific solitary or multiple nodules. In addition, zosteriform-distributed, erysipelas-like, and scarring alopecia presentations have been described. Other descriptions of cutaneous metastatic disease include lesions resembling epidermoid cysts, condyloma acuminatum, or benign soft tissue tumors [1]. Sister Mary Joseph's nodule refers to a metastatic nodule to the umbilicus that is more commonly of gastric origin. It is a rare phenomenon, and it usually portends a poor prognosis [4,14,30].

Carcinoma of the genitourinary systems

Cancer of the urinary tract has a higher incidence in men, with a reported frequency of 2%, versus 1% in women. It is unusual for cutaneous metastases to be the initial sign in patients who have cancer of the urinary tract [31]. Cutaneous metastases have a predisposition for the inguinal and umbilical regions [1]. Clinically, the lesions appear as subcutaneous nodules, although there are reports of lesions that presented as large cutaneous ulcers, suggestive of squamous cell carcinomas [1,31]. A case was reported in which metastatic disease from a transitional cell carcinoma of the bladder presented as a dermatomal erythema mimicking zoster sine herpete (a term used for herpes zoster without the classic vesicular rash) [32].

Prostate cancer does not metastasize to the skin frequently, with an incidence of 0.36% [29]. Morphologically, these cutaneous metastases may appear as firm red to violaceous nodules, and can resemble a cylindroma or a pilar cyst if presenting on the scalp [1].

Skin metastases from carcinomas of the uterine cervix and endometrium are very rare, even in late-stage disease [1,6,33].

Hematologic malignancies that metastasize to the skin

Cutaneous metastasis can also occur in hematologic malignancies, such as leukemia and lymphoma [1,34]. Skin involvement may appear similar for both types of diseases, and the lesions can arise at any time during the course of the disease. Morphologically, the lesions present as macules, papules, plaques, and nodules that are pink, red, and brown to purple [34–36]. They are usually firm and characteristically painless [37]. They may also present as palpable purpura, ulcers, or bullae. The cutaneous manifestations of these disorders are referred to as leukemia and lymphoma cutis.

Leukemia cutis

Leukemia cutis represents dissemination of systemic leukemia to the skin. Its presence is associated with late-stage disease and a poor prognosis [34]. Rarely, the skin involvement may precede the appearance of blasts in the peripheral smear, and when this occurs it is known as "aleukemic leukemia cutis" [38]. The incidence of leukemia cutis ranges from 1% to 50%, with the highest incidence seen in patients who have congenital leukemia, and myeloid leukemias with monocytic differentiation [34,39].

The clinical presentation of leukemia cutis varies depending on the type of leukemia (Table 3). The most frequent locations affected by leukemia cutis include the face, chest, back, scalp, legs, arms, and mucocutaneous surface. Leukemia cutis associated with acute monocytic leukemia generally has the most extensive skin and mucocutaneous involvement [40]. The face and neck are more commonly involved in patients who have chronic lymphocytic leukemia (CLL) and acute lymphocytic leukemia (ALL). Leukemia cutis presents most often as skin- to plum-colored nodules or plaques. In some cases these nodules can ulcerate or form bullae, as has been described in CLL and adult T-cell leukemia. Gum hypertrophy in the oral cavity can be present as well, which can cover the teeth completely [1,40,41]. In acute myelogenous leukemia (AML), cutaneous tumors called

Table 3
Leukemia cutis: morphology and skin distribution

Type of leukemia	Skin morphology	Location
Acute myelocytic leukemia	Papules, nodules, infiltrative plaques, and granulocytic sarcomas	Occur anywhere in the body
Acute monocytic leukemia	Plum-colored papules or nodules	Extensive skin and mucocutaneous involvement
Chronic lymphocytic leukemia	Papules, plaques, and nodules. May present as erythroderma or bullae	Face and neck
Adult T-cell leukemia	Macules, papules, plaques, and ulcerative tumors	Widespread

granulocytic sarcomas can also be seen. Granulocytic sarcomas are pathognomonic of AML, and were formerly called chloromas because of the green hue generated by elevated myeloperoxidase enzyme levels in leukemic cells [42].

In addition to cutaneous nodules, leukemia cutis has also been described to present clinically as arciform lesions or plaques that simulate mycosis fungoides, as well as massive diffuse infiltrations, producing leonine facies. Leukemia cutis has been reported to occur at the site of a previous varicella zoster infection, as well as a skin ulcer caused by leishmaniasis [34,40].

The diagnosis of leukemia cutis is confirmed by biopsy; it can be facilitated by touch preparation of the biopsy specimen [36]. The histologic features of leukemia cutis vary with the type of leukemia. There are typically dense dermal collections of neoplastic and benign inflammatory cells infiltrating collagen bundles, and surrounding adnexal structures [34]. Treatment is targeted to the specific underlying leukemia with chemotherapeutic agents [36]. If persistent skin lesions remain, localized electron beam therapy can be added as an adjunct to systemic treatment, or a bone marrow transplant may be considered [34,36].

Lymphoma cutis

Cutaneous spread of underlying lymphoma is more commonly seen with histiocytic and lymphocytic lymphomas. It can sometimes be difficult to determine if a specific lesion is metastatic or a primary lesion, and this requires a proper staging workup. Although there are other types of lymphoma that involve the skin as primary cutaneous lesions, such as cutaneous T-cell lymphoma, this article will only discuss those that have a primary underlying systemic disease. Some series estimate that skin metastases occur in up to 9.1% of patients who have non-Hodgkin's lymphoma [1].

Cutaneous dissemination in Hodgkin's disease is less common than in non-Hodgkin's lymphoma, with a frequency range of 0.5% to 3.4% [43–46]. The mechanism of cutaneous spread of disease most commonly involves retrograde lymphatic spread distal to the involved lymph nodes. In addition, direct extension from an underlying lymph node and hematogenous dissemination can be seen. The trunk is the most common site of involvement. The clinical presentation of the skin involvement in both Hodgkin's disease and non-Hodgkin's lymphoma is that of firm, raised, smooth, slightly violaceous to erythematous nodules or plaques that range in size from a few millimeters to a few centimeters [1,43]. The nodules may break down, producing ulcers with sharp borders [1,43]. Lymphoma of the skin may look like a gumma of syphilis; it is an indurated plaque sometimes called "lymphoma en cuirasse" or erythema nodosum-like subcutaneous nodules. Lymphoma cutis has also been reported to resemble a penile chancre [1].

Histologically, cutaneous Hodgkin's disease resembles the histology of the affected lymph nodes. The cell infiltrate consists primarily of atypical lymphocytes with occasional eosinophils and plasma cells. Lacunar and Reed-Sternberg cells may also be found, depending on the histologic subtype of the primary disease [43].

Malignancies that directly extend to the skin

Another mechanism of cutaneous spread of malignancy is by way of direct extension. As an example of this kind of spread, This article will discuss Paget's disease of the breast (PDB) and extramammary Paget's disease (EMPD). Although there has been some debate about the pathogenesis of this epidermal malignancy, it is most commonly accepted that the cutaneous findings of PDB and certain cases of EMPD represent the direct extension of an underlying adenocarcinoma.

Paget's disease of the breast

First described in 1974 by Sir James Paget, PDB refers to a form of intraepidermal adenocarcinoma that presents clinically as an eczematous-like process in the nipple-areola complex [15,47]. PDB is associated with an underlying breast cancer, including ductal carcinoma in situ and invasive ductal carcinoma in over 90% of the cases [47,48].

Epidemiology

PDB is present in approximately 0.5% to 4.3% of patients who have breast carcinoma. In addition to an eczematous process overlying the nipple-areola complex, half of patients who have Paget's disease will also have a palpable underlying nodule. Of these patients, half of these will have lymph node metastasis [15]. The peak incidence is between the sixth and seventh decades, with a median of 56 years. PDB is also seen rarely in men, and carries a worse prognosis. There are no known clinical or epidemiologic risk factors associated with PDB [15,47].

Clinical presentation

PDB most commonly presents on the nipple and areola as a well-demarcated, erythematous, exudative, or scaly area with or without an underlying palpable breast nodule. Tiny vesicles on the nipple have also been described in PDB [15]. The nipple is thought to be involved first, and then the lesion spreads to the areola. It rarely involves the surrounding skin. In about 25% of the cases, there is pain, itching, and soreness as presenting symptoms without any objective skin changes. There can be serous or bloody discharge as ulceration and nipple destruction occur [15,49].

Many patients have symptoms for several months before they are diagnosed with PDB. In one study, the duration of time before a correct diagnosis of PDB was made was 6.5 months. Usually PDB is a unilateral disease, but there are cases of bilateral involvement.

Any patient suspected to have PDB should also undergo a careful breast and lymph node examination for underlying masses or lymph node involvement. PDB associated with intraductal carcinoma in situ (DCIS), which accounts for about 50% of all cases, usually does not have a palpable tumor within the breast. The presence of a palpable mass should raise the suspicion of invasive carcinoma [49].

Pathogenesis

The pathogenesis of PDB has been under debate over past years. Once thought to represent an inflammatory process that induced underlying breast carcinoma, it is now understood that PDB represents intraepidermal adenocarcinoma of the breast. The most accepted theory of pathogenesis is that PDB arises via the migration of neoplastic ductal epithelial cells through the breast ductal system to the epidermis of the nipple [49]. This epidermotropic theory has been supported by studies using immunohistochemical staining (IHC) and molecular markers [47]. These studies have shown that Paget's cells and ductal epithelial cells have similar IHC patterns, whereas they differ from the staining pattern of the surrounding keratinocytes. For example, Paget's cells and mammary ductal epithelium stain positive for keratins 8, 18, and 19, whereas the cells of the normal nipple epithelium are negative. In addition, PDB may express molecular markers such as HER-2/neu, cyclin D1, and Ki-67, which are found in aggressive breast cancers with poor prognosis [50–52].

The less-supported theory of the pathogenesis of PDB is the in situ transformation theory, suggesting that keratinocytes within the epidermis of the nipple "transform" into malignant cells. Of mention are Toker cells, which are benign clear cells in the epidermis of the nipple in about 10% of the normal population. They are believed to be ectopic mammary elements within the nipple epithelium. Toker cells share some common imunohistochemical properties with cells of PDB and intraductal carcinoma, such as positive staining for cytokeratin 7 and anti-cytokeratin (CAM 5.2). The in situ transformation theory suggests that cells such as Toker cells may be the origin of intraepidermal PDB without an underlying breast cancer [49,53,54].

Diagnosis

Clinically, PDB can be a difficult diagnosis to make. The differential diagnosis is broad, including common dermatoses such as eczematous dermatitis, dermatophyte infection, psoriasis, and contact dermatitis. Erosive adenomatosis of the nipple may present with an ulcerated lesion of the nipple as well. Once traditional therapies for inflammatory and infectious processes fail, clinicians should consider PBD as a diagnosis and perform a biopsy. Other neoplasms to be considered in the differential diagnosis include Bowen's disease, basal cell carcinoma, and melanotic or amelanotic malignant melanoma [15,49].

The diagnosis of PDB is made with a shave or punch biopsy. It is not necessary to obtain a great amount of dermis because the diagnosis is identified by epidermal changes. Alternatively, one may use a scraping technique similar to the Tzanck smear, using a scalpel to smear material on a slide for cytologic evaluation [15,49]. Given the complexity of the breast ductal system, if a patient also presents with a palpable nodule in the breast, the dermatologist should consider referring the patient to a general surgeon or breast surgeon for biopsy or needle aspirate. Once the diagnosis of PDB is made, mammography may help locate nonpalpable breast masses.

Histology

The hisotologic hallmark for the diagnosis of PDB is the presence of Pagetoid cells, which are large pale cells that are distinct from the surrounding keratinocytes. Pagetoid cells have abundant vacuolated cytoplasm, enlarged hyperchromatic and polymorphic nuclei, and prominent nucleoli. Mitoses may be frequently observed. The cells may be lying singly above the basilar layer of the epidermis, or in small nests that can lie in all levels of the epidermis, in what is called a Pagetoid pattern. This Pagetoid pattern can also be seen in other diseases such as malignant melanoma in situ, and squamous cell carcinoma in situ [15,49].

Immunohistochemical studies can differentiate PDB from its histologic simulators. A panel of antibodies staining for s100 protein, melan A, low and high molecular weight cytokeratins, and carcinoembryonic antigen (CEA) is most helpful. With this panel, PDB will usually stain positive for CEA and low molecular weight keratin. Melanomas will stain positive only for s100 and melan A, whereas squamous cell carcinoma in situ will generally be positive for high molecular weight cytokeratins, sometimes for low molecular weight cytokeratins, and negative for the other antibodies [15].

Treatment

The treatment of patients who has PDB is controversial and depends on the presence or absence of an underlying mass, with surgery as the cornerstone of treatment. Patients who have a palpable mass almost always have an associated underlying invasive carcinoma (75%–100%) and a high rate of axillary lymph node metastasis

(45%–65%). Therefore, the traditional treatment has been for these patients to receive a mastectomy with axillary lymph node dissection. If a patient who has a palpable mass does not have radiologically multifocal disease, more conservative surgery to spare the breast tissue can be considered, followed by radiation treatment and close clinical follow-up. Conservative surgery should be performed cautiously because of higher recurrence rates and multifocal disease [55–57].

For PDB patients who do not have a palpable mass or mammographic abnormalities, the trend is toward more conservative surgical therapy, such as excision of the nipple areola complex, or excision plus radiation. For patients who refuse surgery or are not surgical candidates, radiation treatment is an option. Recent reports also describe topical imiquimod 5% cream as another nonsurgical option [58].

Overall survival is affected by lymph node status and is reported to be 75% to 95% in patients who have negative lymph nodes, and as low as 20% to 25% in patients who have positive lymph nodes. Because the prognosis is determined largely by nodal status, adjuvant therapies to surgery should be based on the final tumor-node-metastasis stage [55,57,59].

Extramammary Paget's disease

EMPD is a less common type of cancer, arising in areas with apocrine glands, including the perianal region, vulva, scrotum, penis, and axilla [15,53,60]. EMPD represents a form of intraepidermal adenocarcinoma that clinically resembles an eczematous dermatitis. It is usually multifocal and fairly widespread at the time of diagnosis. In contrast to PDB, EMPD is associated with an underlying malignancy of an adjunct organ in only 15% to 33% of patients; cancer of the vulva is the most common.

Epidemiology
EMPD is relatively uncommon, and no ethnic, racial, or geographical predisposition has been well-described. It primarily affects middle-aged to elderly women [15].

Clinical presentation
EMPD has a similar clinical presentation to PDB. It appears as an erythematous patch or plaque that may be scaly. Symptoms associated with it include pruritus and pain or burning. It is usually present in the vulva, scrotum, or perianal region. The lesion is only rarely ulcerated, and unlike PDB, there is usually no underlying mass associated with it [15].

Pathogenesis
The pathogenesis of EMPD is controversial. Three clinical types of EMPD have been described, and each may have a different pathogenesis of disease.

The most common type of EMPD has no association with an underlying invasive carcinoma. Some authors believe that this finding supports the theory that the disease originates in the epidermis, similar to the theory that Toker cells give rise to PDB. Other authors argue that it arises from an intraepidermal part of a ductal structure, and some believe that EMPD arises from a duct or gland and spreads upwards to the epidermis.

The second clinical type of EMPD is associated with visceral malignancy, the most common being adenocarcinoma of the anal canal or rectum. This type has also been described to occur with underlying carcinomas of the bladder, cervix, sebaceous glands, and apocrine glands. In this clinical scenario, it is postulated that malignancy lies in the epidermis by way of direct extension from underlying ducts, epithelium, or metastasis. Immunohistochemical staining of this type of EMPD is similar to the primary carcinoma.

The third, and most rare clinical type of EMPD is associated with an underlying sweat gland carcinoma. There exists debate as to how it develops; some authors believe that it originates from epidermal ductal cells and then spreads to the dermis, or that it originates from an underlying sweat gland carcinoma and spreads upwards to the epidermis [15].

Diagnosis
Similar to PDB, the differential diagnosis of EMPD includes common dermatoses such as eczematous dermatosis, dermatophyte infection, and contact dermatitis. Once the skin fails to respond to traditional anti-inflammatory or antifungal therapies, the clinician should perform a shave or punch biopsy for histologic examination to evaluate for EMPD. In addition, squamous cell carcinoma in situ (Bowen's disease) should also be considered.

Histology
The histopathology of EMPD is similar to that of PDB. The presence of large, pale, single, or clustered cells at all levels of the epidermis is characteristic. These cells will stain positively for

mucin in most cases. The histologic differential diagnosis includes malignant melanoma in situ, squamous cell carcinoma in situ, and in some cases, an irritated seborrheic keratosis. Examination by light microscopy can usually differentiate among these diagnoses, and a helpful clue can be the presence of keratohylaine granules within the atypical EMPD cells through the granular cell layer. Immunohistochemical studies often are used to confirm the diagnosis of EMPD, however. As with cases of PDB, a panel of antibodies staining for s100 protein, high and low molecular weight cytokeratins, and CEA can be helpful. EMPD generally stains positive for CEA and low molecular weight cytokeratins, whereas melanoma stains positive for s100, and squamous cell carcinoma in situ stains positive generally for high molecular weight cytokeratins, and sometimes low molecular weight cytokeratins as well.

Immunohistochemical staining has also been helpful to identify the absence or presence of underlying carcinoma in EMPD. The genetic marker for the mucin glycoprotein MUC5AC has been shown to be present almost universally in EMPD disease without underlying carcinoma, whereas it seems to be absent in both mammary and extramammary Paget's disease associated with underlying carcinoma [53]. Gross cystic disease fluid protein-15 has also been found to be present in cases of EMPD without underlying carcinoma [61]. In addition, whereas cytokeratin 7 is positive in most EMPD, cytokeratin 20 positivity has been found only in cases associated with underlying anal carcinoma [62].

Treatment

The treatment of EMPD is directed by the presence or absence of an underlying carcinoma. Therefore, any patient who has a diagnosis of EMPD should have a thorough physical examination and lymph node examination. This should include a pelvic examination if the vulvar area is involved, and a digital rectal examination followed by an examination of the anus and sigmoid colon if the perianal area is involved. The clinician should biopsy any further suspicious lesions to look for underlying carcinoma. If there is underlying malignancy, this needs to be removed in addition to the EMPD.

Surgical therapy via wide local excision is the cornerstone of treatment for EMPD. Mohs micrographic surgery has also been used to decrease the high rate of recurrence. For patients who refuse surgery or are nonsurgical candidates, radiation, chemotherapy, and topical treatments such as 5-flourouracil, retinoids, and more recently, imiquimod, have been used for EMPD [15]. Topical treatments have also been used in conjunction with surgery, both in an attempt to reduce the tumor burden before surgery, and to clear positive surgical margins.

Summary

Cutaneous metastasis from internal malignancies can be difficult to diagnose. Skin lesions can present as skin-colored or erythematous, firm nodules, but other morphologies can occur, such as alopecia neoplastica in breast cancer, and a bleeding nodule on the scalp in renal carcinoma. Clinicians need to be aware of clinical presentations of such metastases, because their detection can help make a primary diagnosis of a disease and restage a patient who has known disease, and may alter treatment strategies.

One should do a thorough skin examination, including the scalp, particularly on all cancer patients, and biopsy any new, persistent skin lesions. PDB and EMPD can represent direct extension of underlying carcinoma to the epidermis, and a workup for underlying malignancy must be considered to assist with treatment planning.

References

[1] Schwartz RA. Cutaneous metastatic disease. J Am Acad Dermatol 1995;33(2):161–82.

[2] Brodland DG, Zitelli JA. Mechanisms of metastasis. J Am Acad Dermatol 1992;27(1):1–8.

[3] Lambert WC, Schwartz RA. Metastasis. J Am Acad Dermatol 1992;27(1):131–2.

[4] Lookingbill DP, Spangler N, Sexton FM. Skin involvement as the presenting sign of internal carcinoma. J Am Acad Dermatol 1990;22(1):19–26.

[5] Cox SE, Cruz PD. A spectrum of inflammatory metastasis to skin via lymphatics: three cases of carcinoma erysipeloides. J Am Acad Dermatol 1994;30(2):304–7.

[6] Hayes AG, Berry AD. Cutaneous metastasis from squamous cell carcinoma of the cervix. J Am Acad Dermatol 1992;26(5):846–50.

[7] Mallon E, Dawber RPR. Alopecia neoplastica without alopecia: a unique presentation of breast carcinoma scalp metastasis. J Am Acad Dermatol 1994;31(2):319–21.

[8] Requena L, Sanchez YE, Nunez C, et al. Epidermotropically metastatic breast carcinomas: rare histopathologic variants mimicking melanoma and Paget's disease. Am J Dermatopathol 1996;18(4): 385–95.

[9] Rosen T. Cutaneous metastases. Med Clin North Am 1980;64(5):885–900.

[10] Hazelrigg DE, Rudolph AH. Inflammatory metastatic carcinoma. Arch Dermatol 1977;113(1):69–70.

[11] Brownstein MH, Helwig EB. Spread of tumors to the skin. Arch Dermatol 1973;107(1):80–6.

[12] Whitaker-Worth DL, Carlone V, Susser WS, et al. Dermatologic diseases of the breast and nipple. J Am Acad Dermatol 2000;43(5):733–51.

[13] Tschen EH, Apisarnthanarax P. Inflammatory metastatic carcinoma of the breast. Arch Dermatol 1981;117(2):120–1.

[14] Lookingbill DP, Spangler N, Helm KF. Cutaneous metastases in patients with metastatic carcinoma: a retrospective study of 4020 patients. J Am Acad Dermatol 1993;29(2):228–36.

[15] Niedt G. Paget's disease. In: Rigel DS, Friedman RJ, editors. Cancer of the skin. 1st edition. China: Elsevier Inc.; 2005. p. 303–9.

[16] Cohen I, Levy E, Schreiber H. Alopecia neoplastica due to breast carcinoma. Arch Dermatol 1961;84: 490–2.

[17] Saaed S, Keehn CA, Morgan MB. Cutaneous metastasis: a clinical, pathological and immunohistochemical appraisal. J Cutan Pathol 2004;31(6): 419–30.

[18] Brownstein MH, Helwig AB. Patterns of cutaneous metastasis. Arch Dermatol 1972;105(6):862–8.

[19] Sidiqqui MA, Zaman MN. Primary carcinoma en cuirasse. J Am Geriatr Soc 1996;44(2): 221–2.

[20] Mullinax K, Cohen JB. Carcinoma en cuirasse presenting as keloids of the chest. Dermatol Surg 2004;30(2):226–8.

[21] Fergusson MA, White BA, Johnson DE, et al. Carcinoma en cuirasse of the scrotum: an unusual presentation of lung carcinoma metastatic to the scrotum. J Urol 1998;160(6):2154–5.

[22] Schwartz RA, Rubenstein DJ, Raventos A, et al. Inflammatory metastatic carcinoma of the parotid. Arch Dermatol 1984;120(6):796–7.

[23] Newcomb WD. Unusual cutaneous metastases in carcinoma of the breast. Lancet 1924;206:1056–7.

[24] Lin JH, Lee JY, Chao SC, et al. Telangiectatic metastatic breast carcinoma preceded by en cuirasse metastatic breast carcinoma. Br J Dermatol 2004; 151(2):506–25.

[25] Waisman M. Carcinoma of the inframammary crease. Arch Dermatol 1978;114(10):1520–1.

[26] Shamai-Lubovitz O, Rothem A, Ben-David E, et al. Cutaneous metastatic carcinoma of the breast mimicking malignant melanoma, clinically and histologically. J Am Acad Dermatol 1994;31(6): 1058–9.

[27] Rubinstein RY, et al. Cutaneous metastatic lung cancer: literature review and report of a tumor on the nose. Ear Nose Throat J 2000;79(2):96–7.

[28] Krathen RA, Orengo IF, Rosen T. Cutaneous metastasis: a meta-analysis of data. South Med J 2003;96(2):164–7.

[29] Mueller TJ, Wu H, Greenberg RE, et al. Cutaneous metastases from genitourinary malignancies. Urology 2004;63(6):1021–6.

[30] Powell FC, Cooper AJ, Massa M, et al. Sister Mary Joseph's nodule: a clinical and histologic study. J Am Acad Dermatol 1984;10(4):610–5.

[31] Schwartz RA, Fleishmann JS. Transitional cell carcinoma of the urinary tract presenting with a cutaneous metastasis. Arch Dermatol 1981;117(8): 513–5.

[32] Jaworsky C, Bergfeld WF. Metastatic transitional cell carcinoma mimicking zoster sine herpete. Arch Dermatol 1986;122(12):1357–8.

[33] Yamamoto T, Ohkubo H, Nishioka K. Cutaneous metastases from carcinoma of the cervix resemble acquired lymphangioma. J Am Acad Dermatol 1994;30(6):1031–2.

[34] Paydas S, Zorludemir S. Leukacmia cutis and leukaemic vasculitis. Br J Dermatol 2000;143(4):773–9.

[35] Jasim ZF, Cooke N, Sommerville JE, et al. Chronic lymphocytic leukaemia skin infiltrates affecting prominent parts of the face and the scalp. Br J Dermatol 2006;154(5):981–2.

[36] Miller MK, Strauchen JA, Nichols KY, et al. Concurrent chronic lymphocytic leukemia cutis and acute myelogenous leukemia cutis in a patient with untreated CLL. Am J Dermatopathol 2001;23(4): 334–40.

[37] Smeena S, James WD, Lynn M. Cutaneous manifestations of cancer. Curr Opin Oncol 1999;11(2): 139–52.

[38] Desch JK, Smoller BR. The spectrum of cutaneous disease in leukemias. J Cutan Pathol 1993;20(5): 407–10.

[39] Garcia-Rio I, Delgado-Jimenez Y, Aragues M, et al. A case of Grover's disease with syringoma-like features and leukemia cutis. J Cutan Pathol 2006; 33(6):443–6.

[40] Su WPD, Buechner SA, Li CY. Clinicopathologic correlations in leukemia cutis. J Am Acad Dermatol 1984;11(1):121–8.

[41] Agnew KL, Ruchlemer R, Catovsky D, et al. Cutaneous findings in chronic lymphocytic leukaemia. Br J Dermatol 2004;150(6):1129–35.

[42] Youssef AH, Zanetto U, Kaur MR, et al. Granulocytic sarcoma (lekaemia cutis) in association with basal cell carcinoma. Br J Dermatol 2006;154(1): 177–204.

[43] Smoller B. Other lymphoproliferative and myeloproliferative diseases. In: Bolognia JL, Jorizzo JL, editors. Dermatology, vol. 2. Philadelphia: Elsevier's Health Sciences; 2003. p. 1943–51.

[44] Smith JL, Butler JJ. Skin involvements in Hodgkin's disease. Cancer 1980;45(2):345–61.

[45] Guitart J, Fretzin D. Skin as the primary site of Hodgkin's disease: a case report of primary Hodgkin's disease and review of its relationship with non-Hodgkin's lymphoma. Am J Dermatopathol 1998;20(2):218–22.

[46] Sioutos N, Kerl H, Murphy SB, et al. Primary cutaneous Hodgkin's disease. Unique clinical morphologic and immunophenotypic findings. Am J Dermatopathol 1994;16(1):2–8.

[47] Dixon FC, Galea MH, Ellis IO, et al. Paget's disease of the nipple. Br J Surg 1991;78(6):722.

[48] Fu W, Mittel VK, Young SC. Paget disease of the breast. Am J Clin Oncol 2001;24(4):397–400.

[49] Jamali FR, Ricci A, Deckers PJ. Paget's disease of the nipple-areola complex. Surg Clin North Am 1996;76(2):365–81.

[50] Fu W, Lobocki CA, Silberberg BK, et al. Molecular markers in Paget disease of the breast. J Surg Oncol 2001;77(3):171–8.

[51] Rosen PP. Letters to the editor. Arch Pathol Lab Med 2002;126:1159.

[52] Anderson JM, Ariga R, Govil H, et al. Assessment of HER-2/Neu status by immunohistochemistry and fluorescence in situ hybridization in mammary Paget's disease and underlying carcinoma. Appl Immunohistochem Mol Morphol 2003;11(2):120–4.

[53] Kuan SF, Montag AG, Hart J, et al. Differential expression of mucin genes in mammary and extramammary Paget's disease. Am J Surg Pathol 2001; 25(12):1469–77.

[54] Marucci G, Betts CM, Golouh R, et al. Toker cells are probably precursors of Paget cell carcinoma: a morphological and ultrastructural description. Virchows Arch 2002;441(2):117–23.

[55] Soini Y. Claudins 2, 3, 4, and 5 in Paget's disease and breast carcinoma. Hum Pathol 2004;35(12): 1531–6.

[56] Sanchez-Carpintero I, Martinez MI, Mihm MC. Clinical and histopathologic observations of the action of imiquimod in an epithelioid hemangioendothelioma and Paget's mammary disease. J Am Acad Dermatol 2006;55(1):75–9.

[57] Lagios MD, Westdahl PR, Rose MR, et al. Paget's disease of the nipple. Cancer 1984;54(3):545–51.

[58] Mirer E, El Sayed F, Ammoury A, et al. Treatment of mammary and extramammary Paget's skin disease with topical imiquimod. J Dermatolog Treat. 2006;17(3):167–71.

[59] Kawase K, Dominick JD, Tucker SL, et al. Paget's disease of the breast: there is a role for breast-conserving therapy. Ann Surg Oncol 2004; 12(5):1–7.

[60] Shieh S, Dee AS, Cheney RT, et al. Photodynamic therapy for the treatment of extramammary Paget's disease. Br J Dermatol 2002;146(6):1000–5.

[61] Kohler S, Smoller BR. Gross cystic disease fluid protein-15 reactivity in extramammary Paget's disease with and without associated internal malignancy. Am J Dermatopathol 1996;18(2):118–23.

[62] Ohnishi T, Watanabbi S. The use of cytokeratin 7 and 20 in the diagnosis of primary and secondary extramammary Paget's disease. Br J Dermatol 142(2);243–7.

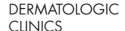
DERMATOLOGIC
CLINICS

ELSEVIER
SAUNDERS

Dermatol Clin 26 (2008) 103–119

Cutaneous Reactions to Chemotherapy: Commonly Seen, Less Described, Little Understood

Rachel E. Sanborn, MD[a],*, David A. Sauer, MD[b]

[a]Division of Hematology and Medical Oncology, Oregon Health and Science University,
3181 S.W. Sam Jackson Park Road, Mail Code L586, Portland, OR 97239-3098, USA
[b]Division of Pathology, Oregon Health and Science University, 3181 S.W. Sam Jackson Park Road,
Mail Code L471, Portland, OR 97239, USA

Over the past several decades, tremendous advances have been accomplished in the design and development of chemotherapeutic and molecularly targeted agents for the treatment of cancer. These advances have led to unprecedented improvements in survival and in quality of life for people suffering from cancer. Unfortunately, the gains in survival through therapy have not come without cost. Myelosuppression is the most common potentially life-threatening complication of chemotherapy, while peripheral neuropathy can compromise quality of life and interfere with the ability to carry out activities of daily living.

Undoubtedly the most common image associated with the idea of cancer and chemotherapy in the mind of the general population is that of hair loss, and the fear of this visible marker of a patient's illness leads to significant trepidation and hesitancy to consider taking chemotherapy. Alopecia is, however, only one example of the diverse ways in which chemotherapy and targeted therapies may affect the skin.

Hyperpigmentation, photosensitivity, acral erythema, and nail dystrophies may provide highly visible and even painful reminders of chemotherapy. Skin rashes from molecularly targeted agents are particularly problematic with certain classes of drugs. As with many nonchemotherapeutic drugs, physicians must vigilantly monitor for rare allergic and idiosyncratic reactions leading to Stevens-Johnson syndrome or toxic epidermal necrolysis. Extravasation of chemotherapy, with resultant severe tissue damage and potential for significant local necrosis, can be particularly devastating for patients.

The pathogenesis of these diverse cutaneous reactions for the most part remains unknown. Despite the large numbers of patients in the United States and worldwide who undergo chemotherapy for a myriad of different malignancies, the mechanisms of most cutaneous reactions remains speculative. Large scientific studies are lacking, and most information regarding the mechanisms of cutaneous reactions exists only in case reports and in anecdotally based limited patient series.

This review will focus on the major categories of cutaneous reactions to chemotherapy and molecularly targeted therapy, with a focus on the pathogenesis underlying the different reactions.

Alopecia

The pathogenesis of hair loss is perhaps the best understood of the cutaneous reactions to chemotherapy. Most chemotherapeutic agents affect cells undergoing mitosis by inducing varying types of DNA damage or by interfering with the function of mitotic spindle formation. Because most hair follicles, particularly those of the scalp, are in the active anagen phase most of the time, chemotherapeutic agents will interrupt replication of the hair matrix cells inducing premature catagen involutionary transformation and resultant weakened hair shafts prone to strand

* Corresponding author.
E-mail address: sanbornr@ohsu.edu (R.E. Sanborn).

0733-8635/08/$ - see front matter © 2008 Elsevier Inc. All rights reserved.
doi:10.1016/j.det.2007.08.006

breakage or cessation of hair shaft formation (Fig. 1) [1–4]. The resulting anagen effluvium first occurs within approximately 7 days of initiation of chemotherapy, with most hair loss occurring within the first 2 months.

It has been postulated that a disruption in the balance of Bcl-2 expression induced by chemotherapy is the etiologic factor leading to growth cessation. This has been correlated in mouse models, in which Bcl-2-overexpressing mice demonstrate increased alopecia, hair follicle dystrophy, and apoptosis after the administration of chemotherapy in comparison to wild-type mice [5]. Table 1 lists those chemotherapeutic agents most commonly associated with alopecia.

Although the traditional chemotherapeutic agents are most commonly associated with alopecia, the new molecularly targeted agents are additional culprits. Sorafenib, a molecularly targeted tyrosine kinase inhibitor against Raf, vascular endothelial growth factor receptor (VEGFR), platelet-derived growth factor receptor (PDGFR), and c-kit, has induced some degree of alopecia in up to half of patients receiving this therapy, with the causative mechanism at this point not understood [6]. As opposed to the skin rash and acral erythema induced by sorafenib, the alopecia does not appear to be dose related [7].

The small proportion of hair follicles in the telogen resting phase (approximately 10%) at the time of initiation of chemotherapy contributes to the incomplete and possibly patchy pattern of hair loss [8]. Ultimately, as these follicles enter the anagen phase during chemotherapy, hair loss will become complete as all hairs are affected. Given that the most rapidly dividing hair follicles exist on the scalp, scalp hair is the most prominently

Table 1
Chemotherapeutic agents most commonly associated with alopecia

Alkylating agents	Carmustine
	Chlorambucil
	Cyclophosphamide
	Dacarbazine
	Ifosfamide
	Mechlorethamine
	Melphalan
	Thiotepa
Anthracyclines	Daunorubicin
	Doxorubicin
	Epirubicin
	Idarubicin
Antimetabolites	Cytarabine
	5-Fluorouracil
	Hydroxyurea
	Methotrexate
Taxanes	Paclitaxel
	Docetaxel
Topoisomerase inhibitors	Irinotecan
	Topotecan
Vinca alkaloids	Vinblastine
	Vincristine
	Vinorelbine
Other mitotic inhibitors	Bleomycin
	Etoposide
	Mitomycin
	Mitoxantrone
Molecularly targeted therapy	Sorafenib

Data from Refs. [1,6,8].

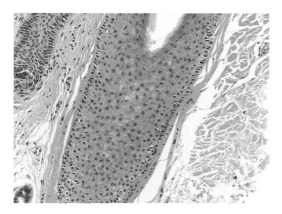

Fig. 1. Premature catagen transformation. Scattered apoptotic bodies (H&E, original magnification ×400).

and rapidly affected. Over time, however, all body hair may be affected, and total alopecia may occur [2,4,9].

There have been no proven methods to prevent hair loss. Cooling of the scalp during chemotherapy infusion was attempted in an effort to decrease blood flow to the region and decrease delivery of chemotherapy to the hair follicles. Scalp-cooling devices were banned by the Food and Drug Administration in 1990 because of lack of efficacy and safety data [2]. Topical minoxidil has met with limited success [10]. At this time, treatment of chemotherapy-induced alopecia remains primarily that of cosmetic and emotional support, with scalp coverings including wigs, hats, and other headwear.

In most patients undergoing chemotherapy, alopecia is temporary, with hair regrowth after withdrawal of the offending agents. Hair may grow back finer or more sparsely than previously. In some patients the texture of the hair may change (ie, previously straight hair may regrow curly) or color may change. The pathogenesis of this color and texture change, and predicting who will be affected, is not currently understood.

Acral erythema

The condition of acral erythema is also referred to as Burgdorf's syndrome, hand-foot syndrome, palmar-plantar erythrodysesthesia, or toxic erythema of the palms and soles. This condition refers to the development of dysesthesia over the palms and soles, followed by swelling and the formation of well-circumscribed erythematous macules [9, 11–13]. These lesions can progress to involve the entire palm and sole, and can involve the dorsal surfaces of hands or feet [1,2,13]. Erythema may be followed by blistering and superficial desquamation, with the bullous variant most commonly associated with cytarabine [1,2,13–15]. Re-epitheliazation can occur after withdrawal of the chemotherapeutic agent. While most commonly associated with hands and feet, involvement of other areas of the body have been reported, including the penis, trunk, and, in a patient who had previously undergone lower extremity amputation, the postamputation stump [16–18].

Histologically, mild epidermal spongiosis and basal vacuolar change, scattered apoptotic keratinocytes, and a sparse superficial perivascular lymphocytic infiltrate are demonstrated (Fig. 2) [3]. Papillary dermal edema and vascular dilatation may also be present [1,9,12,13]. The histologic evaluation may be important to differentiate from similarly appearing syndromes. Of note, the clinical and histologic appearance of acral erythema may be indistinguishable from acute graft-versus-host disease in patients undergoing hematologic transplant [1,12,13,19]. In patients with a concurrent cutaneous reaction such as Sweet syndrome, the development of acral erythema may be masked [20]. Leukocytoclastic vasculitis clinically resembling sorafenib-induced acral erythema has been documented [21].

Numerous chemotherapeutic agents have been associated with acral erythema, with the occurrence associated both with duration of infusion as well as with dosing of drugs [1,15,22–24]. 5-fluorouracil (5-FU) has a low incidence of acral erythema when administered as a bolus, but when given over a prolonged infusion time the incidence increases. Capecitabine, an oral precurser of 5-FU, mimics the prolonged infusion of the agent, and is consequently associated with a higher

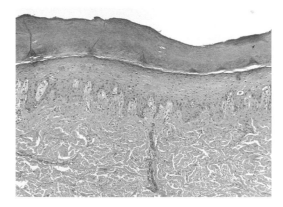

Fig. 2. Acral erythema. Basal vacuolar changes, scattered apoptotic keratinocytes and superficial perivascular lymphocytic infiltrate (H&E, original magnification ×200).

incidence of acral erythema [22]. In a phase II study of breast cancer patients treated with capecitabine, 56% developed acral erythema [22]. Liposomal doxorubicin has been associated with significant acral erythema as a dose-limiting effect [25]. Chemotherapeutic combinations may induce toxicity from either or all agents. In one prospective series, 36% of patients undergoing induction chemotherapy for acute myelogenous leukemia with cytosine arabinoside with daunorubicin or doxorubicin experienced acral erythema [12].

Sorafenib has induced acral erythema in 25% to 60% of patients undergoing therapy [6,7]. Sunitinib, a multitargeted tyrosine kinase inhibitor of VEGFR and PDGFR, may induce acral erythema in 20% of patients undergoing therapy [26]. Table 2 lists the chemotherapeutic agents most commonly associated with acral erythema.

The pathophysiology of acral erythema is not currently known. It has been hypothesized that a direct toxic effect on the skin is to blame, with factors of temperature gradient, difference of thickness of stratum corneum, absence of sebaceous glands and hair follicles, and the higher concentration of eccrine glands all contributing to the relative risk of the palms and soles [1,13]. The varying and unpredictable effects of acral erythema may be because the condition exists as a spectrum of inflammatory and reactive changes that have yet to be fully and accurately characterized [13].

There is no effective method of preventing acral erythema, although pyridoxine (vitamin B6) might be of modest benefit [27]. Withdrawal of the offending agent will allow for healing. Acral

Table 2
Chemotherapeutic agents most commonly associated with acral erythema

Alkylating agents	Cyclophosphamide
	Melphalan
	Thiotepa
Anthracyclines	Daunorubicin
	Doxorubicin (Including liposomal doxorubicin)
	Idarubicin
Antimetabolites	Capecitabine
	Cytarabine
	5-Fluorouracil
	Hydroxyurea
	Methotrexate
Platinum compounds	Cisplatin
Taxanes	Docetaxel
	Paclitaxel
Vinca alkaloids	Vincristine
Other mitotic inhibitors	Bleomycin
	Etoposide
	Mitomycin

Data from Refs. [1,2,13].

erythema may recur with repeat exposure but may be less severe [12]. Dose reductions may alleviate symptoms when continued administration is necessary [17]. Although the lesions typically resolve within 1 to 2 weeks of withdrawal of the agent, persistent dysesthesia and skin changes can occur [28]. This injects a note of caution that the "temporary" effect may be relative and quality of life can be significantly compromised.

Neutrophilic eccrine hidradenitis

Neutrophilic eccrine hidradenitis (NEH; also known as drug-induced eccrine hidradenitis) typically involves the trunk, extremities, head, and neck. The condition may manifest as either a painful or nonpainful macular, papular, plaquing, or pustular erythematous rash, within 1 to 2 weeks of starting chemotherapy, typically in concurrence with a fever [1,8,9]. The rash resolves with desquamation, usually without subsequent hyperpigmentation or scarring [1,9].

Histologically, NEH is characterized by an infiltrate of neutrophils around and within eccrine secretory coils with associated vacuolar degeneration and eccrine epithelial necrosis (Fig. 3) [1,3,8,9,11,29]. Mucinous degradation of the periadnexal fibroadipose tissue may also be present [9]. The disorder has been identified in patients with significant neutropenia, in which case the

dense neutrophilic infiltration is absent, but instead a lymphocytic infiltrate may be identified [1,8]. Apocrine glands can also be affected [30].

Table 3 lists the chemotherapeutic agents most commonly associated with NEH. Separate from chemotherapy, the hematopoietic growth factors G-CSF and GM-CSF may also induce NEH.

The pathogenesis of the condition has not been established. It has been hypothesized that direct toxic effect of the eccrine glands as a result of chemotherapy excretion is to blame [8,31]. However, compared with the large number of eccrine glands, relatively few areas are involved with NEH. The reason for involvement of discrete areas is not understood. Given that the condition may occur even in the presence of significant neutropenia, it is unlikely that a direct neutrophilic effect is the primary etiology [1]. The etiology is likely more complex, as the disorder has been demonstrated as a paraneoplastic syndrome in a patient who did not receive chemotherapy [32].

Therapy is again withdrawal of the offending agent. The condition is self-limiting and does not require therapy. Corticosteroids may have a limited role for painful lesions, but in an immunocompromised patient, the risk of infection must be weighed against potential benefit [33]. Treating recurrent NEH with dapsone has been reported, however the utility of this has yet to be fully established [34].

Epidermal dysmaturation

The term epidermal dysmaturation refers to a constellation of disrupted keratinocyte

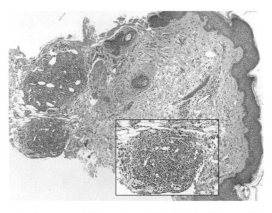

Fig. 3. Neutrophilic eccrine hidradenitis. Neutrophils infiltrating eccrine secretory coils with eccrine epithelial degeneration and necrosis (*inset*) (H&E, original magnification ×50 [inset, ×400]).

Table 3
Chemotherapeutic agents most commonly associated with neutrophilic eccrine hidradenitis

Alkylating agents	Chlorambucil
	Lomustine
Anthracyclines	Daunorubicin
	Doxorubicin
Antimetabolites	Cytarabine
Platinum compounds	Cisplatin
Vinca alkaloids	Vincristine
Other mitotic inhibitors	Bleomycin
	Mitoxantrone

Data from Refs. [1,8,9,31,34].

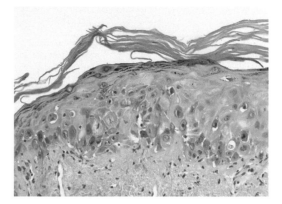

Fig. 4. Epidermal dysmaturation. Disrupted keratinocyte maturation, nuclear pleomorphism, mitoses above the basal layer, and apoptosis (H&E, original magnification ×630).

maturation with altered epidermal polarity, nuclear pleomorphism, mitoses above the basal layer and focal apoptosis (Fig. 4) [3,21]. It may be shown on biopsy to occur in the context of acral erythema, or, in the case of docetaxel, simultaneously with acral erythema or NEH [17,35].

The lesions may consist of scattered discrete maculopapular eruptions [36]. Docetaxel administration has been associated with the development of an erythematous, pruritic, well-demarcated nodule or plaque occurring proximal to the infusion site. These lesions are not associated with extravasation [17,37]. The pathogenesis of the reaction is unknown.

Eccrine squamous syringometaplasia

Eccrine squamous syringometaplasia is characterized by erythematous macules, papules, plaques, or vesicles, developing between 2 days and 5 weeks after chemotherapy. The eruption may be limited or generalized. The clinical picture is similar to neutrophilic eccrine hidradenitis, and in a similar fashion spontaneously resolves without scarring within 4 weeks [1,38].

The histologic pattern is that of squamous metaplasia of the eccrine ducts with relative sparing of the eccrine coils (Fig. 5) [3,38]. There may also be periductal stromal edema and fibroblastic proliferation with minimal epithelial necrosis and apoptosis [1,9]. As opposed to NEH, the upper portion of the eccrine duct is primarily affected, and neutrophilic infiltration is minimal or absent [1,9,31]. With docetaxel administration, eccrine squamous syringometaplasia may occur simultaneously with epidermal dysmaturation [35].

The pathogenesis of the reaction is unknown, but in a similar fashion to NEH, is thought to be secondary to a direct toxic effect upon the eccrine glands as a result of chemotherapy excretion in

sweat [1,9]. Chemotherapeutic agents associated with eccrine squamous syringometaplasia are listed in Table 4.

Hyperpigmentation

Cutaneous hyperpigmentation may manifest with a variety of presentations, and may be caused by numerous chemotherapeutic agents, with discoloration of the skin, mucous membranes, nails, or hair. The mechanism of the toxicity has not been studied or established, but is postulated to be a result of direct toxic effects on melanocytes, stimulating increased melanin secretion [1,8,9]. The histologic appearance may be varied, but may demonstrate a subtle increase in pigmented

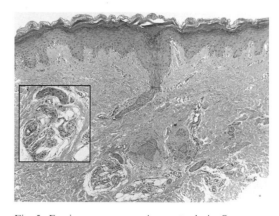

Fig. 5. Eccrine squamous syringometaplasia. Squamous metaplasia of eccrine ducts with sparing of eccrine coils (*inset*) (H&E, original magnification ×100 [inset, ×400]).

Table 4
Chemotherapeutic agents most commonly associated
with eccrine squamous syringometaplasia

Alkylating agents	Cyclophosphamide
Anthracyclines	Daunorubicin
	Doxorubicin
Antimetabolites	Cytarabine
	5-Fluorouracil
	Methotrexate
Platinum compounds	Cisplatin
Taxanes	Docetaxel
Other mitotic inhibitors	Bleomycin
	Etoposide
	Mitoxantrone

Data from Refs. [1,9,31,35].

Table 5
Chemotherapeutic agents most commonly associated
with hyperpigmentation

Alkylating agents	Busulfan
	Cyclophosphamide
	Ifosfamide
	Treosulfan
Anthracyclines	Daunorubicin
	Doxorubicin
Antimetabolites	5-Fluorouracil
	Hydroxyurea
	Methotrexate
Platinum compounds	Cisplatin
Taxanes	Docetaxel
	Paclitaxel
Other mitotic inhibitors	Bleomycin
	Etoposide
	Mitoxantrone

Data from Refs. [1,2,4,8,31,41,43].

melanocytes at the dermal-epidermal junction with melanophages in the papillary dermis, where there is also a sparse superficial and perivascular lymphocytic infiltrate (Fig. 6) [3]. There may also be accompanying spongiosis and focal parakeratosis [39]. Table 5 lists the chemotherapeutic agents most commonly associated with cutaneous hyperpigmentation.

Different chemotherapeutic agents demonstrate characteristic manifestations of hyperpigmentation. Bleomycin may induce hyperpigmentation in up to 20% of patients receiving the agent, with the most common areas of pigmentation occurring over pressure points, including fingers, elbows, or knees, although generalized hyperpigmentation also may occur [8]. Flagellate hyperpigmentation occurs most commonly on the trunk, in a linear-type pattern reminiscent or suggestive of excoriation. Flagellate hyperpigmentation may occur at

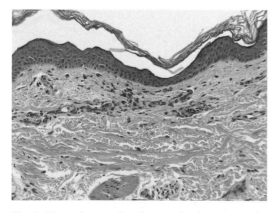

Fig. 6. Hyperpigmentation. Increased melanocytes at the dermal-epidermal junction, dermal melanophages and a sparse superficial lymphocytic infiltrate (H&E, original magnification ×400).

previous sites of minor trauma, including irritation from clothing. The hyperpigmented lesions may be heralded by pruritis, and have been documented to occur in the presence of urticarial plaques, but also have occurred without pruritis [39]. It has been suggested that the mechanism of action of bleomycin hyperpigmentation relates to the absence in skin of an inactivating enzyme for bleomycin, which leads to elevated chemotherapeutic concentrations and thus toxicity [40].

Agents such as busulfan and cyclophosphamide have been associated with a more generalized hyperpigmentation [4,8]. Treosulfan, an alkylating agent with similar structure to busulfan, can cause similar patterns of hyperpigmentation [41]. 5-FU may induce generalized hyperpigmentation as well as discrete hyperpigmentation over veins used in drug infusion [8,42]. Docetaxel has been associated with similar but erythematous supravenous discoloration over the arm receiving the infusion [43]. It may be manifested by well-circumscribed hyperpigmentation over the veins of the extremity through which chemotherapy was infused.

Hyperpigmentation generally fades with withdrawal of the agent. Repeat systemic exposure may induce a recall reaction and flare of previous hyperpigmentation, even when the site of infusion is changed to a different extremity [44]. Reticulate pigmentation in a pattern similar to bleomycin flagellate hyperpigmentation has been seen with docetaxel, leading to the suggestion that the mechanism of toxicity may be similar between the two agents, and the reactivation of tissue toxicity proposed as a contributing factor [44,45].

Chemotherapy and radiation recall and sensitivity reactions

Cutaneous recall reactions are most commonly thought to occur as a result of exposure to the combination of chemotherapy and radiation, with an inflammatory chemotherapy-induced reaction occurring at sites of previous radiation therapy. This may include recall of previous significant, or even mild, sunburn [4,46,47]. Chemotherapeutic agents may also induce recall reactions at sites of previous chemotherapy extravasation, or at locations of previous chemotherapy infusion [19,48]. Table 6 lists the chemotherapeutic agents most commonly associated with chemotherapy and radiation recall.

One case report described tender nodule formation occurring at the location of multiple previous venipuncture sites for chemotherapy infusion in a patient without a history of extravasation. Biopsies demonstrated nonspecific septal and lobular panniculitis, which resolved spontaneously. It was suggested that "microextravasation" that may have occurred at the time of each chemotherapy infusion could have led to subclinical tissue damage that manifested with clinical findings at the time of systemic infusion of 5-FU and gemcitabine [49].

The mechanism of induction of the radiation or chemotherapy recall reaction is not understood. These reactions may manifest years after the initial exposure [4]. It has been proposed that underlying genetic defects induced by the initial

Table 6
Chemotherapeutic agents most commonly associated with chemotherapy and radiation recall

Alkylating agents	Cyclophosphamide
	Melphalan
Anthracyclines	Daunorubicin
	Doxorubicin
Antimetabolites	Cytarabine
	5-Fluorouracil
	Gemcitabine
	Hydroxyurea
	Methotrexate
Taxanes	Docetaxel
	Paclitaxel
Vinca alkaloids	Vinblastine
Other mitotic inhibitors	Bleomycin
	Dactinomycin
	Etoposide
	Mitomycin
Antiestrogens	Tamoxifen

Data from Refs. [1,2,4,9,31,49–54].

toxic insult may predispose the skin to development of the reactions at the time of free-radical formation with the new exposure [46]. The etiology of the reaction may vary with the different chemotherapeutic agents.

Methotrexate has been shown to cause recall of sun or radiation exposure with varying time delays between exposure to chemotherapy and to sun or radiation [50]. The recall reaction may occur with days or weeks between the exposures or sunburns, and may spare chronically sun-exposed areas [51,52]. Photosensitivity has not been shown to occur with simultaneous exposures to methotrexate and radiation, separating the reaction from that of a photosensitizing agent (discussed later [50,52]). Delayed radiation recall has been seen even with tamoxifen, an estrogen agonist/antagonist that is not a standard chemotherapeutic agent [53].

Classically the chemotherapy or radiation recall reaction involves a discrete, well-demarcated area of the skin outlining the previous radiation field. This reaction may become diffuse in patients who have previously received diffuse radiation. One case report details a patient initially treated with whole-body electron beam radiation for leukemia cutis. This was followed by induction chemotherapy with doxorubicin and cytosine arabinoside. The patient developed rapid and widespread radiation recall reaction with resultant toxic epidermal necrolysis [54].

Biopsy specimens may demonstrate follicular hyperkeratosis, follicular pustule formation, dermal sclerosis, and vascular or stromal atypia. Ballooning degeneration of epidermal keratinocytes may be seen on biopsy, as well as a mixed inflammatory infiltrate. Acanthosis and occasional epidermal cell apoptosis may also be seen [46,47].

Separately from a recall effect, concurrent administration of sensitizing chemotherapeutic agents with radiation has been shown to have additive, and sometimes synergistic, therapeutic effects. In addition to rendering the tumor more sensitive to radiation and chemotherapeutic damage, increased toxicity is demonstrated in normal tissues, including the skin. Cutaneous hyperpigmentation can very quickly develop in the setting of combined-modality chemoradiation therapy, which may in some cases be permanent. Sensitizing chemotherapeutic agents include adriamycin, 5-FU, gemcitabine, cisplatin, etoposide, and the taxanes [8,9,42].

Phototoxic dermatitis

Increased sensitivity to sun exposure may be manifested with exposure to multiple chemotherapeutic agents. Sun sensitivity may manifest in a variety of ways, including increased tendency for erythematous sunburn, hyperpigmentation in areas of sun exposure, and rash occurring on sun-exposed skin [42,55,56].

With 5-FU, sun exposure may produce any of the above reactions. In patients with erythematous reaction after even mild sun exposure, the reaction may fade over time, or may be followed by secondary hyperpigmentation [42]. The mechanism of sun sensitivity is not understood, although the combined effects of DNA damage and chemotherapy-induced epidermal thinning have been proposed [42]. In the case of dacarbazine, either the accumulation of the metabolite 2-azahypoxanthine in the skin or a decrease in metabolizing enzymes in the skin leading to drug accumulation have been postulated to induce phototoxic dermatitis through induction of injury to the epidermal cells [57]. Given that vinblastine has been shown to induce significant phototoxic dermatitis shortly after administration, with even minimal sunlight exposure, other mechanisms of toxicity likely contribute that have yet to be elucidated [55]. Severe phototoxic reactions may induce subtotal epidermal necrosis with a sparse superficial and deep dermal infiltrate of lymphocytes (Fig. 7) [3].

Inflammation of actinic keratoses

Preexisting actinic keratoses experience transient inflammation with exposure to certain chemotherapeutic agents. This was first described in patients undergoing therapy with 5-FU [42]. Subsequent to this discovery, 5-FU has been used in the topical therapy of actinic keratoses [58]. Doxorubicin has additionally been identified as a causative agent, as well as sorafenib [59]. In the common situation in which a patient is receiving multiple chemotherapeutic agents simultaneously, identification of a single causative agent may not be possible [58].

It is unclear whether the combination of chemotherapy and sun exposure leads to a more intense local inflammatory reaction or whether a different mechanism is at work to cause the reaction, such as a direct toxic effect on the higher number of cells undergoing DNA synthesis within and around actinic keratoses [42,58]. The inflammation generally improves with the application of topical steroids [31]. Actinic keratosis inflammation does not preclude further chemotherapy administration [1,58].

Extravasation

Extravasation is defined as the leakage of chemotherapeutic drugs into the surrounding tissues. Extravasation injuries remain uncommon, with estimated incidence published in the literature of between 0.1% and 6% in patients receiving chemotherapy [60]. The published rate is likely an underestimation, however, as many cases of extravasation go unreported.

Chemotherapeutic agents are divided into the classification categories of irritants or vesicants, depending on the potential for localized toxicity and tissue damage. Many chemotherapeutic agents may overlap the definitions of irritants or vesicants, and have the capacity to act as either. Table 7 lists chemotherapeutic agents most commonly classified as irritants. Table 8 summarizes chemotherapeutic agents most commonly classified as vesicants.

Irritants

Irritants are defined as agents that produce local inflammation, pain, tightness, or phlebitis either at the site of injection or along the vein. Irritants may induce local sclerosis or hyperpigmentation, but do not induce tissue necrosis. The symptoms of the local reaction after extravasation are typically self-limiting, most commonly without long-term sequelae [1].

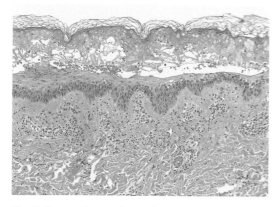

Fig. 7. Severe phototoxic reaction with epidermal necrosis, basal regeneration, and sparse superficial and deep lymphocytic inflammation (H&E, original magnification ×200).

Table 7
Chemotherapeutic agents most commonly classified as irritants

Alkylating agents	Cyclophosphamide
	Ifosfamide
	Melphalan
Antimetabolites	5-Fluorouracil
	Gemcitabine
Platinum compounds	Carboplatin
Taxanes	Docetaxel
	Paclitaxel
Topoisomerase inhibitors	Irinotecan
	Topotecan
Other mitotic inhibitors	Bleomycin
	Etoposide

Data from Refs. [1,60,61].

Although case reports of local interventions including glycerine, chlorhexidine, and dimethyl-sulfoxide (DMSO) have been published for the treatment of docetaxel extravasation, it is not clear that the application of an antidote for irritant extravasation is indicated or more effective than local palliative measures [61].

Vesicants

Vesicants have the ability to induce tissue necrosis, with resultant potential for severe and long-lasting injury and local damage. The full effect of the extravasation injury is not usually immediately apparent; but may evolve over days

Table 8
Chemotherapeutic agents most commonly classified as vesicants

Alkylating agents	Dacarbazine
	Melphalan
Anthracyclines	Daunorubicin
	Doxorubicin (Including liposomal doxorubicin)
	Idarubicin
Antimetabolites	5-Fluorouracil
Platinum compounds	Cisplatin
Taxanes	Docetaxel
	Paclitaxel
Vinca alkaloids	Vinblastine
	Vincristine
	Vinorelbine
Other mitotic inhibitors	Bleomycin
	Dactinomycin
	Etoposide
	Mitomycin

Data from Refs. [1,2,19,60,62,65,69,70].

or weeks. Early local symptoms of a vesicant extravasation resemble those of an irritant extravasation: local pain, erythema, burning, pruritis, or swelling [1,62]. Over the course of the reaction, however, as tissue necrosis evolves and becomes clinically apparent, progressive erythema, discoloration, blistering, or desquamation may develop. The severity of the local reaction may vary both upon the agent extravasated as well as upon the total dose of extravasated material. Published patient series have estimated that only approximately one third of vesicant extravasations will progress to tissue ulceration [63].

The local necrosis may heal with conservative management, leaving minimal long-term sequelae, or may progress to significant eschar formation and tissue ulceration that ultimately require surgical debridement and intervention, with long-term morbidity for the patient. Ulceration after vesicant extravasation is typically marked by delayed healing. Morbidity may consist of cosmetic defects, chronic pain, or loss of function secondary to contractures or neuropathy, even in the absence of ulceration of skin [64]. Repeat infusion of the offending agent, even in another limb, may induce a recall reaction at the site of extravasation [48]. One case of squamous cell carcinoma of the skin was documented at the site of a doxorubicin extravasation 10 years previously [65].

Depending on the total dose of extravasated chemotherapy, and upon the location of the extravasation, necrosis may involve underlying tissues such as nerves, vessels, or tendons. The degree of damage to these underlying structures tends to occur in areas where there is relatively little underlying subcutaneous fat, such as the dorsum of the hand, antecubital fossa, and chest wall.

The pathogenesis of the severe tissue damage of vesicant chemotherapeutic agents is not fully understood. Agents that bind to DNA induce more damage than non-DNA–binding drugs [62,66]. It has been postulated that as cells affected by DNA-binding chemotherapeutic agents die, the agent is taken up by surrounding cells, causing progressive and prolonged local damage [66]. This has particularly been suggested to be the case for the severe tissue damage seen with doxorubicin extravasation [62]. Additionally, the significant free radical formation of vesicant agents are suggested as a potential mechanism of the severe necrotic effect [67].

Treatment of a vesicant extravasation includes immediate cessation of infusion, aspiration of as much extravasated drug as possible through the still-intact catheter, and attempts at aspiration of the extravasated agent in the surrounding tissue. This aspiration may help to limit the extent of tissue damage. Application of cold packs in theory helps to increase degradation of toxic metabolites through vasoconstriction and localization of drug, in addition to providing symptomatic pain relief. Hot packs increase local vasodilation, diluting the extravasated drug. Cold packs should not be administered in the event of extravasation of vinca alkaloids; increased tissue ulceration has been demonstrated in animal models with the use of cold packs [68].

The local application of antidotes to different chemotherapeutic agents is based on very limited data. Sodium thiosulfate is recommended as an effective antidote for mechlorethamine cisplatin [60]. Hyaluronidase has been recommended for extravasation of vinca alkaloids [69]. The mechanism of action in prevention of tissue damage is not fully understood and has not been extensively studied. Hyaluronidase has been suggested to act via temporary breakdown of hyaluronic acid, which holds together tissue planes, and subsequent facilitation of drug dispersement and dilution [64].

Topical application of DMSO has been proposed to help prevent significant tissue necrosis in animal and in human models. The pathophysiology of the interaction is not known, although free-radical scavenging and facilitation of elimination of drug from local tissues are postulated pathways of efficacy [63]. Procedures such as liposuction or saline flushout have been proposed through a single-institution series, but have not met with widespread usage [64].

Dexrazoxane, employed for protection of anthracycline-induced cardiotoxicity, has been evaluated in animal models and demonstrated to be protective against local tissue damage and ulceration in anthracycline extravasation [70]. Potent free-radical scavenging effects are suggested as the mechanism of protection from tissue damage.

Hypersensitivity

Although any drug may induce a hypersensitivity reaction in an individual recipient, certain chemotherapeutic and molecularly targeted agents have a higher incidence of hypersensitivity reactions. The hypersensitivity reactions tend to be type I hypersensitivity reactions, and may range from transient urticaria to a pruritic maculopapular rash to an anaphylactic response [4]. The inciting agent may be either the chemotherapeutic drug itself (such as is the case with asparaginase), or may be secondary to the solubility vehicles (as is the case for paclitaxel, which is dissolved in cremophor [2]). Molecularly targeted antibody agents such as rituximab, cetuximab, and trastuzumab are associated with hypersensitivity reactions in 3.5% to 18% of patients [2,71–73].

The pathogenesis of hypersensitivity reactions is poorly understood, with immune-mediated reactions nonspecifically blamed [2]. Pretreatment prophylaxis with dexamethasone, or a combination of dexamethasone with H1 and H2 blockers, is generally required for patients receiving asparaginase or the taxanes [2]. Despite the incidence of hypersensitivity with the molecularly targeted antibodies, histamine blockers are commonly administered before therapy, but steroid prophylaxis is not routinely required [71–73]. Table 9 summarizes the chemotherapeutic agents most commonly associated with hypersensitivity reactions.

Table 9
Chemotherapeutic agents most commonly associated with hypersensitivity reactions

Alkylating agents	Busulfan
	Chlorambucil
	Cyclophosphamide
	Ifosfamide
	Melphalan
	Thiotepa
Anthracyclines	Daunorubicin
	Doxorubicin
Antiangiogenic agents	Thalidomide
Antimetabolites	Cytarabine
	5-Fluorouracil
	Gemcitabine
	Methotrexate
Molecularly targeted agents	Cetuximab
	Rituximab
	Sorafenib
	Trastuzumab
Nitrogen mustards	Mechlorethamine
Platinum compounds	Carboplatin
	Cisplatin
Taxanes	Docetaxel
	Paclitaxel
Other mitotic inhibitors	Asparaginase
	Bleomycin
	Etoposide
	Mithramycin
	Mitomycin

Data from Refs. [2,4,19,31,71–76,78–80,83,84].

Cutaneous hypersensitivity reactions may additionally manifest along a spectrum of reactions that includes erythema multiforme, Stevens-Johnson syndrome, and toxic epidermal necrolysis (TEN). Erythema multiforme may develop within several weeks of exposure to the chemotherapeutic agent, and may be either localized to an area near the infusion or diffuse [74,75]. The reaction has been seen with the nitrogen mustards, with 5-FU in combination with mitomycin C, and with sorafenib [74–76]. On physical examination, lesions may consist of erythematous papules with central clearing, although macular lesions or bullae may also be seen. Histologic examination demonstrates epidermal cell necrosis within and above the basal layer with vacuolar change and a lichenoid lymphocytic infiltrate which obscures the dermal-epidermal junction (Fig. 8) [3]. Spongiosis, dilation of the dermal vessels, a perivascular infiltrate and fragmentation of the dermal collagen fibers may also be seen [74,75].

Stevens-Johnson syndrome, defined as cutaneous erythema multiforme in addition to involvement of at least two mucosal sites, may occur as an idiosyncratic reaction to a variety of drugs. It has been documented with topical nitrogen mustard, with dense mononuclear cell infiltrate, extensive epidermal keratinocyte necrosis, and dermoepidermal separation [76]. As with erythema multiforme, the pathogenesis of the reaction is not understood, but is associated with a cell-mediated hypersensitivity reaction [76]. In cases of multidrug administration, a single causative agent may not be able to be clearly elucidated, or alternatively the effects of multiple agents may have synergistic activity [77,78].

The antiangiogenic agent thalidomide has been associated with diffuse exfoliative erythroderma as well as with fulminant TEN, the life-threatening condition of epidermal detachment existing as the most severe aspect of the erythema multiforme/Stevens-Johnson/TEN spectrum [79,80]. In TEN there is subepidermal bulla formation with confluent epidermal necrosis (Fig. 9) [3]. Although the mechanism of action of thalidomide induction of TEN is not fully understood, it is the best studied of the chemotherapeutic agents in this regard. The release and action of tumor necrosis factor-α (TNF-α), inducing keratinocyte apoptosis and causing the associated constitutional symptoms including fever, has been postulated as the main culprit of TEN.

As thalidomide is additionally a TNF-α inhibitor, it was examined in a randomized, placebo-controlled trial of patients suffering from TEN. The main end points of the trial were the progression of skin detachment after day 7 of therapy and overall mortality. After 22 patients were randomized, the trial was discontinued early when an unexpected increase in mortality was noted in the thalidomide arm (83% versus the expected 30% rate in the placebo arm). It was suggested in this study that thalidomide had the ability to paradoxically enhance TNF-α production in some situations, thereby increasing the mortality in TEN [81]. Although steroids are commonly employed among therapies for TEN, one institutional series suggested that skin reactions were more

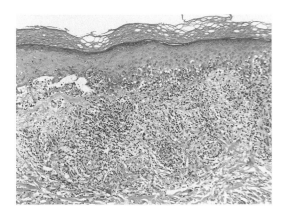

Fig. 8. Erythema multiforme. Epidermal cell necrosis, vacuolar change, and obscuring of the dermal-epidermal junction by a lichenoid lymphocytic infiltrate (H&E, original magnification ×200).

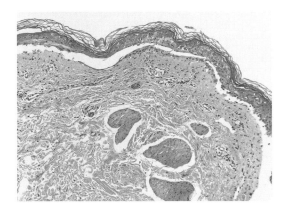

Fig. 9. Toxic epidermal necrolysis. Subepidermal bullae with confluent epidermal necrosis and a sparse perivascular lymphocytic infiltrate (H&E, original magnification ×100).

severe in patients receiving thalidomide in combination with dexamethasone in the treatment of multiple myeloma [82]. Other agents associated with TEN include mithramycin, methotrexate, and cytosine arabinoside [83,84].

Hydroxyurea dermopathy

Hydroxyurea is an oral agent used in the treatment of myeloproliferative disorders, as well as sickle cell disease. The chronicity of these diseases leads to long-term administration of the drug. In addition to lower leg ulcers (typically developing over the malleolar regions and associated with minor trauma), a characteristic dermopathy has been associated with long-term use of hydroxyurea [85–87].

The dermopathy consists of a lichenoid, papular, erythematous, and scaling eruption developing over the hands and feet, occurring several years after starting therapy with hydroxyurea. The dorsal surfaces are affected more commonly than the palms and soles. Histologically, the eruption demonstrates hyperparakeratosis and parakeratosis overlying a thickened epidermis with epidermal cell atypia, mitoses, and necrosis with a sparse lichenoid lymphocytic infiltrate and vacuolar alteration (Fig. 10). There may also be thickening of the basement membrane in chronic reactions [3,87].

The mechanism of the reaction is unknown, but is postulated to be secondary to prolonged cytostatic effects on the epidermal keratinocytes, as well as impairment of cellular repair

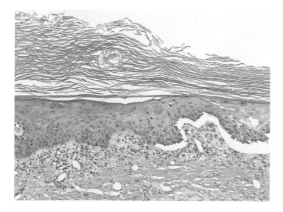

Fig. 10. Hydroxyurea dermopathy. Epidermal hyperplasia, parakeratosis, vacuolar change, lichenoid lymphocytic infiltrate, and epidermal cell atypia, mitoses, and apoptoses (H&E, original magnification ×400).

mechanisms. This may be supported by the development of skin atrophy as the reaction resolves [87].

Targeted therapy

The past decade has been marked with the explosive development of new molecularly targeted agents for the treatment of cancer [88]. Although in theory the development of the targeted drugs was intended to improve therapeutic efficacy while reducing toxicity in comparison to standard chemotherapeutic agents, the novel molecularly targeted agents have demonstrated significant toxicity as well. Cutaneous toxicities of the targeted agents fitting the classic chemotherapeutic toxicity descriptions are discussed in their respective sections of this article. Some targeted therapies have demonstrated more unique cutaneous toxicities and are discussed here.

Perhaps the most widely recognized cutaneous toxicity of molecularly targeted therapy is the acneiform skin rash associated with epidermal growth factor receptor (EGFR) inhibition. A variety of EGFR-targeted agents have been developed, both as intracellular tyrosine kinase inhibitors as well as monoclonal antibodies targeted against the extracellular receptor protein [89–92]. All EGFR-targeted agents are associated with a characteristic papular and pustular rash most commonly located on the face, scalp, chest, and back. The time of onset is typically within 1 to 2 weeks after initiating therapy with an EGFR inhibitor. This may consist of an erythematous papular rash with a pustular component, frequently associated with pruritis and generalized dry skin. The pustules are not preceded by classic comedones as in acne vulgaris, the common form of acne. Painful cracking and fissuring on the hands and feet are common. The rash tends to fade over time. The reasons for the variability of severity and duration of the eruption are poorly understood.

Histologically, the rash is characterized by a perifollicular lymphocytic infiltrate or a suppurative neutrophilic folliculitis [93]. Thinning and compaction of the stratum corneum is demonstrated [94]. While the EGFR-related folliculitis is sterile, a secondary suprainfection may commonly occur. The etiology of the rash is not fully understood, but is thought to be because EGFR is expressed in the skin, including the epidermis and follicles (as well as eccrine and sebaceous glands), resulting in cutaneous EGFR inhibition [93–96]. An EGFR-knockout mouse model demonstrates mice with thin epidermis and disorganized hair follicle formation [97]. Epidermal inhibition of EGFR would be expected to produce epidermal thinning through inhibition of keratinocyte proliferation, however the mechanism by which this inhibition results in the acneiform eruption is not understood [98].

EGFR inhibition can also induce sterile paronychial inflammation. The pathophysiology behind this toxicity beyond EGFR inhibition and impairment of keratinocyte maturation around the nail bed is not understood. The nail bed disruption induced by the paronychial inflammation may lead to painful secondary suprainfection.

The skin rash tends to fade over time even without intervention. Dose reduction of the causative agent may be required for a symptomatic rash or for paronychial inflammation. The rash does not respond to standard acne therapy, although secondary bacterial suprainfection may require antibiotics. Symptomatic management for dry skin is indicated. Symptoms resolve upon withdrawal of the offending agent.

Although the EGFR inhibitors are associated with less alopecia than standard chemotherapeutic agents, alopecia can develop after prolonged use of the agent. Conversely, excessive hair growth may also be seen, especially on the face [99]. This is a particularly problematic cosmetic issue for women, as many hair removal and bleaching methods may aggravate the underlying skin rash [100]. Again, EGFR-knockout mouse models demonstrate hypertrichosis with curly hair and whiskers, and eventual alopecia [97,101,102]. This assists in confirming the direct inhibition of EGFR on the hair follicle as the culprit.

Sorafenib may induce a skin rash separate from the acral erythema. This may be characterized by diffuse erythema, and may progress to desquamation [6]. The mechanism of action is thought to be possibly secondary to indirect EGFR inhibition through interruption of the mitogen-activated protein kinase pathway [21].

Nail dystrophy

Chemotherapeutic agents can cause a variety of nail changes, from hyperpigmentation to ridging of the nail plate to premature separation of the nail plate (onycholysis). Nail hyperpigmentation is most commonly associated with doxorubicin, 5-FU, and cyclophosphamide [42,103,104]. Transverse leukonychia, also known as Beau-Reil lines, are white transverse lines that develop on the nails during chemotherapy. The appearance of the lines seems to correlate with chemotherapy cycles, with solitary or multiple ridges typically spaced 2 to 3 mm apart [31,105].

The histologic appearance of transverse leukonychia is not well described, as patients are generally reluctant to undergo a nail biopsy for what is largely perceived as a cosmetic finding. The lines move distally as chemotherapy is stopped, and resolve with nail outgrowth after cessation of chemotherapy. The pathogenesis of transverse leukonychia has been postulated to be secondary to transient cessation of growth of the nail plate with exposure to chemotherapy [105,106]. Docetaxel, mitoxantrone, doxorubicin, vincristine, and cyclophosphamide have all been implicated as common causative agents, although many patients with nail ridging receive combination regimens, with a single causative agent not clearly defined [107]. Sorafenib has been associated with transverse leukonychia as well.

Onycholysis (separation of the nail plate) tends to occur most commonly on the great toes. Thickening and ridging of the nail may be associated with onycholysis, occurring in the absence of fungal infection, and may result in complete loss of the nail [108,109]. It has been associated with mitoxantrone, as well as with doxorubicin and paclitaxel [108,109]. The pathogenesis of the nail plate separation is not understood, but the condition resolves with cessation of chemotherapy [108]. A correlation with sun exposure to the affected nails has been suggested in one patient series [109].

Summary

Despite the frequency of cutaneous toxicities with chemotherapeutic and molecularly targeted agents used in cancer therapy as well as the stark visibility of these toxicities, little is understood about the pathogenesis of the reactions. Cutaneous toxicities such as acral erythema, hyperpigmentation, and nail dystrophy may occur commonly, yet little is published outside of small patient series and case reports. Many conditions are inadequately histologically described. This is likely because of reluctance on the part of both patients and health care providers to perform a biopsy in a patient already experiencing "enough" toxicity from the cancer and the therapy without an added invasive procedure.

Therapy for the cutaneous toxicities of chemotherapeutic agents remains largely supportive, with withdrawal of the offending agent as the most effective means of alleviating toxicity. Small series or case reports may indicate possible treatment options, but most remain largely unproven. Greater understanding of the pathogenesis of the cutaneous toxicities may lead to more effective and more specific interventions, and may additionally allow for improved delivery of chemotherapy in the treatment of a malignancy.

A greater understanding of the causative mechanisms of cutaneous toxicities, particularly in the case of the molecularly targeted agents, may also improve understanding of intracellular signaling pathways in both the skin and the cancer cells. This understanding may provide not only the knowledge with which to avoid such toxicities in the design of future agents, but also the knowledge with which to more optimally and more lethally target malignant cells.

References

[1] Susser WS, Whitaker-Worth DL, Grant-Kels JM. Mucocutaneous reactions to chemotherapy. J Am Acad Dermatol 1999;40:367–98.

[2] Alley E, Green R, Schuchter L. Cutaneous toxicities of cancer therapy. Current Opinion in Oncology 2002;14:212–6.

[3] Weedon D. Skin pathology. 2nd edition. Edinbugh, UK: Elsevier Science Ltd; 2002.

[4] Hood AF. Cutaneous side effects of cancer chemotherapy. Med Clin North Am 1986;70:187–209.

[5] Muller-Rover S, Rossiter H, Paus R, et al. Overexpression of Bcl-2 protects from ultraviolet B-induced apoptosis but promotes hair follicle regression and chemotherapy-induced alopecia. Am J Pathol 2000;156:1395–405.

[6] Ratain MJ, Eisen T, Stadler WM, et al. Phase II placebo-controlled randomized discontinuation trial of sorafenib in patients with metastatic renal cell carcinoma. J Clin Oncol 2006;16:2505–12.

[7] Strumberg D, Awada A, Hirte H, et al. Pooled safety analysis of BAY 43-9006 (sorafenib) monotherapy in patients with advanced solid tumours: Is rash associated with treatment outcome? Eur J Cancer 2006;42:548–56.

[8] Bolognia JL, Jorizzo JL, Rapini RP, editors. Dermatology. St. Louis (MO): Mosby; 2003.

[9] McKee PH, Calonje E, Granter SR, editors. Pathology of the skin. 3rd edition. St. Louis (MO): Mosby; 2005.

[10] Duvic M, Lemak NA, Valero V, et al. A randomized trial of minoxidil in chemotherapy-induced alopecia. J Am Acad Dermatol 1996;35:74–8.

[11] Remlinger KA. Cutaneous reactions to chemotherapy drugs: The art of consultation. Arch Dermatol 2003;139:77–81.

[12] Demircay Z, Gurbuz O, Alpdogan TB, et al. Chemotherapy-induced acral erythema in leukemic patients: A report of 15 cases. Int J Dermatol 1997;36: 593–8.

[13] Baack BR, Burgdorf WHC. Chemotherapy-induced acral erythema. J Am Acad Dermatol 1991; 24:457–61.

[14] Waltzer JF, Flowers FP. Bullous variant of chemotherapy-induced acral erythema. Arch Dermatol 1993;129:43–4.

[15] Hellier I, Bessis D, Sotto MA, et al. High-dose methotrexate-induced bullous variant of acral erythema. Arch Dermatol 1996;132:590–1.

[16] Sorscher SM. Penile involvement with hand-foot syndrome. Am J Clin Dermatol 2004;5:209–10.

[17] Zimmerman GC, Keeling JH, Burris HA, et al. Acute cutaneous reactions to docetaxel, a new chemotherapeutic agent. Arch Dermatol 1995;131: 202–6.

[18] Lai SE, Kuzel T, Lacouture ME. Hand-foot and stump syndrome to sorafenib. J Clin Oncol 2007; 25:341–6.

[19] Wyatt AJ, Leonard GD, Sachs DL. Cutaneous reactions to chemotherapy and their management. Am J Clin Dermatol 2006;7:45–63.

[20] Cohen PR. Acral erythema: a clinical review. Cutis 1993;51:175–9.

[21] Chung NM, Gutierrez M, Turner ML. Leukocytoclastic vasculitis masquerading as hand-foot syndrome in a patient treated with sorafenib. Arch Dermatol 2006;142:1510–1.

[22] Blum JL, Jones SE, Buzdar AU, et al. Multicenter phase II study of capecitabine in paclitaxel-refractory metastatic breast cancer. J Clin Oncol 1999; 17:485–93.

[23] Hoff PM, Valero V, Ibrahim N, et al. Hand-foot syndrome following prolonged infusion of high doses of vinorelbine. Cancer 1998;82:965–9.

[24] Schey SA, Cooper J, Summerhayes M. The "hand-foot syndrome" occurring with chronic administration of etoposide. Eur J Haematol 1992;48:118–9.

[25] Lotem M, Hubert A, Lyass O, et al. Skin toxic effects of polyethylene glycol-coated liposomal doxorubicin. Arch Dermatol 2000;136:1475–80.

[26] Motzer RJ, Hutson TE, Tomczak P, et al. Sunitinib versus interferon alpha in metastatic renal-cell carcinoma. N Engl J Med 2007;356:115–24.

[27] Vail DM, Chun R, Thamm DH, et al. Efficacy of pyridoxine to ameliorate the cutaneous toxicity associated with doxorubicin containing pegylated (stealth) liposomes: a randomized, double-blind clinical trial using a canine model. Clin Cancer Res 1998;4:1567–71.

[28] Banfield GK, Crate D, Griffiths CL. Long-term sequelae of palmar-plantar erythrodysaeshesia syndrome secondary to 5-fluorouracil therapy. J Royal Society of Med 1995;88:356P–7P.

[29] Flynn TC, Harrist TJ, Murphy GF, et al. Neutrophilic eccrine hidradenitis: a distinctive rash associated with cytarabine therapy and acute leukemia. J Am Acad Dermatol 1984;11:584–90.

[30] Brehler R, Reimann S, Bonsmann G, et al. Neutrophilic hidradenitis induced by chemotherapy involves eccrine and apocrine glands. Am J Dermatopathol 1997;19:73–8.

[31] Koppel RA, Boh EE. Cutaneous reactions to chemotherapeutic agents. Am J Med Sci 2001; 321:327–35.

[32] Pierson JC, Helm TN, Taylor JS, et al. Neutrophilic eccrine hidradenitis heralding the onset of acute myelogenous leukemia. Arch Dermatol 1993;129:791–2.

[33] Bernstein EF, Spielvogel RL, Topolsky DL. Recurrent neutrophilic eccrine hidradenitis. Br J Dermatol 1992;127:529–33.

[34] Shear NH, Knowles SR, Shapiro L, et al. Dapsone in prevention of recurrent neutrophilic eccrine hidradenitis. J Am Acad Dermatol 1996;35:819–22.

[35] Eich D, Scharffetter-Kochanek, Eich HT, et al. Acral erythrodysesthesia syndrome caused by intravenous infusion of docetaxel in breast cancer. Am J Clin Oncol 2002;25:599–602.

[36] Chun Y-S, Chang SN, Oh D, et al. A case of cutaneous reaction to chemotherapeutic agents showing epidermal dysmaturation. J Am Acad Dermatol 2000;43:358 60.

[37] Chu C-Y, Yang C-H, Yang C-Y, et al. Fixed erythrodysaesthesia plaque due to intravenous injection of docetaxel. Br J Dermatol 2000;142:808–11.

[38] Valks R, Fraga J, Porras-Luque J, et al. Chemotherapy-induced eccrine squamous syringometaplasia: a distinctive eruption in patients receiving hematopoietic progenitor cells. Arch Dermatol 1997;133:873–8.

[39] Rubeiz NG, Salem Z, Dibbs R, et al. Bleomycin-induced urticarial flagellate drug hypersensitivity reaction. Int J Dermatol 1999;38:140–1.

[40] Lindae ML, Hu CH, Nickoloff BJ. Pruritic erythematous linear plaques on the neck and back. Arch Dermatol 1987;12:393–8.

[41] Scheulen ME, Hilger RA, Oberhoff C, et al. Clinical phase I dose escalation and pharmacokinetic study of high-dose chemotherapy with treosulfan and autologous peripheral blood stem cell transplantation in patients with advanced malignancies. Clin Cancer Res 2000;6:4209–16.

[42] Falkson G, Schulz EJ. Skin changes in patients treated with 5-fluorouracil. Br J Dermatol 1962; 74:229–36.

[43] Schrijvers D, Van den Brande J, Vermorken JB. Supravenous discoloration of the skin due to docetaxel treatment. Br J Dermatol 2000;142:1069–70.

[44] Prussick R, Thibault A, Turner ML. Recall of cutaneous toxicity from fluorouracil. Arch Dermatol 1993;129:644–5.

[45] Allen BJ, Parker D, Wright AL, et al. Reticulate pigmentation due to 5-fluorouracil. Int J Dermatol 1995;34:219–20.

[46] Smith KJ, Germain M, Skelton H. Histopathologic features seen with radiation recall or enhancement eruptions. J Cutan Med Surg 2002;6:535–40.

[47] Ee H-L, Yosipovitch G. Photo recall phenomenon: an adverse reaction to taxanes. Dermatology 2003; 207:196–8.

[48] Shapiro J, Richardson GE. Paclitaxel-induced "recall" soft tissue injury occurring at the site of previous extravasation with subsequent intravenous treatment in a different limb. J Clin Oncol 1994; 12:2237 8.

[49] Stratman EJ. Chemotherapy recall reactions. J Am Acad Dermatol 2002;46:797.

[50] Mallory SB, Berry DH. Severe reactivation of sunburn following methotrexate use. Pediatrics 1986; 78:514–5.

[51] Westwick TJ, Sheretz EF, McCarley D, et al. Delayed reactivation of sunburn by methotrexate: sparing of chronically sun-exposed skin. Cutis 1987;39:49–51.

[52] Korossy KS, Hood AF. Methotrexate reactivation of sunburn reaction. Arch Dermatol 2981; 117: 310–1.

[53] Parry BR. Radiation recall induced by tamoxifen. Lancet 1992;340:49.

[54] Solberg LA, Wick MR, Bruckman JE. Doxorubicin-enhanced skin reaction after whole-body electron-beam irradiation for leukemia cutis. Mayo Clin Proc 1980;55:711–5.

[55] Breza TS, Halprin KM, Taylor R. Photosensitivity reaction to vinblastine. Arch Dermatol 1975;111: 1168–70.

[56] Vogler WR, Huguley CM, Kerr W. Toxicity and antitumor effect of divided doses of methotrexate. Arch Intern Med 1965;115:285–93.

[57] Treudler R, Georgieva J, Ceilen CC, et al. Dacarbazine but not temozolomide induces phototoxic dermatitis in patients with malignant melanoma. J Am Acad Dermatol 2004;50:783–5.

[58] Johnson TM, Rapini RP, Duvic M. Inflammation of actinic keratoses from systemic chemotherapy. J Am Acad Dermatol 1987;17:192–7.

[59] Lacouture ME, Desai A, Soltani K, et al. Inflammation of actinic keratoses subsequent to therapy with sorafenib, a multitargeted tyrosine-kinase inhibitor. Clin Exp Dermatol 2006; 31:783–5.

[60] Ener RA, Meglathery SB, Styler M. Extravasation of systemic hemato-oncological therapies. Ann Oncol 2004;15:858–64.

[61] Berghammer P, Pohnl R, Baur M, et al. Docetaxel extravasation. Support Care Cancer 2001; 9:131–4.

[62] Rudolph R, Larson DL. Etiology and treatment of chemotherapeutic agent extravasation injuries: a review. J Clin Oncol 1987;5:1116–26.

[63] Bertelli G, Gozza A, Forno GB, et al. Topical dimethylsulfoxide for the prevention of soft tissue injury after extravasation of vesicant cytotoxic drugs: a prospective clinical study. J Clin Oncol 1995;13:2851–5.

[64] Gault DT. Extravasation injuries. Br J Plast Surg 1993;40:91–6.

[65] Lauvin R, Miglianico L, Hellegouarc'h R. Skin cancer occurring 10 years after the extravasation of doxorubicin. N Engl J Med 1995;332:754.

[66] Sauerland C, Engelking C, Wickham R, et al. Vesicant extravasation part 1: mechanisms, pathogenesis, and nursing care to reduce risk. Oncol Nurs Forum 2006;33:1134–41.

[67] Vargel I, Erdem A, Ertoy D, et al. Effects of growth factors on doxorubicin-induced skin necrosis: documentation of histomorphological alterations and early treatment by GM-CSF and G-CSF. Ann Plast Surg 2002;49:646–53.

[68] Bertelli G. Prevention and management of extravasation of cytotoxic drugs. Drug Saf 1995;12:245–55.

[69] Bertelli G, Dini D, Forno GB, et al. Hyaluronidase as an antidote to extravasation of vinca alkaloids: clinical results. J Cancer Res Clin Oncol 1994;120:505–6.

[70] Langer SW, Sehested M, Jensen PB. Dexrazoxane is a potent and specific inhibitor of anthracycline-induced subcutaneous lesions in mice. Clin Cancer Res 2000;6:3680–6.

[71] Saltz LB, Meropol NJ, Loehrer PJ, et al. Phase II trial of cetuximab in patients with refractory colorectal cancer that expresses the epidermal growth factor receptor. J Clin Oncol 2004;22:1201–8.

[72] Cunningham D, Humblet Y, Siena S, et al. Cetuximab monotherapy and cetuximab plus irinotecan in irinotecan-refractory metastatic colorectal cancer. N Engl J Med 2004;351:337–45.

[73] Bonner JA, Harari PM, Giralt J, et al. Radiotherapy plus cetuximab for squamous-cell carcinoma of the head and neck. N Engl J Med 2006;354:567–78.

[74] Brauer MJ, McEvoy BF, Mitus WJ. Hypersensitivity to nitrogen mustards in the form of erythema multiforme. Arch Intern Med 1967;120:499–503.

[75] Spencer HJ. Local erythema multiforme-like drug reaction following intravenous mitomycin C and 5-fluorouracil. J Surg Oncol 1984;26:47–50.

[76] MacGregor JL, Silvers DN, Grossman ME, et al. Sorafenib-induced erythema multiforme. J Am Acad Dermatol 2007;56:527–8.

[77] Brodsky A, Aparici I, Argeri C, et al. Stevens-Johnson syndrome, respiratory distress and acute renal failure due to synergic bleomycin-cisplatin toxicity. J Clin Pharmacol 1989;29:821–3.

[78] Lee TC, Hook CC, Long HJ. Severe exfoliative dermatitis associated with hand ischemia during cisplatin therapy. Mayo Clin Proc 1994;69:80–2.

[79] Horowitz SB, Stirling AL. Thalidomide-induced toxic epidermal necrolysis. Pharmacotherapy 1999;19:1177–80.

[80] Rajkumar SV, Gertz MA, Witzig TE. Life-threatening toxic epidermal necrolysis with thalidomide therapy for myeloma. N Engl J Med 2000;343:972–3.

[81] Wookenstein P, Latarjet J, Roujeau J-C, et al. Randomised comparison of thalidomide versus placebo in toxic epidermal necrolysis. Lancet 1998;352:1586–9.

[82] Hall VC, El-Azhary RA, Bouwhuis S, et al. Dermatologic side effects of thalidomide in patients with multiple myeloma. J Am Acad Dermatol 2003;48:548–52.

[83] Purpora D, Ahern MJ, Silverman N. Toxic epidermal necrolysis after mithramycin. N Engl J Med 1978;299:1412.

[84] Ozkan A, Apak H, Celkan T, et al. Toxic epidermal necrolysis after the use of high-dose cytosine arabinoside. Pediatr Dermatol 2001;18:38–40.

[85] Nguyen TV, Margolis DJ. Hydroxyurea and lower leg ulcers. Cutis 1993;52:217–9.

[86] Kennedy BJ, Smith LR, Goltz RW. Skin changes secondary to hydroxyurea therapy. Arch Dermatol 1975;111:183–7.

[87] Daoud MS, Gibson LE, Pittelkow MR. Hydroxyurea dermopathy: a unique lichenoid eruption complicating long-term therapy with hydroxyurea. J Am Acad Dermatol 1997;36:178–82.

[88] Druker BJ, Tamura S, Buchdunger E, et al. Effects of a selective inhibitor of the Abl tyrosine kinase on the growth of Bcr-Abl positive cells. Nat Med 1996;2:561–6.

[89] Kris MG, Natale RB, Herbst RS, et al. Efficacy of gefitinib, an inhibitor of the epidermal growth factor receptor tyrosine kinase, in symptomatic patients with non-small cell lung cancer: a randomized trial. JAMA 2003;290:2149–58.

[90] Fukuoka M, Yano S, Giaccone G, et al. Multi-institutional randomized phase II trial of gefitinib for previously treated patients with advanced non-small-cell lung cancer. J Clin Oncol 2003;21:2237–46.

[91] Shepherd FA, Pereira JR, Cuileanu T, et al. Erlotinib in previously treated non-small-cell lung cancer. N Engl J Med 2005;353:123–32.

[92] Mendelsohn J. Epidermal growth factor inhibition by a monoclonal antibody as anticancer therapy. Clin Cancer Res 1997;3:2703–7.

[93] Busam KJ, Capodieci P, Motzer R, et al. Cutaneous side-effects in cancer patients treated with the antiepidermal growth factor receptor antibody C225. Br J Dermatol 2001;144:1169–76.

[94] Van Doorn R, Kirtschig G, Scheffer E, et al. Follicular and epidermal alterations in patients treated

with ZD1839 (Iressa), an inhibitor of the epidermal growth factor receptor. Br J Dermatol 2002;147: 598–601.

[95] King LE, Gates RE, Stoscheck CM, et al. The EGF/TGF alpha receptor in skin. J Invest Dermatol 1990;94(Supp 6):164S–70S.

[96] Perez-Soler R, Delord JP, Halpern A, et al. HER1/ EGFR inhibitor-associated rash: Future directions for management and investigation outcomes from the HER1/EGFR inhibitor rash management forum. Oncologist 2005;10:345–56.

[97] Hansen LA, Alexander N, Hogan ME, et al. Genetically null mice reveal a central role for epidermal growth factor receptor in the differentiation of the hair follicle and normal hair development. Am J Pathol 1997;150:1959–75.

[98] Segaert S, Van Cutsem E. Clinical signs, pathophysiology and management of skin toxicity during therapy with epidermal growth factor receptor inhibitors. Ann Oncol 2005;16:1425–33.

[99] Dueland S, Sauer T, Lund-Johansen F, et al. Epidermal growth factor receptor inhibition induces trichomegaly. Acta Oncol 2003;42:345–6.

[100] Morse L, Calarese P. EGFR-targeted therapy and related skin toxicity. Semin Oncol Nurs 2006;22: 152–62.

[101] Threadgill DW, Dlugosz AA, Hansen LA, et al. Targeted disruption of mouse EGF receptor: effect of genetic background on mutant phenotype. Science 1995;269:230–4.

[102] Du X, Tabeta K, Hoebe K, et al. Velvet, a dominant EGFR mutation that causes wavy hair and defective eyelid development in mice. Genetics 2004; 166:331–40.

[103] Pratt CB, Shanks EC. Hyperpigmentation of nails from doxorubicin. JAMA 1974;228:460.

[104] Shah PC, Rao KR, Patel AR. Cyclophosphamide induced nail pigmentation. Br J Dermatol 1978; 98:675–80.

[105] Llombart-Cussac A, Pivot X, Spielmann M. Docetaxel chemotherapy induces transverse superficial loss of the nail plate. Arch Dermatol 1997;133: 1466–7.

[106] Slee PH. Nail changes after chemotherapy. N Engl J Med 1997;337:168.

[107] Chapman S, Cohen PR. Transverse leukonychia in patients receiving cancer chemotherapy. South Med J 1997;90:395–8.

[108] Makris A, Mortimer P, Powles TJ. Chemotherapy-induced onycholysis. Eur J Cancer 1996;32A: 374–5.

[109] Hussain S, Anderson DN, Salvatti ME, et al. Onycholysis as a complication of systemic chemotherapy: report of five cases associated with prolonged weekly paclitaxel therapy and review of the literature. Cancer 2000;88:2367–71.

Dermatol Clin 26 (2008) 121–159

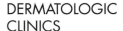

Cutaneous Reactions Related to Systemic Immunomodulators and Targeted Therapeutics

Lisa A. Hammond-Thelin, MD

6126 Amble Trail, San Antonio, TX 78249, USA

The past decade has been remarkable in the field of oncology for the fulfillment of the promise of molecularly targeted therapeutics. As with any new class of agents, investigators eagerly awaited tumor regressions and, hopefully, improvements in survival with these drugs. What was not anticipated was the extent and characteristics of skin rashes and other dermatologic events that presented with the initial use of gefitinib, erlotinib, and cetuximab. In fact, the anti–epidermal growth factor receptor (EGFR) therapy–induced effect may be an entirely new dermatologic entity [1]. The initial reactions to this novel rash included dismay due to its prominence, especially on the face. However, as more data and studies matured showing that rash correlates with response and survival, what was once a "negative issue" has become, with some agents, a "positive issue" with both patients and physicians eagerly waiting for the first manifestations of the EGFR inhibitor (EGFRI)-induced rash. Other dermatologic toxicity that has become more prominent with the arrival of molecularly targeted agents includes paronychia, pigmentation issues, skin fissures, and calluses. Other events not previously seen as a result of cytotoxic therapy include acral erythema and subungual splinter hemorrhages. These are depicted in Table 1, which shows the distribution of these toxicities among the different molecularly targeted agents. Clearly, the issue of dermatologic toxicity in oncology with the novel molecularly targeted agents and systemic immunomodulators has never been more at the forefront of discussion then it is now. Skin toxicity

with these agents results in more time-consuming patient management issues that require patient education and challenging treatment issues, give insight into what may be happening at the physiologic level, and may be predictive of response. All of these issues will be reviewed in the following text.

Epidermal growth factor receptor pathway inhibitors

Introduction

The development of EGFRIs has primarily focused on two classes: monoclonal antibodies such as cetuximab and pamitumumab that target the extracellular ligand-binding domain of the EGFR, and the small molecule tyrosine kinase inhibitors, such as erlotinib and gefitinib, that target the EGFR intracellularly. A further distinction among the EGFR inhibitors can be made based on whether they predominantly inhibit the EGFR or are a dual human epidermal growth factor receptor (HER) 1/2 or pan-HER inhibitor such as lapatinib or EKB569 and canertinib, respectively (Table 2). Data suggest that there may ultimately be differences in administration schedules and toxicities such as rash among these agents that relates to their intrinsic differences. For instance, matuzumab and cetuximab participate in antibody-dependent cellular cytotoxicity, based on their immunoglobulin G1 (IgG1) backbone, while pamitumumab (IgG2) does not [2]. To date agents approved by the Food and Drug Administration (FDA) include cetuximab, pamitumumab, erlotinib, and gefitinib, the latter has subsequently had its use restricted. An alternate approach to inhibiting the EGFR is by using an

---

The author has either served as a consultant or received honoraria from the following companies: Amgen, AstraZeneca, Genentech, OSI Pharmaceuticals.

E-mail address: lisa-hammond-md@satx.rr.com

doi:10.1016/j.det.2007.08.010

Table 1
Dermatologic toxicities associated with novel systemic immunomodulators and targeted therapeutics

Dermatologic toxicity	Agent or class of agents									
	EGFRIs	Sorafenib	Sunitimib	Imatinib	Dasatinib	Bortezomib	Thalidomide	Lenalidomide	m-TOR inhibitors	Bevacizumab
Novel follicular rash	++								+	?+ 1 case report
Cutaneous vasculitic rash				+						
IGD						+	+	+		
Rash, nonspecific			+ transient yellow discoloration	+	+	+	+	+		+
Paronychia	+	+	+							
Nail dystrophia			+						+	
Acral erythema/HFS	+	++	++							
Subungual splinter hemorrhages		++	+	Rare						
Calluses		++	+							
Skin hypopigmentation or hyperpigmentation	+			++						
Hair depigmentation			+							
Hair repigmentation				+						
Skin fissures	+									

Abbreviations: EGFRIs, epidermal growth factor receptor inhibitors; IGD, interstitial granulomatous dermatitis.

agent that inhibits a broad range of kinases in an effort to inhibit 2 or more signaling pathways. The cutaneous adverse effects with these less specific inhibitors, such as vandetanib [3,4], are less well characterized but appear to be similar to the typical EGFR effect seen with the pure HER-directed agents.

Epidermal growth factor receptor in skin

While the EGFR is maximally expressed in the basal layer of the epidermis it is also present in the dermal papilla, the epithelium of hair follicles, and eccrine and sebaceous sweat glands [5]. This receptor is important in the normal differentiation and development of skin follicles and keratinocytes; abnormal expression of EGFR has been implicated in hyperproliferative epidermal disorders and tumor development [6]. To date, the exact mechanistic pathway by which EGFR inhibition elicits the now infamous EGFRI-induced rash is unknown. There is evidence that inflammation may not be just a secondary effect of EGFRIs, as these agents may also alter the immune system by unblocking cutaneous chemokine production leading to leukocyte chemostasis and infiltration in the skin [7].

The "novel" epidermal growth factor receptor inhibitor-induced rash

Given the distribution of EGFR, it is not surprising that modulation of this receptor would evoke dermal effects. To date these dermal effects are similar regardless of the agent administered, indicating that dermatologic toxicity is a class effect [8]. The most prevalent dermal effect is a skin rash that has been inconsistently described in the literature (Fig. 1A, B). The terminology for this rash has not been standardized and one must be aware that "rash," "acne," "acne-like rash," "acneiform skin reaction," "acneform rash," "acneiform follicular rash," "maculopapular skin rash," and "monomorphic pustular lesions" all refer to the same adverse entity. In initial phase I studies, oncologists lacking dermatologic expertise started to apply these terms to a rash that "looked like acne." However, the EGFRI-induced rash lacks the true features of acne, that is microcomedones and comedones are not present. In fact, a review of the literature shows only two patients who have been reported to actually have comedones associated with this follicular rash [9]. However, despite a number of large studies the actual distribution of the rash is poorly detailed in the literature

[10–12] and it is actually in smaller studies and case reports that a more comprehensive description is provided (Table 3) [13–38]. This skin rash most frequently occurs on the face but also appears on the scalp, upper chest, and back and less frequently on the extremities [8,39,40]; however, the true incidence of extremity rash may be underestimated.

The skin rash typically presents within the first 2 weeks after starting an EGFRI [7,8,41], is dose dependent, may improve in some patients with continuation of therapy [12,41–44], and typically resolves spontaneously after treatment is completed [45]. However, one report notes that nearly half of the patients with cetuximab-induced rash continue with rash beyond 28 days or completion of one course. While the EGFRI-induced rash is typically of grade 1 to 2 severity, occasionally, more severe grade 3 dermatologic effects, such as development of an impetigo honey-combed crust appearance, have been noted [1,46]. Recently it has been suggested that the incidence of secondarily infected rash may be more frequent than previously recognized [1]. This is difficult to assess as a review of published data shows a paucity of culture data on pustules of EGFRI-induced rashes for assessment of secondary infection and colonizing bacteria (Table 4) [47–50].

Similarities and contrasts between this novel rash and typical acne vulgaris have been sought. The literature, for the most part, does not address the issue of acne scarring with EGFRIs. While a few investigators comment that permanent acne scarring has not been observed [7], dramatic scarring, erythema, and postinflammatory hyperpigmentation after a severe follicular eruption due to EGFRI-induced therapy has been reported in two patients [51,52]. Moderate acne scarring was also observed in a third patient by this author. The issue of geographic location has been discussed but poorly documented; one report states that rash was possibly worse in geographic areas with high heat and humidity [7,8]. It is also unclear if a history of acne predisposes patients to more severe rashes. One report shows no apparent association of severity of this rash with skin type or history of acne [53]. Another report states that patients with oilier skin or those more prone to acne may expect a more severe rash and a higher incidence of pustules [8].

Interesting variants or characteristics of this rash have been reported. Hemorrhagic papules with crusts or follicular papules with a hemorrhagic quality have been described in four patients treated with cetuximab [40,45]. Another case

Table 2
Classes of epidermal growth factor receptor inhibitors

Class of EGFR inhibitor		Type of receptor inhibition	HER receptor inhibited				Additional receptors targeted	Rash as adverse event	US FDA status (approved, indication, investigational)
Name	Type		HER-1	HER-2	HER-3	HER-4			
Monoclonal antibodies									
Cetuximab	Chimeric IgG1	Extracellular domain	+					Yes	Approved. CRC: Irinotecan refractory or intolerant metastatic; Head and neck cancer: in combination with radiation in locally advanced disease; single agent in recurrent or metastatic disease
Matuzumab	Humanized IgG1	Extracellular domain	+					Yes	Investigational
Panitumumab	Humanized IgG2	Extracellular domain	+					Yes	Approved. CRC: EGFR + metastatic failing fluoropyrimidine-, oxaliplatin-, irinotecan-containing regimens
Nimotuzumab	Humanized	Extracellular domain	+					No	Investigational

Tyrosine kinase	Reversible	Irreversible			
Erlotinib	+			Yes	Approved NSCLC: advanced, refractory Pancreatic cancer: locally advanced, unresectable, or metastatic
Gefitinib	+			Yes	Approved NSCLC: locally advanced (IIIB) or metastatic after failure of both platinum and docetaxel; relabeled with restrictions[a]
Lapatinib	+			Yes	Investigational
EKB569		+		Yes	Investigational
Canertinib		+		Yes	Investigational
Multikinase Inhibitor					
Vandetanib	+		VEGFR-2 RET	Yes	Investigational: orphan drug status for follicular, medullary, anaplastic, localized advanced and metastatic papillary thyroid cancer

Abbreviations: CRC, colorectal cancer; EGFR, epidermal growth factor receptor; FDA, Food and Drug Administration; Ig, immunoglobulin; NSCLC, non-small cell lung cancer; RET, rearranged during transfection; VEGFR, vascular endothelial growth factor receptor.

[a] Restricted for patients who previously or currently receiving and benefiting from gefitinib as of June 17, 2005 and for previously enrolled patients or new patients in non-Investigational New Drug (IND) clinical trials approved by the IRB before June 17, 2005.

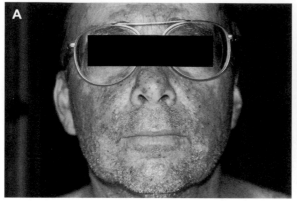
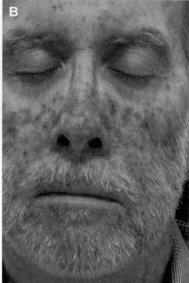

Fig. 1. (*A*, *B*) Photographs of patients with the typical EGFRI-induced novel follicular rash on face and neck.

report notes lack of rash development in a prior radiation field of a patient treated with erlotinib who otherwise had a diffuse rash [54]. In addition, pain is a feature of this novel rash, especially in patients who have erythema and inflammation [1]. Standard analgesia is recommended in these instances. If pain is localized or becomes more severe, then a diagnosis of cellulitis should be entertained.

Correlation between rash and response/survival

A riveting feature of the EGFRI-induced rash is the possibility of its use as a surrogate end point. Numerous studies with both monoclonal antibodies and small molecule tyrosine kinase inhibitors (TKIs) demonstrate a correlation between this acneiform rash/skin toxicity with tumor response, time to tumor progression, and overall survival [55–59]. This indicates that rash may be a method to identify tumors with signaling pathways that are more susceptible to inhibition by EGFRIs. While this relationship has been established for cetuximab and erlotinib, it is more ambiguous with gefitinib. A number of studies demonstrate that those patients who do not develop rash have a poorer prognosis. However, lack of rash does not necessarily preclude response, as documented recently with nimotuzumab and with gefitinib. While rash is not a side effect of nimotuzumab [60,61], in the case of

gefitinib, durable radiographic regressions and symptom improvement have been observed in the absence of rash and diarrhea [58]. Speculation as to why the skin is spared with nimotuzumab include that it has different pharmacokinetic properties (longer half-life and a higher area under the curve) [62] and a lower magnitude affinity to EGFR than cetuximab. Also, it is a humanized antibody with a larger proportion of human sequence and has been obtained by humanizing a murine antibody elicited against the EGFR of human placenta in contrast to cultured cells [63]. The evaluation of rash as a surrogate marker continues, as it would allow selection of those patients most likely to respond to the potential of the rash inducing EGFRIs.

Dose-to-rash strategy

The observation that development of skin rash correlates with improved tumor assessment parameters has led to studies evaluating "dose-to-rash" strategies. Two studies have been initiated in this setting. One evaluates increasing doses of erlotinib in patients with non–small cell lung cancer [64]. A second study randomizes colorectal cancer patients with no rash or grade 1 rash to continue with cetuximab/irinotecan at current recommended doses or increase the dose of cetuximab [65]. If this strategy indeed becomes standardized in the community oncology practice, well-defined guidelines as to when to start treatment for rash and with what agents, whether single-agent, combination or sequential, will assist in maximizing patient dose by minimizing drug interruptions and dose reductions.

However, while this strategy appears attractive, preclinical data show mutated EGFR is completely inhibited at lower concentrations of gefitinib than those with wild-type EGFR [66]. These data support the clinical findings that doubling the dose of gefitinib only leads to more diarrhea, skin toxicity, grade 3 and 4 toxicity, dose reductions, and treatment discontinuations but not response [58]. Further evaluation of this dose-to-rash strategy is under way to confirm or refute its validity.

Histologic assessment

Histologic assessment of biopsies of rashes induced by anti-EGFR-targeted therapy predominantly reveal a neutrophilic infiltration (see Table 4) [39]. Neutrophils are especially increased around the hair follicle and sweat gland [67]. While overall skin thickness remains unchanged with anti-EGFR therapy, the stratum corneum becomes thinner and the normal basketweave appearance is lost [68]. Hair follicles become enlarged and are blocked by excess keratinocytes [8,39,68]. The intrafollicular collection of neutrophils resembles an infectious folliculitis; whether this is a superinfectious phenomenon is unclear. Suppurative inflammation is hypothesized to result from mechanical rupture of the follicle as a result of excessive hyperkeratosis, follicular plugging, and subsequent obstruction of the follicular ostium [53]. Skin biopsy after 1 week of therapy with cetuximab reveals an increase in Kip1 expression suggesting that rash results from interference of downstream signaling of EGFR and that one of the likely modulators is the negative growth regulator Kip1, which leads to G1 cell cycle arrest [53].

Atypical epidermal growth factor receptor inhibitor-associated rashes

As more experience with EGFRIs is obtained, other cutaneous effects have been noted. While the typical EGFRI-induced rash has been interpreted as a direct result of interference with pilosebaceous follicle homeostasis, Tscharner and colleagues [69] reported a case that clinically and histologically resembled a transient acantholytic dermatosis following a second course of cetuximab. Another atypical rash, necrolytic migratory erythema (glucagonoma)-like skin lesions, was reported by Trojan and colleagues [70] in a 55-year-old female with NSCLC and a history of livedo reticularis after exposure to single-agent gefitinib. Withdrawal of gefitinib and treatment with oral steroids led to improvement of this rash, which was assessed as possibly gefitinib related although the history of prior livedo reticularis was acknowledged.

Sycosis and pyoderma gangrenosum–like lesions were observed in a 55-year-old male with NSCLC treated with gefitinib 250 mg/d [71]. Approximately 7.5 months after starting gefitinib, despite systemic and topical antibiotics, papules and pustules on the upper lip coalesced to form sycosis vulgaris–like lesions. In addition, an erythematous lesion on the hypogastrium ulcerated after gefitinib was held. This lesion disappeared 1 month after gefitinib dose reduction. No biopsies were performed because of patient refusal. A purpuric drug eruption that was possibly gefitinib induced was reported in a 76-year-old female after 2 months of gefitinib [72]. This presented as ecchymosis on the buttocks and soles of feet, with ulceration and hemorrhage due to a fissure, and petechiae on the legs. Histologic evaluation revealed subcorneal pustules with lymphocytes and neutrophils, diffuse extravasation of erythrocytes, perivascular lymphocyte infiltration, edema and dilated capillaries compatible with leukocytoclastic vasculitis. Gefitinib dosing ceased and betamethasone was started with subsequent development of paronychia. In 10 days, the purpura subsided to brown pigmentation and the sole ulceration reepithelialized. Because of the severity of these symptoms, gefitinib was not rechallenged. The author proposes that gefitinib induced a direct or indirect disorder in the capillaries leading to leukocytoclastic vasculitis [72].

Issues with assessing rash

A number of factors have precluded optimal management of EGFRI cutaneous adverse events and include that cutaneous toxicity has been relatively uncommon with traditional cytotoxic agents and initial classification and grading of anti-EGFR–induced skin rashes by clinical investigators in early trials was inconsistent [73]. There has also been lack of a standardized terminology to describe the rash; lack of an adequate grading system of the rash in the initial development of these agents; lack of expert dermatologic

Table 3
Frequency, severity, and distribution of epidermal growth factor receptor inhibitor-induced rashes

Author	Drug	N	Tumor type	Dose of EGFRI, mg	% Rash	No./grade (Gr) of severe rashes	Reported frequency of distribution of rash			
							Face/ Scalp/Neck	Shoulders/ trunk	Arms/Legs	Genital mucosa
Nemunaitis et al [15]	Canertinib	32	Solid tumors	300–560 po/d	Rash/acne 56/44	2 Gr 3	Not reported			
Garland et al [81]	Canertinib + docetaxel	26	Solid tumors	45–70 IV/d × 14dq21d	50	0	Not reported			
Calvo et al [16]	Canertinib	24	Solid tumors	250–300 po qd × 7dqowk	83	1 Gr 2[a] 2 Gr 3	"face in periorifacial distribution, upper trunk"			
Campos et al [17]	Canertinib	53	Ovarian cancer	50 poqd × 21q28d	36	1 Gr 3/4	Not reported			
		52		200 poqd × 21q28d	58	4 Gr 3/4				
Cunningham et al [55]	Cetuximab	329	CRC	400/250 IV qwk	80	26 (9.4% cetuximab/ irinotecan; 5.2% cetuximab)	Not reported			
Jacot et al [45]	Cetuximab	9	Solid tumors	400/250 IV qwk	67	NR	55%	44%	0%	0%
Saltz et al [12]	Cetuximab	57	CRC[b]	400/250 IV qwk	86	10 Gr 3	"predominantly on upper face and torso"			
Micantonio et al [47]	Cetuximab	1	CRC	NR	100	1 Gr 3	100%	100%	100%	0%
Chan et al [18]	Cetuximab + carboplatin	60	NSP	400/250 IV qwk	83	7 Gr 3	Not reported			
Burtness et al [19]	Cetuximab + cisplatin	58	H&N	NR	NR	16% Gr 3	Not reported			
Bonner et al [20]	Cetuximab/xrt	211	H&N	400/250 IV qwk	87	8 Gr 3	Not reported			
Baselga et al [21]	Cetuximab + cisplatin	96	H&N	400/250 IV qwk	72	2 Gr 3, 1 Gr 4	Not reported			

Herbst et al [22]	Cetuximab + cisplatin	131	H&N	400/250 IVqwk	70	5 Gr 3	Not reported			
Gutzmer et al [82]	Cetuximab ± irinotecan	2	CRC/H&N	NR	100	2 severe	100%	100%	50%	0%
Kimyai-Asadi et al [40]	Cetuximab + irinotecan	1	CRC	520 mg IV/wk	100	1 Gr 3	100%	100%	100%	0%
Molinari et al [23]	Cetuximab	13	CRC	400/250	85%	31%	85%	NR	23% lower back or extremities	0%
Erlichman et al [24]	EKB569 I	30	Solid tumors	25–125 po/d× 14q28d	60	2 Gr 3	Not reported			
	EKB569 C	29	Solid tumors	25–100 po/ d × 28d	83	0				
Souliers et al [13]	Erlotinib	115	H&N squamous cell carcinoma	150 po/d	79c	11 Gr 3; 1 Gr 4	Not reported			
Perez-Soler et al [84]	Erlotinib	57	NSCLC	150 po/d	75d	1 Gr 3	Not reported			
Hidalgo et al [41]	Erlotinib	40	Solid tumors	25–200 po/d	59	0	"face in periorifacial distribution and upper trunk"			
Shepherd et al [25]	Erlotinib	485	NSCLC	150 po/d	76	9 Gr 3-5	Not reported			
Townsley et al [78]	Erlotinib	38	CRC	150 po/d	90	4 Gr 3	Not reported			
Philip et al [26]	Erlotinib	38	HCC	150 po/d	84	5 Gr 3	Not reported			
Gatzemeier et al [27]	Erlotinib + cisplatin + gemcitabine	1172	NSCLC	150 po/d	NR	10% Gr 3,4	Not reported			
Herbst et al [28]	Erlotinib + carboplatin + paclitaxel	526	NSCLC	150 po/d	62	7.2% Gr 3	Not reported			
Hainsworth et al [29]	Erlotinib + bevacizumzb	63	RCC	150 po/d	100	8 Gr 3	Not reported			
Matheis et al [30]	Gefitinib	3	NSCLC	250 po/d	100	NS	100%	100%	66%c	
West et al [31]	Gefitinib	136	BAC	500 po/d	82	14 Gr 3 2 Gr 4	Not reported			0%
Jacot et al [45]	Gefitinib	20	Solid tumors	250/500 po/d	55	NR	82%	64%	5%	5%

(continued on next page)

Table 3 (*continued*)

Author	Drug	N	Tumor type	Dose of EGFRI, mg	% Rash	No./grade (Gr) of severe rashes	Reported frequency of distribution of rash			
							Face/ Scalp/Neck	Shoulders/ trunk	Arms/Legs	Genital mucosa
Baselga et al [32]	Gefitinib	88	Solid tumors	150–1000 po/d	65	6 Gr 3	Not reported			
Herbst et al [10]	Gefitinib + paclitaxel + carboplatin	342	NSCLC	250 po/d	Rash/acne 58/20[h]	4.7% Gr 3	Yes; most frequent	Yes; less frequent	Yes; less frequent	Vaginal dryness and itching; discomfort on urination due to perineal dryness
		342	NSCLC	500 po/d	Rash/acne 69/26	14.6% (13.7 Gr 3)				
Kris et al [58]	Gefitinib	102[f]	NSCLC	250 po/d	62[g]	0	"face, neck, and trunk"			
		114[f]	NSCLC	500 po/d	75[g]	5 Gr 3				
Fukuoka et al [11]	Gefitinib	103	NSCLC	250 po/d	Rash/acne 46.6/13	1	Not reported			
		106	NSCLC	500 po/d	Rash/acne 68.8/14	9 Gr 3	Not reported			
Giaccone et al [33]	Gefitinib + gemcitabine + cisplatin	362	NSCLC	250 po/d	Rash/acne 44/18	5%	Not reported			
		358	NSCLC	500 po/d	Rash/acne 57/28	18%				
Rich et al [34]	Gefitinib	55	GBM	50–1000 po/d	60: 100 no EIA 54 + EIA	No EIA: 1 Gr 3 + EIA: 4 Gr 3, 3 Gr 4	Not reported			

Study	Drug	N	Tumor	Dose	Rash	Grade	Comment
Rothenberg et al [35]	Gefitinib	56	CRC	250 po/d	43	0	Not reported
Park et al [14]	Gefitinib	54	CRC	500 po/d	83	4 Gr 3	Not reported
	Gefitinib	111	NSCLC	250 po/d	Rash/acne 61/20	1 Gr 3	Not reported
Burris et al [36]	Lapatinib	67	Solid tumors	500-1600 po/d	31[i]	1 Gr 3	Not reported
Vanhoefer et al [37]	Matuzumab	22	Solid tumors	400-2000 IV/wk	Acneiform 64; Epidermolysis 32	0	Not reported
Rowinsky et al [38]	Pamitumumab	88	RCC	1-2.5 mg/kg IV/w	68%-100% by dose level	NS	"face in periorificial distribution and upper trunk"

Abbreviations: BAC, bronchiolaviolar cancer; CRC, colorectal cancer; EIA, enzyme-inducing antieleptics; GBM, glioblastoma multiforme; H&N, head and neck cancer; HCC, hepatocellular carcinoma; IV, intravenous; NSCLC, non-small cell lung cancer; NSP, nasopharyngeal carcinoma; po, by mouth; q, every; RCC, renal cell carcinoma.

[a] grade 2 rash severe due to intolerability.

[b] EGFR-positive CRC.

[c] Rash nos + dermatitis + acne.

[d] Rash + dermatitis + acne.

[e] 1 patient with typical pustular lesions, 1 patient with excema craquele.

[f] Numbers from those patients evaluable for safety.

[g] Dermatologic side effects in one category "rash, pruritus, dry skin and acne"; separate "rash" not given.

[h] Data from Table 5 skin reactions by grade: rash or acne category.

[i] Rash = rash/acne/dermatitis acneiform.

Table 4
Histologic and culture data from skin biopsies of patients treated with epidermal growth factor receptor inhibitors

| | | | | Histologic and culture data | | | | | |
| | | | | Skin biopsy results | | | Rash stain/culture results | | |
Author/ref	N with rash/N total	Drug	Time (post-drug)	Site of biopsy	Histologic findings	IHC Results	Site	Stain	Microorganisms
Busam et al [53]	10/10	Cetuximab	Day 8	Chest	4 superficial folliculitis 4 florid suppurative folliculitis 2 focal intraepidermal acantholysis	↑ interfollicular epidermal keratinocytes (↑ Kip1) (n = 4)	Forehead	Negative	All initially negative; *S. aureus* in some persistent lesions
Albanell et al [68]	65	Gefitinib	Day 28	Upper thorax & supraclavicular area	Stratum corneum thinner Most samples lacked hair follicle Few: keratin plugs, microorganisms in dilated infundibula Acute neutrophilic folliculitis Some prominent lichenoid changes	↓ P-EGFR, MAPK, KPI ↑ Kip1, apoptosis	NR	NR	NR
Kimyai-Asadi et al [40]	1/1	Cetuximab	1 wk	NR	Neutrophilic suppurative folliculitis	NR	NR	Negative	NR
Malik et al [48]	?/28	Erlotinib	Day 28	Upper back (surveillance biopsies)	No acute folliculitis Superficial perivascular & periadnexal chronic inflammatory infiltrate Hair follicles associated with chronic lymphocytic infiltrate 1 prominent follicular plug with microorganisms	Dose-related up-regulation of p27 Non-dose related decrement in P-EGFR	NR	NR	NR

Baselga et al [32]	57/88; 44 skin biopsies, 34 paired	Gefitinib	Approx day 28	Clinically normal skin area	Stratum corneum: basket-weave lost; foci of parakeratosis. Basal layer epidermis: focal mononuclear infiltrates; vacuolar degeneration; apoptotic keratinocytes. Keratin plugs & microorganisms in dilated infundibula. Acute folliculitis	Decrement in P-EGFR and MAPK. Increment in phospho-STAT3, Ki67, p27^{KIP1}	NR	NR	NR
Jacot et al [45]	55%/20 67%/9 6 skin biopsies	Gefitinib Cetuximab	NR	NR	5 superficial florid neutrophilic suppurative folliculitis. Neutrophilic infiltrate around infundibula w/rupture of epithelial lining	NR	NR	Negative	6 cultures negative
Van Doorn et al [9]	3/3	Gefitinib	Day 5–12	2 biopsies of pustular lesions	Purulent folliculitis, follicle destruction, perifollicular granuloma, dermal edema, vasodilation	NR	NR	1 +; 2-	1 + Propionibacterium acnes; 2 negative
Fernandez-Galar et al [49]	1/1	Gefitinib	Day 7[a]	Active lesion	Stratum corneum: orthokeratotic hyperkeratosis. Epidermis: lymphocyte exocytosis basal layer w/hydropic degeneration. Dermal papillae: dense infiltrate lymphocytes/neutrophils; perifollicular dense multinucleated giant cells/macrophages	Direct immunofluorescence: negative for immunoglobulins, fibrinogen, complement	NR	Negative	Negative

(continued on next page)

Table 4 (continued)

| Author/ref | N with rash/N total | Drug | Time (post-drug) | Histologic and culture data | | | | Rash stain/culture results | | |
| | | | | Skin biopsy results | | | | | | |
				Site of biopsy	Histologic findings	IHC Results	Site	Stain	Microorganisms
Monti et al [90]	2/2	Cetuximab	A few days	Pustular lesion	Extension of suppurative folliculitis into the infundibula Intraepithelial pustules	NR	NR	NR	NR
Micantonio et al [47]	1/1	Cetuximab	1 wk	Pustular lesion neck	Neutrophilic folliculitis Perifollicular dense inflammatory infiltrate lymphocytes, neutrophils, multinucleated giant cells w/follicle destruction	NR	Pustular lesion	NR	No bacteria, no fungi
Hammoud et al [50]	4/4	Gefitinib (n = 2) Cetuximab (n = 1) Canertimib (n = 1)	Day 7	Papules and pustules	Acute suppurative folliculitis	NR	Nasal lesion and pustules	NR	2 cultures + S. aureus 2 cultures negative
Matheis et al [30]	3/3	Gefitinib	Day 9–30	Pustules, site of bx NS	Perifollicular infiltrate, dilated follicles, keratin debris, hyperkeratosis, atrophic sebaceous glands	NR	Pustules (n = 2) Cyst that became inflamed (n = 1)	Gram + cocci (n = 1) Gram – rods, + coccobacilli (n = 1)	Pustules: Culture negative (n = 1) Culture + coag - staph (n = 1) Cyst: Lactobacilli +
Vanhoefer et al [37]	14/22	Matuzumab	21 at day 28; 1 at 5 mos	NR	Stratum corneum: thinning; loss of basket-wave configuration	D P-EGFR, pMAPK, Ki-67 I p27^{Kip1}, pSTAT3 No change: TGF-a; total EGFR in interfollicular epidermis	NR	NR	NR

Abbreviations: IHC, immunohistochemistry; Kip 1, interfollicular epidermal keratinocytes; KPI, keratinocytes proliferation index; MAPK, mitogen-actvated protein kinase; NR, not reported; P-EGFR, phosphorylated EGFR; TGF-a, transforming growth factor alpha.

[a] Skin rash started day 7, patient referred to dermatology 2 months later due to persistence of rash.

input in early development of these agents; and lack of studies formally evaluating the efficacy of agents used to treat rash. As the number of these agents entering the clinic has increased and the treatment indications for these agents has expanded, more attention has been focused on this issue. The dilemma of an inadequate grading system was apparent in the study by Messersmith and colleagues [74] in which three patients had severe rashes necessitating cessation of erlotinib for 3, 14, and 17 days. However, per the Common Toxicity Criteria grading, these rashes were only grade 2, as they covered less than 50% of the body surface area. Since the conduct of this study, the National Cancer Institute Common Toxicity Criteria version 3 has been instituted in which acneiform rash is graded as a separate category with grade 2 defined as "intervention indicated" and grade 3 as "associated with pain, disfigurement, ulceration, or desquamation" [75].

Management of rash—active

To date, optimal management of the anti-EGFR–induced skin rash has not been established. A number of different agents have been used in this setting, however no randomized clinical trials have been performed. These agents include oral and topical corticosteroids, retinoids, topical and oral antibiotics, benzyl peroxide, alpha hydroxyl acids, and topical immunomodulatory agents. Table 5 [46,76,77] contains a compilation of a literature review looking at reports, opinions, and recommendations as to what has been tried. A number of reports, especially those conducted early in the development of EGFRIs, state that the maneuvers tried were not efficacious or did not substantially affect the course of the rash [12]; in others, a general statement such as "minocycline enabled most patients to continue study medication" appears [78]. These reports have been excluded from Table 4 in an effort to focus on reports that provide more specific treatment recommendations.

In general, there appear to be divergent opinions with regard to the use of topical and oral corticosteroids. Some clinicians state that although they may be useful in mild rashes, they appear to be ineffective in advanced or severe rashes. Other clinicians have already incorporated them into treatment algorithms [79,80]. Caution has been urged regarding the use of corticosteroids in the setting of the EGFRI-induced rash because of the following concerns: corticosteroids

induce or aggravate acne, acneiform eruptions, rosacea, and telangiectasia; systemic steroids may interfere with the antibody-dependent cytotoxic action of the monoclonal antibodies; and there is a risk of corticosteroid induced atrophy and pigment changes. Significant differences were not noted between patients receiving gefitinib with and without corticosteroids, although the percentage of patients receiving concomitant steroids is not given and the total sample size is small (n = 20) [45]. There are also data showing that administration of dexamethasone with canertinib with docetaxel does not result in exacerbation of rash [81].

The use of retinoids to treat EGFRI-induced rashes has also been controversial. Less data exist in the literature to support retinoid use compared with corticosteroids and antibiotics and comedones are not a feature of the EGFRI rash. In addition there is concern that the skin-drying effects of retinoids may exacerbate the EGFRI rash. Also, it is unknown whether there are any interactions between the antitumor properties of EGFR inhibitors and retinoids. Finally, the therapeutic effects of isotretinoin require 6 to 8 weeks, which limits its use for acute toxicity. However, positive anecdotal results have been reported with isotretinoin. Van Doorn and colleagues [9] noted that while follicular eruption responded favorably to tretinoin treatment in one patient, scaling of the skin worsened. Gutzmer and colleagues [82] report successful use of topical metronidazole gel to the face and oral isotretinoin in two patients treated with cetuximab. A 63-year-old male with colorectal cancer (CRC) receiving concomitant irinotecan had complete resolution of almost all pustules on the face, trunk, and extremities and remained on isotretinoin for 6 months after initiation with a partial tumoral response. The second patient, a 37-year-old female with laryngeal cancer had resolution of pustules on the face, scalp, and upper chest with only remaining erythematous macules on the face after 4 months with stable disease.

A number of antibiotics have been incorporated into the management of the EGFRI-induced rash including tetracycline and its derivatives, cephalosporins, clindamycin, erythromycin, and metronidazole. There appears to be a regional divergence with regard to choice of antibiotic use with our European colleagues favoring fusidic acid cream, a steroidal antibiotic used in Europe for the treatment of cutaneous *Staphylococcus aureus* infections. With topical antibiotics, it is

Table 5
Published results, opinions, and recommendations regarding treatment of the epidermal growth factor receptor inhibitor-induced rash

	Class of agents used to treat EGFRI-induced rash								
	Corticosteroids		Retinoids	Antibiotics		Benzoyl peroxide	Alpha hydroxyl acids	Topical immuno-modulatory agents	Other
Author/ref	Topical	Oral		Topical	Oral (doses in mg/d)[a]				
Perez-Soler et al [1]	Ineffective in advanced, severe rash; ± clobetasol propionate mild face rash	NA	Not recommended	Muciprocin: S. aureus + or impetigo	Not recommended for routine use	Not recommended	Need evaluation	No data available; warrants investigation	
Segaert and Van Cutsem [65]	No, unless eczema present	Not recommended unless eczema present	Not recommended	Mild/grade 1 rash Cream: metronidazole; Gel/lotion: erythromycin; clindamycin	Grade 2: Minocycline 100 Lymecycline 300 Doxycycline 100 Grade 3: Minocycline 200 Lymecycline 600 Doxycycline 200	Gel or cream recommended for face	Not recommended	NA	Salicylic acid in alcoholic lotion (chest/back) Topical menthol Oral antihistamine
Busam et al [53]	No consistent clinical improvement	NA	NA	No consistent clinical improvement	No consistent clinical improvement	NA	NA	NA	
Fox [51]	Recommends finite therapeutic trial	Topicals preferred	Lack of data	Little to no effect	Consider minocycline, tetracycline	Minimally helpful	Lack of data	Consider tacrolimus ointment, pimecrolimus cream	

Rothenberg and Hochster [93]	NA	Hydrocortisone (face) Clobetasol and betametha-sone (non-face)	NA	1st line: clindamycin or erythromycin gel	2nd line: tetracycline erythromycin cephalosporin	Yes: 2.5% concentration rather than usual 5%	NA	NA
Garey et al [80]	Grade 3 macular rash	Grade 1–2 macular rash	NA	Grade 1 pustular rash: clindamycin gel	Grade 2–3 pustular rash	NA	NA	NA
Cortesi et al [76]	Not needed with early intervention	Grade 2 rash: betametazone 0.122% cream	NA	Grade 2 rash: gentamicin 0.166% cream tid	Not needed with early intervention	Grade 1: 0.025% cream bid upon presentation erythema	NA	NA
Gutzmer et al [82]	NA	NA	Oral Isotretinoin 30–40 mg active; 20 mg/d maintenance	0.75% metronidazole gel 1% erythromycin	NA	NA	NA	2% triclosan in unguentum leniens
Jacot et al [45]	NA	Corticoid cream	NA	4% erythromycin solution econozole cream	Systemic fusidic acid PCN lymecycline	Gel: 2 partial resolutions w/o treatment interruption	NA	NA	Povidone iodine Hexamidine solution
Segaert et al [83]	NA	NA	Mild-mod rash: Topical adapalene 0.1 gel/cream	Mild-mod: erythromycin Clindamycin Metronidazole cream	Mod-severe: Systemic > 12 wks Minocycline 100 Lymecycline 300 Doxycycline 50–100	Mild-mod rash: NA	Some potential, need studies	Salicylic acid in alcoholic lotion (chest/back) Topical menthol cream
Van Doorn et al [9]	NA	NA	Tretinoin 0.025% bid; rash improved, skin scaling worsened	NA	Minocycline 100	Minocycline 100 NA	NA	NA

(continued on next page)

Table 5 (*continued*)

Author/ref	Corticosteroids		Retinoids	Antibiotics			Alpha hydroxyl acids	Topical immuno-modulatory agents	Other
	Topical	Oral		Topical	Oral (doses in mg/d)[a]	Benzoyl peroxide			
Shah et al [95]	Variable response	Variable response	Not recommended	Clindamycin 1%	Tetracycline 250 mg qid Minocycline 100 mg bid	5% gel	NA	Pimecrolimus cream 1% some success	NA
Messersmith et al [74]	NA	NA	NA	NA	Minocycline Keflex for 1 grade 2 cellulitis	NA	NA	NA	Topical silvadene
Herbst et al [8]	Effective in more intense flare-ups; oral methyl prednisolone	NA	Some response with tretinoin	Clindamycin gel	minocycline	NA	NA	NA	Hydroxyzine
Sundermeyer[b] et al [46]	NA	NA	Systemic isotretinoin has worked, routine use NR	Metronidazole Erythromycin clindamycin	Minocycline 100–200 Doxycycline 100–200	Recommended	NA	NA	Topical salicylic acid
Alexandrescu et al [77]	NA	NA	NA	NA	NA	NA	NA	NA	Colloidal oatmeal lotion in 10 patients: 6 CR; 4 PR

Hannoud et al [50]	NA	NA	NA	Doxycycline 100 mg/d	Recommended in combination with antibiotics, mean response 2 wk	NA	NA
Monti et al [90]	NA	NA	4% colloidal sulfur galenic cream	NA	NA	NA	NA
Molinari et al [23]	NA	NA	NA	Doxycycline Fusidic acid	Recommended	NA	NA
Matheis et al [30]	Triamcinolone 0.1% compounded with Eucerin 50:50 for eczema (craquele & asteatotic) bid × 1 mo	NA	Metronidazole cream 0.75% bid × 2 wks	Doxycycline 100 mg bid Minocycline 100 mg bid Selenium sulfide 10% + sulfa 5% wash qd × 2 wks	NA	NA	

To date, no evidence-based guidelines exist.

Abbreviations: bid, twice daily; CR, complete response; NA, not addressed in cited article; PR, partial response; q, every; qid, four times daily.

a Unless otherwise specified.

b These agents improved symptom clearing of secondary skin infections.

recommended that when the acneiform rash is fading or becoming scaly that alcoholic lotions or gels be switched to a cream base [65]. General recommendations include use of these agents for 2 weeks outside of a clinical trial and if no improvement, conclude treatment is ineffective and discontinue it [1]. It is also recommend that pustules be cultured at the early onset of rash to determine if *S. aureus* is present. In the setting of pain it is recommended that analgesia be used before dose reduction of EGFRI [1].

Recommendations on the cosmetic treatment of this rash suggest that makeup should not aggravate the rash and that it should be removed with a hypoallergenic liquid cleanser. The use of emollients to counter skin dryness is highly recommended.

Management of rash—preventive

To date, published data on preventive measures is scarce to nonexistent, which is not surprising given the lack of understanding of so many features of this rash. Reported recommendations include protective clothing and sunscreen when outdoors due to sunlight-induced skin rash exacerbation; bath oil or shower oil instead of gels or soaps; tepid water to wash; and use of emollient creams. Prevention results have been reported in two CRC patients treated with cetuximab and irinotecan [45]. Both patients were treated prophylactically with 4% erythromycin solution topically and systemic fusidic acid. While both patients experienced facial erythema, no pustular lesions developed. In addition, recommendations favor the use of intranasal muciprocin once daily to prevent secondary infection [1]. Another effort aimed at subsequent rash prevention was reported by Micantonio and colleagues [47] in a patient with a cetuximab-induced cycle 1 grade 3 rash. This rash only partially resolved with fusidic acid cream in cycle 1 but was successfully prevented in cycle 2 with tetracycline derivatives with only "slight erythema" noted on exam.

Treatment algorithms are beginning to appear in the literature to allow patients to continue receiving therapy without dose interruption or drug discontinuation [79]. Indeed, patient education on early intervention to avoid dose delays or discontinuation because of skin toxicity may become as critical for EGFRI therapy as the management of chemotherapy-related diarrhea. Preliminary data show that early treatment of gefitinib-induced mild and moderate dermatologic

events may prevent worsening of skin lesions and maintain patient treatment compliance [76]. Complete disappearance of grade 1 erythematous lesions occurred in 89% of cases, and in 10 cases of folliculitis there was a 50% complete resolution rate with an additional 4 patients having improvement to grade 1 (see Table 4 for treatment regimen).

When to refer to a dermatologist?

At this time there are no firm recommendations as to when to refer patients with an EGFRI-induced rash to a dermatologist. Perez-Soler and colleagues [1] suggest referral for lesions with an uncharacteristic appearance or distribution; necrosis, blistering, or petechial/pruritic lesions; or atypical dermatological manifestations unrelated to rash. Garey and colleagues [80] recommend referral for any grade 3 rash while Segaert and colleagues [83] recommend patients with the rare grade 4 EGFRI rash be treated in a specialized burn care unit. While many patients with cancer typically experience a wide range of side effects from agents used to treat their cancer, the nature and location of the EGFRI-induced rash is such that even grade 1 toxicity has led to patient request for withdrawal from treatment [11]. Thus, input from a dermatologist early in the treatment may be beneficial in controlling rash so maximal drug is administered.

Other epidermal growth factor receptor inhibitor cutaneous adverse events

Other EGFRI cutaneous adverse events, which typically are of mild severity, include pruritis, dry skin, fissures, erythema, paronychia, nasal ulcers, vaginal dryness, hyperpigmentation, and trichomegaly or abnormal hair growth, predominantly of eye lashes, and telangiectasia [11,13,84–87]. In addition, three cases of hand-foot syndrome associated with gefitinib were recently reported [88]. Skin fissures have been noted not only on the hands and feet but also on the nasolabial fold. Paronychia and pruritis are the most significant of these dermatologic adverse events from a treatment perspective.

Paronychia is characterized by inflammation and tenderness around the nails, in-grown nails, proliferation of granulation tissue, and formation of granuloma-type lesion [53,89]. EGFRI-induced paronychia may be due to skin fragility as epidermal changes observed with cetuximab include thinning of the stratum corneum and reduced keratinocyte proliferation rates [53]. Paronychia typically occurs later than the acneiform rash, usually within weeks to months after initiation of anti-EGFR therapy [8,53,86,90]. Chang and colleagues [91] reported paronychia of the fingers was more common than the toes, that paronychia accompanied skin rash, and that a paronychial biopsy revealed no evidence of folliculitis. Paronychia have frequently been complicated by painful periungual abscesses. Infection does not seem to play a consistent role with *S. aureus* cultured in only some patients and paronychia not responsive to antistaph antibiotics [53,92].

Treatment of paronychia has been successful with the following agents or regimens: oral antibiotics (minocycline [91] and doxycycline [92]) or antifungals; 4% colloidal sulfur galenic cream with AlCl3 galenic gel as astringent for pain control [90]; a drying paste containing the antiseptic chlorhexidine, an anti-yeast (nystatin), and in severe cases a topical corticosteroid [65]; soaks and cushioning of affected areas (eg, 1 part vinegar:3 parts water for 20 minutes twice daily [93]); and temporary discontinuation of the EGFRI. In one patient, rapid and almost complete resolution of inflammation occurred with use of doxycycline. This was attributed to the anti-inflammatory properties of doxycycline, which down-regulates proinflammatory cytokines (tumor necrosis factor [TNF]-α, interleukin [IL]-1β), and that tetracycline has the most potent anti-matrix metalloproteinase activity [94].

While rash typically resolves quickly, paronychial lesions have taken several months for complete healing after drug therapy stopped [12] and, despite these measures, paronychia can recur with retreatment [91]. While the nail fold inflammation induced by EGFR inhibitors mimics the clinical picture of an ingrown nail, partial nail bed excision has been unsuccessful [65]. On the other hand, weekly silver nitrate treatment for pyogenic granuloma has been successful [83].

Pruritis can be chronic and, despite treatment with antihistamines such as diphenhydramine and hydroxyzine hydrochloride, at times results have been less than impressive. Occasionally, pruritis can reach grade 3 severity requiring discontinuation of drug [84].

Dry skin or xerosis has typically been mild with an incidence of 35% and may be associated with scaly skin and pruritis, particularly on the arms and legs and in areas of previous rash [89]. Recommendations for treatment of dry skin include bland emollients such as Eucerin cream (Beiersdorf, Jobst, Germany), Cetaphil cream (Galderma,

Lausanne, Switzerland), and aquaphor (Beiersdorf) healing ointment [95]. Xerosis can develop into chronic asteatotic eczema [65]. Secondary infection may occur most commonly with *S. aureus* infections and rarely with herpes simplex virus. A severe case is illustrated by a 75-year-old man with advanced squamous cell carcinoma of the lung who presented with a generalized cutaneous xerosis and fine scaling after 3 months of gefitinib 250 mg/day [96]. After 10 days of treatment with topical corticosteroids and emollients the eruption became almost an erythrodermic exfoliative dermatitis with severe xerosis, scaling, and fissures with a parchment-like appearance that involved most of the body surface area. Laboratory studies showed prerenal uremia. Abdominal skin biopsy revealed a compact parakeratotic hyperkeratosis of the stratum corneum, a dense inflammatory infiltrate of lymphocytes, neutrophils, and nuclear dust around the hair follicles compatible with an acute folliculitis. The patient expired from cardiopulmonary arrest 2 weeks after the cutaneous and renal toxicity appeared.

Fissures have been successfully treated with propylene glycol 50% solution under plastic occlusion, salicylic acid 10% ointment, hydrocolloid dressing, and flurandrenolone tape or liquid cyanoaceylate glue [95]. Symptomatic relief of fissures has been noted with Bag Balm (Dairy Association Co., Rock Island, Quebec, Canada).

Hyperpigmentation of the skin occurred in 10% of patients treated with gefitinib in one report [91]. Most patients who developed this also had acneiform lesions and sunlight was found to accentuate the pigmentation. Bleaching creams have not been helpful and hyperpigmentation has diminished over time [65]. Prevention with either avoidance of sun exposure or use of sun blocks is recommended. Hyperpigmentation may relate to functional alterations or a postinflammatory process in melanocytes resulting in enhanced pigment transfer to basal keratinocytes or to dermal macrophages. Further studies are warranted to elucidate the mechanism of both hyperpigmentation and paronychia development [91].

EGFR inhibitors have various effects on facial and body hair. Trichomegaly presented after 5 months, 10 weeks and affected both eyelids (3) and eyebrows (1 patient) in one report. Bouche and colleagues [85] reported that 1 month after stopping cetuximab, the eyelashes had returned to normal. In comparison, scalp hairs become fine, brittle, and may curl. In general, mild hair loss on the scalp, arms, and legs occurs, although hypertrichosis has been noted on the face and female lip [65]. Telangiectasia develop on the face, ears, chest, back, and limbs, usually close to a follicular pustule [65]. They usually fade over months but leave a residual hyperpigmented area. In addition, a recent publication discussed the long-term effects, at 1 year, of EGFRI therapy including frontal alopecia in woman and growth of facial hair [97]. Abnormally long and thick hair growth distributed diffusely on the chest after 1 year of cetuximab has been reported in association with a persistent grade 3 folliculitis [98].

The three cases of grade 1 to 2 hand-foot syndrome (HFS) were observed in patients treated with gefitinib [88]. While all three had been previously treated with liposomal doxorubicin, only one patient had previously experienced HFS. The dose of gefitinib in these three patients was 250 mg twice daily (n = 2) and 250 mg daily (n = 1). The authors suggest this gefitinib-related HFS may be a "recall reaction."

Epidermal growth factor receptor inhibitor rash-related issues: future directions

Because of the numerous challenging dermatologic issues associated with EGFRI therapy, a number of groups, such as the HER1/EGFR Inhibitor Rash Management Forum, have formed to help formulate suggestions and guidelines regarding all aspects of this rash including treatment, pathology, and etiology [1]. In addition, recommendations address issues such as grading, nomenclature, assessment of rash, and prevention. For instance, it is recommended that future clinical trials testing the effectiveness of topical agents be designed such that one side of the face/body is treated for a week, with perhaps an emollient on the other side. There is only one report in the literature documenting efforts in this area. A patient with a cetuximab-induced rash was treated with 0.2% hydrocortisone valerate on the right half of the face and 0.1% tazarotene cream on the left [99]. One week later, while there was improvement on both sides of the face; the improvement was greater on the side treated with the hydrocortisone cream. However, to date, incorporation of this design in the clinical trial setting has not been reported, making it difficult to assess the true effectiveness of a given agent since these rashes have a propensity to improve in time without treatment.

Despite the previously discussed changes to the CTC grading system, the prevailing opinion is that it remains inadequate and it remains difficult to interpret and compare study results of published EGFRI trial data. Because of the frustration with standard tools for grading skin toxicity and their generally agreed on lack of applicability to the EGFRI-induced rash, different groups have started to formulate their own methods for grading these rashes [1,53,80]. Another issue is that the current grading system was designed for intermittently administered agents and acute toxicities with dose-limiting toxicity restriction to cycle 1; this scenario may no longer be prudent because of the chronic administration of novel targeted therapeutics and the nature of their toxicities [100]. Thus, a necessary transformation in the methods of assessing and grading these rashes is under way, which hopefully will yield a standardized tool that can be incorporated into treatment algorithms for these agents [101].

In addition, as further expertise with this novel rash is garnered, novel methods of treating the rash may be developed. Possibilities include agents that reverse EGFR inhibition in the skin only, agents that block cytokine kinase cascades contributing to rash, and early treatment of secondary infections based on culture results [1]. An alternative strategy would be to develop agents that are as effective as the currently approved ones but do not cause rash. The preliminary data with nimotuzumab indicate this may be a feasible strategy; however, this is a long-term approach and the issue remains that patients in the clinic today are experiencing EGFRI-induced dermatologic events.

The potential for patient selection based on the number of cytosine-adenine (CA) repeats in intron 1 of EGFR is under investigation. Preclinically, there is greater sensitivity to gefitinib in cell lines with a shorter number of CA repeats and a higher frequency of rash in patients whose skin biopsies have short CA segments in EGFR exon 1 [102]. Additional support of this theory is found in the gefitinib studies in which Asian patients with short CA repeat segments [103,104] were more sensitive to EGFR inhibitors [11,14] and experienced more toxicity than non-Asian patients [11]. Data such as this may enable identification of those patients who would require early institution of preventative measures.

Non-epidermal growth factor receptor multikinase inhibitors

The Ras/Raf/mitogen-activated protein kinase (MAPK) pathway lies downstream of the EGFR and upon phosphorylation leads to activation of Ras, Raf, and MAP/ERK kinase (MEK) and MAPK. This signaling cascade has been the target for novel anticancer strategies that recently proved successful with the approval of sunitinib and sorafenib.

Sunitinib

Sunitinib, an indolinone, selectively targets VEGFR-2, Flt-3, and PDGFR-β at submicromolar concentrations, in decreasing order of potency [105]. Sunitinib was recently approved for the treatment of gastrointestinal stromal tumors (GIST) after progression or intolerance to imatinib and was also granted accelerated approval for the treatment of patients with advanced renal cell carcinoma. The adverse-event profile includes skin toxicity that is attributed to a direct anti-VEGFR and/or PDGFR effect on dermal epithelial cells and reversible hair depigmentation associated with modulation of tyrosinase-related protein 1 genes and tyrosinase related to the kit signaling pathway [106–108].

Skin toxicity generally appears after 3 to 4 weeks of treatment. However, a transient yellow skin discoloration is observed after 1 week of therapy at doses of 50 mg/d or higher and is associated with yellow coloration of urine because of excretion of the drug and metabolites. In fact, this skin discoloration is one of the most common adverse events in a recent trial (n = 132) [109]. HFS with and without bullous lesions was observed at doses 75 mg/d or higher. Histologic evaluation showed dermal vascular modifications with slight endothelial changes in grade 1 to 2 HFS and more pronounced vascular alterations with scattered keratinocytes, necrosis, and intraepidermal cleavage in grade 3 HFS and peribullous lesions. The incidence of HFS in a phase II study in renal cell carcinoma (n = 106) was 15% of which 7% were grade 3 [110]. Robert and colleagues [97] actually use the term "acral erythema" to describe the sunitinib-induced HFS/PPE (palmar plantar erythrodysesthesia) as they suggest that the multikinase effect is distinct from the classic HFS. In fact, the term "acral erythema" has begun to replace "HFS" to denote a separate dermatologic entity. Specifically, the kinase inhibitor-induced acral erythema is more localized and hyperkeratotic than classic HFS. Paresthesia and dysesthesia precede or accompany the symmetric erythematous areas on palms and soles. Formal treatment algorithms remain to be developed for acral erythema.

Various degrees of hair depigmentation, described as "gray coloration," occurred in 60% to 64% of patients treated with sunitinib. This typically occurred after 5 to 6 weeks of treatment and resolved 2 to 3 weeks after cessation of treatment [106,111]. Hair depigmentation in men with facial hair occurred earlier at 2 to 3 weeks. Occasionally, succession of depigmented and normally pigmented bands correlated with "on" and "off" periods of treatment. Scalp skin biopsies revealed that pigment had disappeared without any other hair shaft abnormality and that hair follicle–associated melanocytes were present indicating that migration and survival of melanocytes was not affected [112]. Moss and colleagues [113] also noted that the repigmented bands of patient hair evident during rest periods off sunitinib are sometimes darker than the original patient hair color.

To date, the incidence of rash with sunitinib has been low, approximately 3%, and moderate, only reaching grade 2 intensity [110].

Sorafenib (Bay 439006)

Another multikinase inhibitor recently approved for the treatment of advanced renal cell carcinoma is sorafenib. In addition, the European Commission has approved sorafenib as an orphan drug for the treatment of hepatocellular carcinoma. Sorafenib is primarily a dual-action RAF kinase and VEGFR-2 inhibitor, but also inhibits PDGFR-β, Flt-3, and c-Kit [114]. The cutaneous adverse effects of sorafenib include rash and desquamation, and HFS/acral erythema (Table 6) [115–124]. Skin toxicity is typically mild to moderate and resolves with treatment interruptions and/or dose reduction. While skin rash occurs in 14% to 38% of patients, actual descriptions of sorafenib-induced rash are rare in the literature. Robert and colleagues [97] describe a rash that typically occurs on the face and scalp, arises after 1 to 2 weeks of drug, is erythematous and squamous in the mediofacial area and scalp, and resembles a classic moderate seborrheic dermatitis. Interestingly, scalp dysesthesia may precede or be associated with this rash. The facial erythema may be aggravated by hot temperatures and usually improves or resolves after several weeks of treatment. No standard treatment has been reported, although 2% topical ketoconazole or topical steroids may alleviate rash symptoms. Scalp biopsies revealed compact, eosinophilic stratum corneum with loss of usual basket-weave configuration.

Table 6
Dermatologic toxicities associated with sorafenib

| Author | Tumor type | Single-agent? | N | Dose, mg | Schedule | Overall derm tox | Dermatologic adverse event | | | | | | | | | |
| | | | | | | | Hand Foot Syndrome/AE | | Rash/desquamation | | Pruritis | | Alopecia | | Other skin reactions | |
							All (%)	Grade 3-4 (%)	All (%)	Grade 3-4 (%)	All	Grade 3-4 (%)	All	Grade 3-4 (%)	All (%)	Grade 3-4 (%)
Awada et al [115]	Solid tumors	Yes	44	50 qd–800 bid	qd ×21q28d	71%	19 (43)	5 (11)	(37)	(5)	(34)	(2)	(30)	0	NR	NR
Strumberg et al [118]	Solid tumors	Yes	69	50 qd–800 bid	Varied weekly	41%	16 (23)	4 (6)	18 (26)	0	NR	NR	11 (16)	2 (3)	5 (7)	0
Ratain et al [120]	RCC	Yes	202[a]	400 bid	Daily	NR	125 (62)	27 (13)	134 (66)	5 (2)	NR	NR	107 (53)	0	87 (43)/187 (93)[b]	0/34 (17)[b]
Moore et al [117]	Solid tumors	Yes	41	50 q4d–600 bid	qd ×28q35d	NR	(22)	(10)	(15)	(0)	(29)	0	(17)	0	(17)	0
Clark et al [116]	Solid tumors	Yes	19	100–800 bid	qd ×7dq14d	NR	NR	NR	6 (32)	2 (11)	4 (21)	0	NR	NR	NR	NR

First author	Tumor type	Sorafenib monotherapy	No. of patients	Dose	Schedule											
Eisen et al [121]	Melanoma	Yes	37[a]	400 bid	Daily	NR	(35)	(10.8)	(51)	(5.4%)	NR	NR	(35.1)	0	(49)	0
Escudier et al [122]	RCC	Yes	769[a]	400 bid	Daily	NR	27%		34%		NR	NR				
Abou-Alfa et al [123]	HCC	Yes	137	400 bid	Daily	NR	42 (31)	7 (5)	23 (16.8)	1 (0.7)	NR	NR	14 (10.2)	0	NR	NR
Richly et al [124]	Solid tumors	No: doxorubicin	34	100–400 bid	Daily	74%	15 (44)	4 (12)	1 (3)	0	NR	NR	9 (26)	0	NR	NR
Siu et al [119]	Pancreatic cancer	No: gemcitabine	42	100–400 bid	Daily	NR	15 (36)	(4.8)	19 (42)	(2.8)	NR	NR	NR	NR	10 (24)	0
Awada et al [125]	Solid tumors	No: capecitabine	35	200–400 bid	Daily	NR	31 (89)	10 (29)	7 (20)	0 (0)	NR	NR	12 (34)	0	NR	NR

Abbreviations: bid, twice daily; AE, acral erythema; HCC, hepatocellular carcinoma; NR, not reported; q, every; RCC, renal cell carcinoma.

[a] Includes placebo group.

[b] Reported as "derm skin, other/derm/skin."

The acral erythema described with sunitinib is less frequent with sorafenib. HFS appears to be dose-dependent and is more frequent at doses of 400 mg or higher twice daily. A recent prospective study evaluating the cutaneous side effects of sorafenib, treated HFS with salicylic-containing topical agents for chemical exfoliation of skin, topical corticosteroids twice daily for more severe inflammation with painful erythema, and analgesics to relieve pain [97]. Sorafenib has been combined with another HFS-inducing agent capecitabine in a phase I study (see Table 6) [125]. In this study, HFS was not only the most frequent toxicity overall but also the most frequent dose-limiting toxicity. At the phase II dose level of sorafenib 400 mg twice daily and capecitabine 1250 mg/m^2/day, well below capecitabine's approved single-agent dose of 2500 mg/m^2, two patients experienced grade 3 HFS. Clearly, dosing of multikinase inhibitors with capecitabine and other agents that cause HFS will need to be done cautiously. The incidence of hyperkeratosis (callus formation) is more common with sorafenib than sunitinib (Fig. 2). Recommended treatment options for hyperkeratosis include the topical exfoliating products Kerasol or Keralac [111]. The incidence of alopecia and pruritus is 27% and 19%, respectively.

Since Raf, a target for sorafenib, is a downstream effector of EGFR, Strumberg and colleagues [126] investigated the relationship between skin toxicity and time to tumor progression (TTP). In data pooled from four sorafenib dose–escalation trials (n = 179), those patients with skin toxicity (rash or HFS)/diarrhea (grade ≥ 2) had a significantly longer TTP then patients

without toxicity ($P < .05$) in those patients treated close to the recommended phase II dose of 300 to 600 mg twice daily. However, the pooled data for all doses of sorafenib (<100 to 800 mg twice daily) showed no significant difference in TTP between those categories. Further evaluation of the relationship between sorafenib skin toxicity and treatment end points is under way.

Novel multikinase inhibitor toxicity: subungual splinter hemorrhages

Painless subungual splinter hemorrhages have also been reported with sorafenib and sunitinib (Fig. 3). This adverse event has typically not been observed with other kinase inhibitors and appears to be a sorafenib and sunitinib drug–related event. It has been proposed that inhibition of VEGFR may prevent physiologic repair of delicate spiral capillaries in the nail bed when traumatized, thus explaining the lack of this effect with other kinase inhibitors [127]. However, this has not been a described effect of the VEGFR inhibitor bevacizumab. Splinter hemorrhages have been observed with sunitinib at 2 to 4 weeks in 30% of patients [127], in more than 60% of patients treated with sorafenib, and are typically more commonly seen under the fingernails than toenails. They are described as straight black or red lines that appear under the distal nail within the first 2 months of therapy and resolve spontaneously [128]. These events do not appear to be dose-related, are not associated with thrombotic or embolic events, and have not been reported with other kinase inhibitors. Subungual splinter hemorrhages may

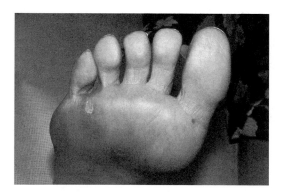

Fig. 2. Hyperkeratosis (callus formation) in a patient being treated with sorafenib. (*Reprinted from* Wood L. Managing the side effects of sorafenib and sunitinib. Commun Oncol 2006;3:558–2; with permission.)

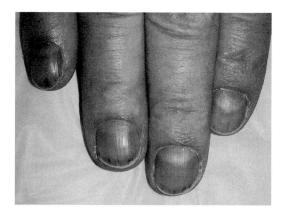

Fig. 3. Subungual hemorrhage (splinter hemorrhage) in a patient treated with sorafenib. (*Reprinted from* Wood L. Managing the side effects of sorafenib and sunitinib. Commun Oncol 2006;3:558–62; with permission.)

directly reflect the anti-VEGFR properties of these agents and nail bed examination and monitoring may be a method of evaluating the antiangiogenesis effects of these agents [127]. The appearance of these splinter hemorrhages do not necessitate treatment or dose modifications.

Combinations of multikinase inhibitors

Data regarding dermatologic toxicity with combinations of multikinase inhibitors is beginning to appear. Two of seven patients treated with the maximum tolerated dose of sorafenib (400 mg twice daily) and erlotinib (150 mg daily) presented within the first 7 days of combined therapy with erythema multiforme–like rash with edematous plaques and targetoid lesions [129]. Neither of these events was dose-limiting. This combination will be assessed in phase II studies and it will be interesting to further evaluate the dermatologic toxicity profile as drugs that target numerous different kinase inhibitors are administered together.

BCR-ABL tyrosine kinase inhibitors

The three BCR-ABL tyrosine kinase inhibitors used in the clinic are imatinib, dasatinib, and nilotinib. Nilotinib is currently only available on an expanded access clinical trial, and limited data are available on its cutaneous effects; therefore, the cutaneous effects of imatinib and dasatinib will be the focus of this section.

Imatinib

Imatinib mesylate is an oral drug approved for treatment of chronic myeloid leukemia and GIST [130,131]. In addition to potently inhibiting the BCR-ABL tyrosine kinase, imatinib inhibits c-kit and PDGFR tyrosine kinases.

The incidence of mild to moderate cutaneous adverse events was between 7% and 21% in initial studies [132]. However, later reports by Valeyrie and colleagues [133] and Van Oosterom and colleagues [134] note rashes of 66.7% and 55%, respectively. This increased incidence is attributed to study design by Valeyrie and colleagues, as theirs is the first study to solely focus on imatinib-induced cutaneous reactions and was performed at a single center. These mild to moderate adverse cutaneous events have predominantly consisted of nonspecific macular eruptions with only rare well-defined rashes presenting themselves [132,133]. Imatinib cutaneous reactions appear to be dose dependent,

possibly indicating that they are related to the drug's pharmacologic effect and not a hypersensitivity reaction [132]. Recently a review of 942 patients with GIST treated with imatinib was conducted to identify prognostic factors for toxicity [135]. This revealed that the risk for rash was higher in older patients and in those with smaller lesions. More severe or recently reported imatinib cutaneous effects include acute generalized exanthematous pustulosis [136,137], a mycosis-fungoides-like reaction [138], Stevens-Johnson syndrome [139], erosive oral lichenoid reactions [140], and hypopigmented vitiligo-like patches and generalized lightening of the skin (see Table 6) [141–144].

In general, hypopigmentation occurs in sun-exposed areas, appears in the first month of imatinib therapy, persists during drug therapy, and is reversible and dose related (Fig. 4). One episode of hypopigmentation of the penis has been reported [144]. In contrast to the EGFRI rash, the presence of hypopigmentation does not predict leukemic cell response or clinical outcome, with only two of six patients achieving a complete cytogenetic response in one series [143]. Although to date, hypopigmentation has predominantly been noted in African Americans, it is likely that this reflects a more pronounced change in skin color rather than a true ethnic effect [143]. In one report, hypopigmentation was documented by a colorimeter and demonstrated progressive increment in the L* (relative lightness) value with corresponding decrement in the b* (indicator of tanning) value [141].

The proposed mechanism for hypopigmentation is the inhibition of the melanocyte c-kit

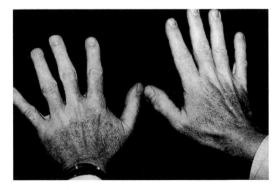

Fig. 4. Hypopigmentation of the digits, which developed several months after initiation of imatinib. (*From* Raanani P, Goldman JM, Ben-Bassat I. Depigmentation in a chronic myeloid leukemia patient treated with STI-571. J Clin Oncol 2002;20:869–70; reprinted with permission from the American Society of Clinical Oncology.)

receptor tyrosine kinase by imatinib [144]. Both c-kit and its ligand stem cell factor (SCF) participate in the regulation of normal pigmentation [145,146]. The proposed signal transduction mechanism responsible for imatinib-induced hypopigmentation involves microphthalmia (Mi), a basic helix-loop-helix leucine zipper (bHLHZip) transcription factor phosphorylated by MAP kinase at a serine residue (S73) that transactivates the tyrosine pigmentation gene promoter and affects pigment production [147].

Treatment recommendations for hypopigmentation include avoidance of sun exposure, use of sun block, and use of tinted cosmetic products and self-tanning topical preparations [143]. While not formally tested in imatinib-induced hypopigmentation, tretinoin treatment of hypopigmented macules in photo-damaged skin of elderly patients has been successful and might prove useful in the current setting [148].

In addition, another pigmentation phenomenon has been observed with imatinib, that of repigmentation of gray hair. This was observed in 9 of 133 patients and occurred after a median of 5 months (range, 2 to 14 months) of treatment with imatinib [149].

Dasatinib

Clinical experience with dasatinib remains limited compared with imatinib, as it was just recently approved for imatinib-resistant or intolerant chronic myelogenous leukemia (CML) and Philadelphia chromosome positive acute lymphocytic leukemia (Ph+ALL). The dermatologic incidence of rash with dasatinib is 26%, pruritis 8%, and acne 5% [150]. Two cases of panniculitis in patients with CML have been reported [151]. In both cases the patients had previously been treated with imatinib without cutaneous side effects. Fever with painful subcutaneous nodules with overlying erythema presented during the fourth week of dasatinib in one case and after 3 months in the other. Both were biopsied and revealed lobular panniculitis with massive infiltration by polymorphonuclear leukocytes. While one patient was successfully retreated, albeit with prednisone that was never successfully tapered, the second rash was not steroid sensitive. Speculation as to why these dasatinib effects occurred in patients with no prior imatinib-related cutaneous events include inhibition of a tyrosine kinase by dasatinib that was not inhibited by imatinib and that dasatinib may have more

completely inhibited a common target, ABL, or platelet-derived growth factor receptor β [151].

Proteosome inhibitors

Bortezomib is a dipeptidyl boronic acid that is a potent selective and reversible inhibitor of the 26S proteosome that leads to blockage of NF-KB signaling and apoptosis [152,153]. Bortezomib has been approved for the treatment of multiple myeloma after failure of at least two prior therapies [154]. Rash and desquamation were initially reported as an infrequent and usually mild adverse event [155–160] with grade 3 events occurring at doses higher than the recommended dose [161]. However, Yang and colleagues [162] observed an overall rash/desquamation incidence of 58% of which four (33%) of these were grade 3. These rashes were described as violaceous; morbiliform; associated with pruritis and erythema; and were located on the face, trunk, and extremities. The median time to onset was 11 days (range, 10 to 27 days) and rash resolved with intravenous dexamethasone and diphenhydramine. Three of four patients were dose reduced and the fourth was not retreated because of progressive disease. Grade 3 typical bortezomib rashes have been observed less frequently in adult phase II studies and in a pediatric phase I study [163–166].

There have also been reports of atypical rashes with this agent. Orlowski and colleagues [155] report a grade 2 maculopapular rash during cycle 1 in a patient treated with bortezomib 1.04 mg/m^2 that showed a perivascular lymphocytic/eosinophilic infiltrate with prominent dermal mucin deposition felt to represent an unusual hypersensitivity reaction. This rash resolved spontaneously, reappeared in cycle 2 in a more confluent appearance with associated dyspnea and arthritis, and resolved with steroids.

A more interesting atypical rash was recently reported in an overview by Gerecitano and colleagues (Fig. 5) [167], although case reports had previously appeared in the literature [168,169]. This rash in the Gereticano and colleagues series is described as a unique erythematous maculopapular rash diagnosed as a bortezomib-induced cutaneous vasculitis in 26 of 140 patients [167]. In contrast to the previously described bortezomib rashes, this cutaneous vasculitic rash typically appeared after at least two courses of bortezomib, usually during the third or fourth course and after the third or fourth

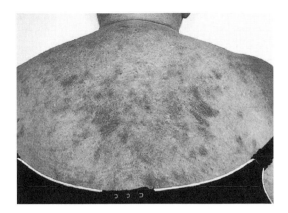

Fig. 5. Photograph of a patient with typical bortezomib-associated cutaneous vasculitic rash. Erythematous maculopapular rash on the trunk and proximal extremities. (*Reprinted from* Gerecitano J, Goy A, Wright J, et al. Drug-induced cutaneous vasculitis in patients with non-Hodgkin lymphoma treated with the novel proteasome inhibitor bortezomib: a possible surrogate marker of response? Br J Hematol 2006;134:391–8; with permission.)

dose. Typically, a nonpurpuric erythematous macular popular rash appeared on the chest, back, proximal extremities, and, less commonly, on the buttocks and was mildly pruritic. The rash appeared within days of drug infusion and resolved about 5 to 7 days after the last dose of drug, was not dose dependent, and dose reduction did not preempt recurrence of rash on rechallenge. Biopsies performed in six patients revealed a perivascular lymphocytic infiltrate without evidence of lymphoma compatible with a non-necrotizing vasculitis. No systemic vasculitis or hypersensitivity reaction or peripheral eosinophilia was noted in these patients. Interestingly, in this series of patients the response rate in the 26 patients with rash was 73% compared with 33% in those patients without rash. The odds ratio for response given the development of rash was 4.6 ($P = .001$). The authors conclude that after initially holding treatment in patients and subsequently treating through rash, that it is probably safe to continue bortezomib in patients with cutaneous restricted vasculitis [167].

Immunomodulatory drugs

This class of drugs suppresses angiogenesis, down-regulates growth signals such as IL-6, inhibits TNF-α, interrupts cell adhesion, and stimulates immune cells such as T and NK cells

[170]. Two of these drugs, lenalidomide and thalidomide, are currently used in the oncology setting. Both are approved for multiple myeloma. In addition, lenalidomide is approved for the treatment of 5q deletion subtype of myelodysplastic syndrome. Lenalidomide is 50,000-fold more potent in vitro versus the parent compound at inhibiting TNF-α, and it is not teratogenic in vitro in models that are sensitive to the teratogenic effect of thalidomide [171,172]. However, the dermatologic effects of lenalidomide are less well characterized because there has been less experience with this agent compared with thalidomide.

The predominant dermatologic changes observed with IMIDs include pruritus (42% L) and rash not otherwise specified (NOS) (16% T, 36% L). However, one review noted that minor to moderate skin eruptions were noted in nearly 50% of patients taking thalidomide alone or with dexamethasone, a higher prevalence than previously reported [173]. Rashes have been described as morbilliform, seborrheic, maculopapular, and nonspecific dermatitis. Rashes typically occur during the first month of therapy, but late-onset rashes may occur up to 4 months. It does not appear that dexamethasone significantly altered the onset of rash. Atypical IMID-related cutaneous adverse events are listed in Table 7 [174]. One report details three rare severe skin reactions (erythroderma, erythema multiforme, and toxic epidermal necrolysis) in patients who received both thalidomide with dexamethasone, which precluded further administration of drug [175–177]. In addition, one episode of toxic epidermal necrolysis syndrome had previously been reported with thalidomide listed as the causative agent [178]. One lenalidomide-induced grade 1 skin rash had the appearance of radiation recall erythema 6 months after previous radiotherapy [179].

In addition, patients treated with these agents have developed interstitial granulomatous dermatitis (IGD) characterized by annular plaques on the trunks and extremities with infiltrates of lymphocytes, histiocytes, eosinophils, and palisading degenerated collagen noted on biopsy [180]. These dermatologic changes resolved with cessation of drug administration. IGD may represent a reactive phenomenon with a histopathological spectrum depending on when in the course of the manifestations the biopsy is performed. Chu and colleagues hypothesize that the underlying pathogenesis may be related to an immune complex disorder resulting in ischemia and collagen degeneration [181].

Table 7
Reports of atypical cutaneous adverse effects observed with imatinib

Author	Event	Tumor type	# pts	Gender	Age	Race	IM dose, mg	Time of onset	Description	Ancillary study	Treatment of event	Result
Brouard et al [136]	AGEP	CML	1	NR	NR	NR	NR	NR	Scarlatiniform erythema with nonfollicular pustules confined to flexural areas	NA	NA	NA
Schwarz et al [137]	AGEP	CML	2	2F	42, 50	2 white	600 qd	12 wks, 3 mos	Generalized except palms, scalp, soles, mucocutaneous	Cultures negative (-), CRP↑, no vasculitis	Imatinib stopped	Reversible (2), atrophic residues (1)
Clark et al [138]	Mycosis-fungoides like	GIST	1	F	57	NR	400 bid	2 wks	Centripetal, macular, pruritic, diffuse skin eruption	CD4:CD8 1:1	Triamcinolone cream Hydroxyzine	Resolved after 1 y
Hsiao et al [139]	Stevens-Johnson	CML	1	M	42	NR	600 qd	1 wk	Generalized pruritic morbilliform erythematous rash. Erosions: oral, conjunctival, mucosal.	Mild perivascular lymphohistiocytic infiltration in dermis[a]	Methylprednisolone Pentoxyfylline	Improved, recurred with 1 dose imatinib rechallenge, residual chronic cicatrizing conjunctivitis
Lim et al [140]	Erosive oral lichenoid reaction	CML	1	F	72	White	400 qd	12 wks	Buccal mucosa and dorsum of tongue	Diffuse lichenoid infiltrate; DIF: negative	Drug withdrawal	Resolution; no rechallenge
Brazzelli et al [141]	Hypopigmentation	CML	1	M	17	White	400 qd	5 mos	Hypopigmentation bilateral popliteal notches, generalized lightening of skin	Wood lamp + Colorimeter +	NA	NA

Author	Reaction	Cancer	n	Sex	Age	Race	Dose	Time	Clinical description	Systemic symptoms	Management	Outcome
Hasan et al [142]	Hypopigmentation	GIST	1	M	70	Black Nigerian	600 qd	3 mos	Hypopigmentation distal fingers	NA	NA	NA
Tsao et al [143]	Hypopigmentation	CML	6	4F, 2M	32-77	6 African American	400-800 qd	At initiation (2) 1st month (1) 3rd month (1)	Generalized (3) Hands (3) Face (2) Torso (2) Upper arms (1) Neck (1)	NA	Dose reduction (1) Dose interruption (1)	Reversible (2)
Raanani et al [144]	Hypopigmentation	CML	1	M	52	White	400-600 qd	6 mos	Hypopigmentation bilateral distal hands and penis	NA	NA	NA
Valeyrie et al [133]	Hypopigmentation	CML	7	NS	NS	Ethnically pigmented	400-600 qd[b]	15 d-3 mos	Hypo- and hyperpigmented lesions cheeks (1 pt)	NA	NA	NA
	Psoriasiform rash	CML	4	NS	NS	NS	NS	1-7 mos	Scalp, arms, trunk maculopapules	NA	NA	NA
	Exfoliative dermatitis	CML	1	NS	NS	NS	600 mg/c	Day 13	Erythematous/purpuric maculopapules w/nonfollicular pustules	NA	Drug held Topical steroids	Resolution in 15 days, no rechallenge
Le Nouail et al [174]	DRESS	CML	1	F	78	NR	"low-dose"	7 wks	Macular/pruritic progressive to generalized skin eruption	Hypereosinophilia; staph. Aureus bacteremia	Imatinib held Hydrea started Antibiotics and topical steroids	Good response

Abbreviations: AGEP, Acute generalized exanthematous pustulosis; bid, twice daily; CML, chronic myelogenous leukemia; CRP, C-reactive protein; DIF, direct immunofluorescence; DRESS: drug reaction with eosinophilia and systemic symptoms; F, female; GIST, gastrointestinal stromal tumor; M, male; NA, not addressed; NR, not reported; NS, not specified though statistics in general pool; pt, patient; q, every; qid, four times a day.

a Performed at beginning of rash.

b At end of dermatologic follow-up Imatinib dose 100-800 (±116 SD).

In the event of mild grade 1 to 2 skin rash, thalidomide should be held until toxicity resolves to baseline or to less than grade 1 and then restarted at a 50% reduction. However, further dosing of thalidomide should be aborted for severe skin reactions such as Stevens-Johnson and toxic epidermal necrolysis syndrome [182]. Preventive measures have been described to minimize the risk of skin rash including avoidance of drugs that cause skin reactions like trimethoprim/sulfamethoxazole (TS) and allopurinol. However, this is problematic because of the role of TS in *Pneumocystis carinii* prophylaxis in those patients on concomitant thalidomide and high-dose dexamethasone [183]. In addition, Ghobrial and Rajkumar [182] recommend that thalidomide doses should not exceed 200 mg/d when given with dexamethasone; however, Singhal and Mehta [183] point out the lack of relationship between thalidomide dose and dexamethasone skin reactions.

Immunosuppressant macrolides: m-TOR inhibitors

The novel mammalian target of rapamycin (mTOR) kinase inhibitors act by binding to the immunophilin FKBP [184]. This complex inhibits mTOR kinase activity inducing changes in proteins downstream of mTOR leading to G1 phase cell cycle arrest [185]. The three rapamycin analogs in clinical development are CCI-779 (temsirolimus), RAD001 (everolimus), and AP23573. The administration of these agents on an intermittent schedule does not result in immunosuppression but dermatologic adverse events have proven to be dose limiting.

Rash has actually been the most common side effect of CCI-779 ranging in incidence from 51% to 76% in phase II studies [186–189]. In fact, maculopapular rash was the most frequent reason for treatment discontinuation (five patients) in one study with a dose-escalation design [190]. This rash to date has not been extensively described. It typically ranges in size from 5 to 10 cm, predominantly appears on the face and neck, occurs during the first few weeks of treatment, and reverses spontaneously [188,190].

Other dermatologic effects include grade 1 to 2 herpes lesions, acne-like rash, eczematous reactions, dry skin, pruritis, and nail disorders. The acne-like rash occurs on the face and trunk, is typically grade 1 to 2, biopsy shows accumulation of neutrophils in the dermis and epidermis, and is reversible with topical steroids [190]. However, this rash was severe and difficult to manage in two renal allograft recipients treated with sirolimus and required drug discontinuation [191].

Do vascular endothelial growth factor inhibitors cause the novel follicular rash? Bevacizumab case report

The angiogenesis inhibitor bevacizumab has been noted to cause an exfoliative dermatitis in 3% to 19% of patients [192]. Other dermatologic events ranging in frequency from 2% to 32% include alopecia, dry skin, nail disorder, skin discoloration, and skin ulcer. In the literature, an unspecified rash has been noted rarely following infusion of bevacizumab [193–195]. However, recently a bevacizumab rash, reminiscent of the EGFRI-induced rash, was described as "red papillary nodules on the chest, back, forehead and around the eyes" [196]. This rash was temporally associated with bevacizumab administration and correlated with response. More pronounced dermatologic events are noted with sorafenib, which also inhibits the VEGFR, suggesting that bevacizumab also has the potential to elicit dermatologic toxicity.

Summary

The development of molecular targeted agents has clearly improved the treatment armamentarium with improved responses and survival in a number of different malignancies. At the same time, the frequency, severity, and characteristic manifestation of adverse dermatologic events has changed in oncology patients as a result of these agents. Further evaluation and investigation of these agents into the mechanism of action, their tissue distribution, characteristics of the adverse events, and management guidelines for some of these events, such as the follicular rash, are needed. The fascinating results showing that rash, and possibly other dermatologic effects, is associated with response and other end points with some of these agents makes management issues even more urgent to optimize drug therapy for these patients.

References

[1] Perez-Soler R, Delord JP, Halpern A, et al. HER1/EGFR inhibitor-associated rash: future directions for management and investigation outcomes from

the HER1/EGFR inhibitor rash management forum. Oncologist 2005;10:345–56.

[2] Damjanov N, Meropol NJ. Epidermal growth factor receptor inhibitors for the treatment of colorectal cancer: a promise fulfilled? Oncology 2004;18: 479–88.

[3] Miller KD, Trigo JM, Wheeler C, et al. A multicenter phase II trial of ZD6474, a vascular endothelial growth factor receptor-2 and epidermal growth factor receptor tyrosine kinase inhibitor in patients with previously treated metastatic breast cancer. Clin Cancer Res 2005;11:3369–76.

[4] Holden SN, Eckhardt SG, Basser R, et al. Clinical evaluation of ZD6474, an orally active inhibitor of VEGF and EGF receptor signaling, in patients with solid, malignant tumors. Ann Oncol 2005;16: 1391–7.

[5] Yano S, Kondo K, Yamaguchi M, et al. Distribution and function of EGFR in human tissue and the effect of EGFR tyrosine kinase inhibition. Anticancer Res 2003;23:3639–50.

[6] Stoscheck CM, Nanney LB, King LE Jr. Quantitative determination of EGF-R during epidermal wound healing. J Invest Dermatol 1992;99:645–9.

[7] Mascia F, Mariani V, Girolomini G, et al. Blockade of the EGF receptor induces a deranged chemokine expression in keratinocytes leading to enhanced skin inflammation. Am J Pathol 2003; 163:303–12.

[8] Herbst RS, LoRusso PM, Purdom M, et al. Dermatologic side effects associated with gefitinib therapy: clinical experience and management. Clin Lung Cancer 2003;4:366–9.

[9] Van Doorn R, Kirtschig G, Scheffer E, et al. Follicular and epidermal alterations in patients treated with ZD1839 (Iressa), an inhibitor of the epidermal growth factor receptor. Br J Dermatol 2002;147: 598.

[10] Herbst RS, Giaccone G, Schiller JH, et al. Gefitinib in combination with paclitaxel and carboplatin in advanced non-small-cell lung cancer: a phase III trial-INTACT 2. J Clin Oncol 2004;22:785–94.

[11] Fukuoka M, Yano S, Giaccone G, et al. Multi-institutional randomized phase II trial of gefitinib for previously treated patients with advanced non-small cell lung cancer. J Clin Oncol 2003;21: 2237–46.

[12] Saltz LB, Meropol NJ, Loewer PJ, et al. Phase II trials of cetuximab in patients with refractory colorectal cancer that express the epidermal growth factor receptor. J Clin Oncol 2004;22:1201–8.

[13] Soulieres D, Senzer NN, Vokes EE, et al. Multicenter phase II study of erlotinib, an oral epidermal growth factor receptor tyrosine kinase inhibitor, in patients with recurrent or metastatic squamous cell cancer of the head and neck. J Clin Oncol 2004;22:77–85.

[14] Park J, Park BB, Kim JY, et al. Gefitinib (ZD1839) monotherapy as a salvage regimen for previously

treated advanced non-small cell lung cancer. Clin Cancer Res 2004;10:4383–8.

[15] Nemunaitis J, Eiseman J, Cunningham C, et al. Phase I clinical and pharmacokinetic evaluation of oral CI-1033 in patients with refractory cancer. Clin Cancer Res 2005;11:3846–53.

[16] Calvo E, Tolcher AW, Hammond LA, et al. Administration of CI-1033, an irreversible pan-erbB tyrosine kinase inhibitor, is feasible on a 7-day on, 7-day off schedule. Clin Cancer Res 2004;10: 7112–20.

[17] Campos S, Hamid O, Seiden MV, et al. Multicenter, randomized phase II trial of oral CI-1033 for previously treated advanced ovarian cancer. J Clin Oncol 2005;23:5597–604.

[18] Chan ATC, Hsu MM, Goh BC, et al. Multicenter, phase II study of cetuximab in combination with carboplatin in patients with recurrent or metastatic nasopharyngeal carcinoma. J Clin Oncol 2005;23: 3568–76.

[19] Burtness B, Goldwasser MA, Flood W, et al. Phase III randomized trial of cisplatin plus placebo compared with cisplatin plus cetuximab in metastatic recurrent head and neck cancer: an Eastern Cooperative Oncology Group Study. J Clin Oncol 2005; 23:8646–54.

[20] Bonner JA, Harari PM, Giralt J, et al. Radiotherapy plus cetuximab for squamous-cell carcinoma of the head and neck. N Engl J Med 2006;354: 567–78.

[21] Baselga J, Trigo JM, Bourhis J, et al. Phase II multicenter study of the antiepidermal growth factor receptor monoclonal antibody cetuximab in combination with platinum-based chemotherapy in patients with platinum-refractory metastatic and/or recurrent squamous cell carcinoma of the head and neck. J Clin Oncol 2005;23:5568–77.

[22] Herbst RS, Arquette M, Shin DM, et al. Phase II multicenter study of the epidermal growth factor receptor antibody cetuximab and cisplatin for recurrent and refractory squamous cell carcinoma of the head and neck. J Clin Oncol 2005;23:5578–87.

[23] Molinari E, De Quatrebarbes J, Andre T, et al. Cetuximab-induced acne. Dermatology 2005;211: 330–3.

[24] Erlichman C, Hidalgo M, Boni JP, et al. Phase I study of EKB-569, an irreversible inhibitor of the epidermal growth factor receptor, in patients with advanced solid tumors. J Clin Oncol 2006;24: 2252–60.

[25] Shepherd FA, Pereira JR, Ciuleanu T, et al. Erlotinib in previously treated non-small-cell lung cancer. N Engl J Med 2005;353:123–32.

[26] Philip PA, Mahoney MR, Allmer C, et al. Phase II study of erlotinib (OSI-774) in patients with advanced hepatocellular cancer. J Clin Oncol 2005; 23:6657–63.

[27] Gatzemeier U, Pluzanska A, Szczesna A, et al. Results of a phase II trial of erlotinib (OSI-774)

combined with cisplatin and gemcitabine (GC) che-motherapy in advanced non-small cell lung cancer (NSCLC) [abstr#7010]. Proc Am Soc Clin Oncol 2004;23:617.

[28] Herbst RS, Prager D, Herman R, et al. TRIBUTE: a phase III trial of erlotinib hydrochloride (OSI-774) combined with carboplatin and paclitaxel che-motherapy in advanced non-small cell lung cancer. J Clin Oncol 2005;23:5892–9.

[29] Hainsworth JD, Sosman JA, Spigel DR, et al. Treatment of metastatic renal cell carcinoma with combination of bevacizumab and erlotinib. J Clin Oncol 2005;23:7889–96.

[30] Matheis P, Socinski MA, Burkhart C, et al. Treat-ment of gefitinib-associated folliculitis. J Am Acad Dermatol 2006;55:710–3.

[31] West HL, Franklin WA, McCoy J, et al. Gefitinib therapy in advanced brochioalveolar carcinoma: Southwest Oncology Group Study S0126. J Clin Oncol 2006;24:1807–13.

[32] Baselga J, Rischin D, Ranson M, et al. Phase I safety, pharmacokinetic, and pharmacodynamic trial of ZD1839, a selective oral epidermal growth factor receptor tyrosine kinase inhibitor, in patients with five selected solid tumor types. J Clin Oncol 2002;20:4292–302.

[33] Giaccone G, Herbst RS, Manegold C, et al. Gefiti-nib in combination with gemcitabine and cisplatin in advanced non-small-cell lung cancer: a phase III trial—INTACT 1. J Clin Oncol 2004;22:777–84.

[34] Rich JN, Reardon DA, Peery T. Phase II trial of gefitinib in recurrent glioblastoma. J Clin Oncol 2004;22:133–42.

[35] Rothenberg ML, LaFleur B, Levy DE, et al. Ran-domized phase II trials of the clinical and biological effects of two dose levels of gefitinib in patients with recurrent colorectal adenocarcinomas. J Clin Oncol 2005;23:9265–74.

[36] Burris HA, Hurwitz HI, Dees EC, et al. Phase I safety, pharmacokinetics, and clinical activity study of lapatinib (GW572016), a reversible dual inhibitor of epidermal growth factor receptor tyrosine ki-nases, in heavily pretreated patients with metastatic carcinomas. J Clin Oncol 2005;23:5305–13.

[37] Vanhoefer U, Tewes M, Rojo F, et al. Phase I study of the humanized antiepidermal growth factor re-ceptor monoclonal antibody EMD72000 in pa-tients with advanced solid tumors that express the epidermal growth factor receptor. J Clin Oncol 2004;22:175–84.

[38] Rowinsky EK, Schwartz GH, Gollob JA, et al. Safety, pharmacokinetics, and activity of ABX-EGF, a fully human anti-epidermal growth factor receptor monoclonal antibody in patients with met-astatic renal cell cancer. J Clin Oncol 2004;22:3003–15.

[39] Perez-Soler R. Can rash associated with HER1/EGFR inhibition be used as a marker of treatment outcome? Oncology 2003;17(Suppl 12):23–8.

[40] Kimyai-Asadi A, Jih MH. Follicular toxic effects of chimeric anti-epidermal growth factor receptor antibody cetuximab used to treat human solid tumors. Arch Dermatol 2002;138:129–31.

[41] Hidalgo M, Siu LL, Nemunaitis J, et al. Phase I and pharmacologic study of OSI-774, an epidermal growth factor receptor tyrosine kinase inhibitor, in patients with advanced solid malignancies. J Clin Oncol 2001;19:3267–79.

[42] Ranson M, Hammond L, Ferry D, et al. ZD1839, a selective oral epidermal growth factor receptor-tyrosine kinase inhibitor is well tolerated and active in patients with solid, malignant tumors: results of a phase I trial. J Clin Oncol 2002;20:2240–50.

[43] Herbst R, Maddox AM, Rothenberg ML, et al. Selective oral epidermal growth factor receptor tyrosine kinase inhibitor ZD1839 is generally well-tolerated and has activity in non-small-cell lung cancer and other solid tumors: results of a phase I trial. J Clin Oncol 2002;20:3815–25.

[44] Schoffski P, Lutz MP, Folprecht G, et al. Cetuximab (C225) plus irinotecan (CPT-11) plus infusional 5-FU-folinic acid (FA) is safe and active in meta-static colorectal cancer (MCRC), that expresses epi-dermal growth factor receptor (EGFR). Proc Am Soc Clin Oncol 2002;21:1599.

[45] Jacot W, Bessis D, Jorda E. Acneiform eruption in-duced by epidermal growth factor receptor inhibi-tors in patients with solid tumors. Br J Dermatol 2004;151:238.

[46] Sundermeyer ML, Lessin SR, Meropol NJ. Tar-geted therapies in colorectal cancer: complications and management. Current Colorectal Cancer Re-ports 2006;2:125–33.

[47] Micantonio T, Fargnoli MC, Ricevuto E, et al. Ef-ficacy of treatment with tetracyclines to prevent acneiform eruption secondary to cetuximab ther-apy. Arch Dermatol 2005;141:1173–4.

[48] Malik SN, Siu L, Rowinsky EK, et al. Pharmaco-dynamic evaluation of the epidermal growth factor receptor inhibitor OSI-774 in human epidermis of cancer patients. Clin Cancer Res 2003;9:2478–86.

[49] Fernandez-Galar M, Espana A, Lopez-Picazo JM. Acneiform lesions secondary to ZD1839, an inhib-itor of the epidermal growth factor receptor. Clin Exp Dermatol 2004;29:138.

[50] Hannoud S, Rixe O, Bloch J, et al [Skin signs associ-ated with epidermal growth factor inhibitors]. Ann Dermatol Venereol 2006;133:239–42 [in French].

[51] Fox LP. Pathology and management of dermato-logic toxicities associated with anti-EGFR therapy. Oncology 2006;20:26–34.

[52] Hammond LA, Figueroa J, Schwartzberg L, et al. Feasibility and pharmacokinetic (PK) trial of ZD1839 (IRESSA), an epidermal growth factor re-ceptor tyrosine kinase inhibitor (EGFR-TKI), in combination with 5-fluorouracil (5-FU) and leuco-vorin (LV) in patients with advanced colorectal can-cer [a(#544)]. Proc Am Soc Clin Oncol 2001;20:137.

[53] Busam KJ, Capodieci P, Motzer R, et al. Cutaneous side-effects in cancer patients treated with the antiepidermal growth factor receptor antibody C225. Br J Dermatol 2001;144:1169–76.

[54] Mitra SS, Simcock R. Erlotinib induced skin rash spares skin in previous radiotherapy field. J Clin Orthod 2006;24(16):e28–9.

[55] Cunningham D, Humblet Y, Siena S, et al. Cetuximab monotherapy and cetuximab plus irinotecan in irinotecan-refractory metastatic colorectal cancer. N Engl J Med 2004;351:337–45.

[56] Clark GM, Perez-Soler R, Siu L, et al. Rash severity is predictive of increased survival with erlotinib HCl [abstr#786]. Proc Am Soc Clin Oncol 2003;22: 196.

[57] Saltz L, Kies M, Abbruzzese JL, et al. The presence and intensity of the cetuximab-induced acne-like rash predicts increased survival in studies across multiple malignancies [abstr#817]. Proc Am Soc Clin Oncol 2003;22:204.

[58] Kris MG, Natale RB, Herbst RS, et al. Efficacy of gefitinib, an inhibitor of the epidermal growth factor receptor tyrosine kinase, in symptomatic patients with non-small-cell lung cancer: a randomized trial. JAMA 2003;290:2149–58.

[59] Cohen EEW, Rosen F, Stadler WM, et al. Phase II trial of ZD1839 in recurrent or metastatic squamous cell carcinoma of the head and neck. J Clin Oncol 2003;21:1980–7.

[60] Ramos TC, Figueredo J, Catala M, et al. Treatment of high-grade glioma patients with the humanized anti-epidermal growth factor receptor (EGFR) antibody h-R3. Cancer Biol Ther 2006; 5(4):375–79.

[61] Allan D. Nimotuzumab: evidence of clinical benefit without rash. Oncologist 2005;10(9):760–1.

[62] Crombet T, Torres L, Neninger E, et al. Pharmacological valuation of humanized anti-epidermal growth factor receptor, monoclonal antibody h-R3, in patients with advanced epithelial-derived cancer. J Immunother 2003;26:139–48.

[63] Crombet T, Osorio M, Cruz T, et al. Use of the humanized anti-epidermal growth factor receptor monoclonal antibody h-R3 in combination with radiotherapy in the treatment of locally advanced head and neck cancer patients. J Clin Oncol 2004; 22(9):1646–54.

[64] Mita CA, Schwartz G, Mita MM, et al. A pilot, pharmacokinetic (PK), and pharmacodynamic (PD) study to determine the feasibility of intrapatient dose escalation to tolerable rash and the activity of maximal doses of erlotinib (E) in previously treated patients with advanced non-small cell lung cancer (NSCLC) [abstract#3045]. Proc Am Soc Clin Oncol 2005;23(16S):203S.

[65] Segaert S, Van Cutsem E. Clinical signs, pathophysiology and management of skin toxicity during therapy with epidermal growth factor receptor inhibitors. Ann Oncol 2005;16:1425–33.

[66] Pao W, Miller V, Zakowski M, et al. EGF receptor gene mutations are common in lung cancers from "never smokers" and are associated with sensitivity of tumors to gefitinib (Iressa) and erlotinib (Tarceva). Proc Natl Acad Sci U S A 2004;101:13306–11.

[67] Bunn PA, Franklin W. Epidermal growth factor receptor expression, signal pathway, and inhibitors in non-small cell lung cancer. Semin Oncol 2002; 29(Suppl 14):38–44.

[68] Albanell J, Rojo F, Averbuch S, et al. Pharmacodynamic studies of the epidermal growth factor receptor inhibitor ZD1839 in skin from cancer patients: histopathologic and molecular consequences of receptor inhibition. J Clin Oncol 2002;20:110–24.

[69] Tscharner GG, Buhler S, Borner M, et al. Grover's disease induced by cetuximab. Dermatology 2006; 213(1):37–9.

[70] Trojan A, Jacky E, Follath F, et al. Necrolytic migratory erythema (Glucagonoma)-like skin lesions induced by EGF-receptor inhibition. Swiss Med Wkly 2003;133:22.

[71] Sagara R, Kitami A, Nakada T, et al. Adverse reactions to gefitinib (Iressa): revealing sycosis- and pyoderma gangrenosum-like lesions. Int J Dermatol 2006; [published online].

[72] Kurokawa I, Endo K, Hirabayashi M. Purpuric drug eruption possibly due to gefitinib. Int J Dermatol 2005;44:167–8.

[73] Lenz HJ. Anti-EGFR mechanism of action: antitumor effect and underlying cause of adverse events. Oncology 2006;20:5–13.

[74] Messersmith WA, Laheru DA, Senzer NN, et al. Phase I trial of irinotecan, infusional 5-fluorouracil, and leucovorin (FOLFIRI) with erlotinib (OSI-774): early termination due to increased toxicities. Clin Cancer Res 2004;10:6522–7.

[75] National Cancer Institute. Common terminology criteria for adverse events, version 3.0. Bethesda (MD): National Cancer Institute; 2003.

[76] Cortesi E, Cerato DP, D'Auria G, et al. Management of cutaneous adverse effects during treatment with ZD1839 in advanced non-small cell lung cancer (NSCLC): surprising efficacy of early local treatment [a7100]. Proc Am Soc Clin Oncol 2004; 23:638.

[77] Alexandrescu DT, Vaillant JG, Dasanu CA. Effect of treatment with a colloidal oatmeal lotion on the acneform eruption induced by epidermal growth factor receptor and multiple tyrosine-kinase inhibitors. Clin Exp Dermatol 2006; [Epub].

[78] Townsley CA, Major P, Siu LL, et al. Phase II study of erlotinib (OSI-774) in patients with metastatic colorectal cancer. Br J Cancer 2006;94:1136–43.

[79] Rhee J, Oishi K, Garey J, et al. Management of rash and other toxicities in patients with epidermal growth factor receptor-targeted agents. Clin Colorectal Cancer 2005;5(Suppl 2):S101–6.

[80] Garey JS, Oishi KJ, Burke B, et al. Treatment of skin rash in a phase II study of cisplatin, docetaxel,

and erlotinib in patients with advanced head and neck cancer: a prospective algorithmic approach [a8231]. Proc Am Soc Clin Oncol 2006;23:786S.

[81] Garland LL, Hidalgo M, Mendelson DS, et al. A phase I and pharmacokinetic study of oral CI-1033 in combination with docetaxel in patients with advanced solid tumors. Clin Cancer Res 2006;12:4274–82.

[82] Gutzmer R, Werfel T, Mao R, et al. Successful treatment with oral isotretinoin of acneiform skin lesions associated with cetuximab. Br J Dermatol 2005;153:849.

[83] Segaert S, Tabernero J, Chosidow O, et al. The management of skin reactions in cancer patients receiving epidermal growth factor receptor targeted therapies. J Dtsch Dermatol Ges 2005;3:599.

[84] Perez-Soler R, Chachaoua A, Hammond L, et al. Determinants of tumor response and survival with erlotinib. J Clin Oncol 2004;22:3238–47.

[85] Bouche O, Brixi-Benmansour H, Bertin A, et al. Trichilomegaly of the eyelashes following treatment with cetuximab. Ann Oncol 2005;16:1171–2.

[86] Boucher KW, Davidson K, Mirakhur B, et al. Paronychia induced cetuximab, an antiepidermal growth factor receptor antibody. J Am Acad Dermatol 2002;45:632–3.

[87] Dueland S, Sauer T, Lund-Johansen F, et al. Epidermal growth factor receptor inhibition induces trichomegaly. Acta Oncol 2003;42:345–6.

[88] Razis E, Karina M, Karanastassi S, et al. Three case reports of hand-foot syndrome with gefitinib. Cancer Invest 2006;24:514–6.

[89] Lee MW, Seo CW, Kim SW, et al. Cutaneous side effects in non-small cell lung cancer patients treated with Iressa (ZD1839), an inhibitor of epidermal growth factor. Acta Derm Venereol 2004;83:116508.

[90] Monti M, Mancini LL, Ferrari B, et al. Complications of therapy and a diagnostic dilemma case. Case 2. Cutaneous toxicity induced by cetuximab. J Clin Oncol 2003;21:4651–3.

[91] Chang GC, Yang TY, Chen KC, et al. Complications of therapy in cancer patients. J Clin Oncol 2004;22:4646–8.

[92] Suh KY, Kindler HL, Medenica M, et al. Doxycycline for the treatment of paronychia induced by the epidermal growth factor receptor inhibitor cetuximab. Br J Dermatol 2006;154:191–2.

[93] Rothenberg M, Hochster H. Treatment of colorectal cancer. Expert Insights 2005;3:1–4.

[94] Golub LM, Lee HM, Ryan ME, et al. Tetracyclines inhibit connective tissue breakdown by multiple non-antimicrobial mechanisms. Adv Dent Res 1998;12:12–26.

[95] Shah NT, Kris MG, Pao W, et al. Practical management of patients with non-small-cell lung cancer treated with gefitinib. J Clin Oncol 2005;23:165–74.

[96] Pascual JC, Belinchon I, Sivera F, et al. Severe cutaneous toxicity following treatment with gefitinib (ZD1839). Br J Dermatol 2005;153:1222.

[97] Robert C, Soria JC, Spatz A, et al. Cutaneous side-effects of kinase inhibitors and blocking antibodies. Lancet 2005;6:491–500.

[98] Montagut C, Grau JJ, Grimalt R, et al. Abnormal hair growth in a patient with head and neck cancer treated with the anti-epidermal growth factor receptor monoclonal antibody cetuximab. J Clin Oncol 2005;23:5273–5.

[99] Moss JE, Burtness B. Cetuximab-associated acneiform eruption. N Engl J Med 2005;353:e17.

[100] Stadler WM. New targets, therapies, and toxicities: lessons to be learned. J Clin Oncol 2006;24:4–5.

[101] Normolle D, Lawrence T. Designing dose-escalation trials with late-onset toxicities using the time-to event continual reassessment method. J Clin Oncol 2006;24:4426–33.

[102] Perea S, Oppenheimer D, Amador M, et al. Genotypic bases of EGFR inhibitors pharmacological actions [abstract#3005]. Proc Am Soc Clin Oncol 2004;23:196.

[103] Liu WW, Innocenti F, Chen P, et al. Inter-ethnic differences in the allelic distribution of human epidermal growth factor receptor intron 1 polymorphism. Clin Cancer Res 2003;9:1009–12.

[104] Zhou Q, Kibat C, Cheung YB, et al. Pharmacogenetics of the epidermal growth factor receptor (EGFR) gene in Chinese, Malay, and Indian populations [abstract#3019]. Proc Am Soc Clin Oncol 2004;23:199.

[105] Mendel DB, Laird AD, Xin X, et al. In vivo antitumor activity of SU11248, a novel tyrosine kinase inhibitor targeting vascular endothelial growth factor and platelet-derived growth factor receptor inhibitors: determination of a pharmacokinetic/pharmacodynamic relationship. Clin Cancer Res 2003;9: 327–37.

[106] Faivre S, Delbado C, Vera K, et al. Safety, pharmacokinetic, and antitumor activity of SU11248, a novel oral multitargeted tyrosine kinase inhibitor, in patients with cancer. J Clin Oncol 2006;24: 25–35.

[107] O'Farrell AM, Foran JM, Fiedler W, et al. An innovative phase I clinical study demonstrates inhibition of FLT3 phosphorylation by SU11248 in acute myeloid leukemia patients. Clin Cancer Res 2003;9: 5465–76.

[108] Fiedler W, Serve H, Dohner H, et al. A phase I study of SU11248 in the treatment of patients with refractory or resistant acute myeloid leukemia (AML) or not amenable to conventional therapy for the disease. Blood 2005;105:986–93.

[109] Demetri GD, van Oosterom AT, Garrett CR, et al. The efficacy and safety of sunitinib in patients with advanced gastrointestinal stromal tumor after failure of imatinib: a randomized controlled trial. Lancet 2006;368:1329–38.

[110] Motzer RJ, Rini BI, Bukowski RM, et al. Sunitinib in patients with metastatic renal cell carcinoma. JAMA 2006;295:2516–24.

[111] Wood L. Managing the side effects of sorafenib and sunitinib. Community Oncology 2006;3:558–62.

[112] Robert C, Spatz, Faivre S, et al. Tyrosine kinase inhibition: grey hair. Lancet 2003;361:1056.

[113] Moss KG, Toner GC, Cherrington JM, et al. Hair depigmentation is a biological readout for pharmacological inhibition of kit in mice and humans. J Pharmacol Exp Ther 2003;307:476–80.

[114] Wilhelm SM, Carter C, Tang LY, et al. Bay439006 exhibits broad spectrum oral antitumor activity and targets the RAF/MEK/ERK pathway and receptor tyrosine kinase involved in tumor progression and angiogenesis. Cancer Res 2004;64:7099–109.

[115] Awada A, Hendlisz A, Gil T, et al. Phase I safety and pharmacokinetics of BAY-439006 administered for 21 days on/7 days off in patients with advanced refractory solid tumours. Br J Cancer 2005; 92:1855–61.

[116] Clark JW, Eder JP, Ryan D, et al. The safety and pharmacokinetics of the multi-targeted tyrosine kinase inhibitor (including Raf kinase and VEGF kinase), BAY 43-9006, in patients with advanced, refractory solid tumors. Clin Cancer Res 2005;11: 5472–80.

[117] Moore MJ, Hirte HW, Siu L, et al. Phase I study to determine the safety and pharmacokinetics of the novel Raf kinase and VEGFR inhibitor BAY43-9006, administered for 28 days on/7 days off in patients with advanced, refractory solid tumors. Ann Oncol 2005;16:1688–94.

[118] Strumberg D, Richly H, Hilger RA, et al. Phase I clinical and pharmacokinetic study of the novel Raf kinase and vascular endothelial growth factor receptor inhibitor BAY43-9006 in patients with advanced refractory solid tumors. J Clin Oncol 2005; 23:965–72.

[119] Siu L, Awada A, Takimoto CH, et al. Phase I trial of sorafenib and gemcitabine in advanced solid tumors with an expanded cohort in advanced pancreatic cancer. Clin Cancer Res 2006;12:144–51.

[120] Ratain MJ, Eisen T, Stadler WM, et al. Phase II placebo-controlled randomized discontinuation trial of sorafenib in patients with metastatic renal cell carcinoma. J Clin Oncol 2006;24:2505–12.

[121] Eisen T, Ahmad T, Flaherty KT, et al. Sorafenib in advanced melanoma: a phase II randomized discontinuation trial analysis. Br J Cancer 2006;95: 581–6.

[122] Escudier B, Szczylik C, Eisen T, et al. Randomized phase III trial of the Raf kinase and VEGFR inhibitor Sorafenib (Bay 43-9006) in patients with advanced renal cell carcinoma (RCC). Proc Am Soc Clin Oncol 2005;23:4510a.

[123] Abou-Alfa GK, Schwartz Lisa, Ricci S, et al. Phase II study of sorafenib in patients with advanced hepatocellular carcinoma. J Clin Oncol 2006;24: 4293–300.

[124] Richly H, Henning BF, Kupsch P, et al. Results of a phase I trial of sorafenib (Bay-439006) in combination with doxorubicin in patients with refractory solid tumors. Ann Oncol 2006;17: 866–73.

[125] Awada A, Gil T, Vanhamme J, et al. A phase I study of sorafenib in combination with capecitabine in patients with advanced solid tumors [abstr#98]. Proc 18th EORTC-NCI-AACR Symposium Molec Targets Cancer Ther 2006;4:33.

[126] Strumberg D, Awada A, Hirte H, et al. Pooled safety analysis of BAY43-9006 (Sorafenib) monotherapy in patients with advanced solid tumors: is rash associated with treatment outcome? Eur J Cancer 2006;42:548–56.

[127] Robert C, Faivre S, Raymond E, et al. Subungual splinter hemorrhages: a clinical window to inhibition of vascular endothelial growth factor receptors? Ann Intern Med 2005;143:313–4.

[128] Autier J, Escudier B, Spatz A, et al. A prospective study of the cutaneous side-effects of sorafenib, a novel multikinase inhibitor [abstr#105]. Proc 18th EORTC-NCI-AACR Symposium Molec Targets Cancer Ther 2006;4:35.

[129] Duran I, Hotte SJ, Chen EX, et al. Dual inhibition of the MAPK pathway by combination targeted therapy: a phase I trial of Sorafenib (SOR) and erlotinib (ERL) in advanced solid tumors [abstr#550]. Proc 18th EORTC-NCI-AACR Symposium Molec Targets Cancer Ther 2006;4:167.

[130] Druker BJ, Talpaz M, Resta DJ, et al. Efficacy and safety of a specific inhibitor of the BCR-ABL tyrosine kinase in chronic myeloid leukemia. N Engl J Med 2001;344:1031–7.

[131] Druker BJ, Sawyers CL, Kantarjian H, et al. Activity of a specific inhibitor of the BCR-ABL tyrosine kinase in the blast crisis of chronic myeloid leukemia. N Engl J Med 2001;344:1038–42.

[132] Brouard M, Sauart JH. Cutaneous reactions to STI571. N Engl J Med 2001;345:618–9.

[133] Valeyrie L, Bustuji-Garin S, Revuz J, et al. Adverse cutaneous reactions to imatinib (STI571) in Philadelphia chromosome-positive leukemias: a prospective study of 54 patients. J Am Acad Dermatol 2003;48:201–6.

[134] Van Oosterom AT, Judson I, Verweij J, et al. Safety and efficacy of imatinib (STI571) in metastatic gastrointestinal stromal cancers: a phase I study. Lancet 2001;358:1421–3.

[135] Glabbeke MV, Verweij J, Casali PG, et al. Predicting toxicities for patients with advanced gastrointestinal stromal tumours treated with imatinib: a study of the European Organization for Research and Treatment of Cancer, the Italian Sarcoma Group, and the Australasian Gastro-Intestinal Trials Group (EORTC-ISG-AGITG). Eur J Cancer 2006; [Epub ahead of print].

[136] Brouard M, Prins C, Mach-Pascual S, et al. Acute generalized exanthematous pustulosis associated with STI571 in a patient with chronic myeloid leukemia. Dermatology 2001;203:57–9.

[137] Schwarz M, Kreuzer KA, Baskaynak G, et al. Imatinib-induced acute generalized exanthematous pustulosis (AGEP) in two patients with chronic myeloid leukemia. Eur J Haemtol 2002;69:254–6.

[138] Clark SH, Duvic M, Prietol VG. Mycosis fungoides-like reactions in a patient treated with Gleevec. J Cutan Pathol 2003;30:279–81.

[139] Hsiao LT, Chung HM, Lin JT, et al. Stevens-Johnson syndrome after treatment with STI571: a case report. Br J Hematol 2002;117:620–2.

[140] Lim DS, Muir J. Oral lichenoid reaction to imatinib (STI571, Gleevec). Dermatology 2002;205:169–71.

[141] Brazzelli V, Roveda E, Prestinari F, et al. Vitiligo-like lesions and diffuse lightening of the skin in a pediatric patient treated with imatinib mesylate: a noninvasive colorimetric assessment. Pediatr Dermatol 2006;23(2):175–8.

[142] Hasan S, Dinh K, Lombardo F, et al. Hypopigmentation in an African patient treated with imatinib mesylate: a case report. J Natl Med Assoc 2003; 95:722–4.

[143] Tsao AS, Kantarjian H, Cortes J, et al. Imatinib mesylate causes hypopigmentation in the skin. Cancer 2003;98:2483–7.

[144] Raanani P, Goldman JM, Ben-Bassat I. Depigmentation in a chronic myeloid leukemia patient treated with STI-571. J Clin Oncol 2002;20:869–70.

[145] Grichnik JM, Burch JA, Burchette J, et al. The SCF-KIT pathway plays a critical role in the control of normal human melanocyte homeostasis. J Invest Dermatol 1998;111:233–8.

[146] Longley BJ, Carter EI. SCF-KIT pathway in human epidermal melanocyte homeostasis. J Invest Dermatol 1999;113:139–40.

[147] Hemesath TJ, Price ER, Takemoto C, et al. MAP kinase links the transcription factor Micropthalmia to c-Kit signalling in melanocytes. Nature 1998; 391:298–301.

[148] Pagroni A, Kligman AM, Sadiq I, et al. Hypopigmented macules of photodamaged skin and their treatment with topical tretinoin. Acta Derm Venereol 1999;79:305–10.

[149] Etienne G, Cony-Makhoul P, Mahon FX. Imatinib mesylate and gray hair. N Engl J Med 2002;347:446.

[150] Fda.gov/ohrms/dockets/AC/06/briefing/2006-4220-B1-01BristolMyersSquibb-background.pdf.

[151] Assouline S, Laneuville P, Gambacorti-Passerini C. Panniculitis during dasatinib therapy for imatinib-resistant chronic myelogenous leukemia. N Engl J Med 2006;354:2623–4.

[152] Orlowski RZ. The role of the ubiquitin-proteosome pathway in apoptosis cell death differ. Cell Death Differ 1999;6:303–13.

[153] Grimm LM, Osborne BA. Apoptosis and the proteosome. Prob Cell Differ 1999;23:209–28.

[154] Kane RC, Bross PF, Farrell AT, et al. Velcade: U.S. FDA approval for the treatment of multiple myeloma progressing on prior therapy. Oncologist 2003;8:508–13.

[155] Orlowski RZ, Stinchcombe TE, Mitchell BS, et al. Phase I trial of the proteosome inhibitor PS-341 in patients with refractory hematologic malignancies. J Clin Oncol 2002;20:4420–7.

[156] Adams J. Proteosome inhibition in cancer: development of PS-341. Semin Oncol 2001;28:613–9.

[157] Papandreou CN, Daliani DD, Nix D, et al. Phase I trial of the proteosome inhibitor bortezomib in patients with advanced solid tumors with observations in androgen-independent prostate cancer. J Clin Oncol 2004;22:2108–21.

[158] Shah MH, Young D, Kindler HL, et al. Phase II study of the proteosome inhibitor bortezomib (PS-341) in patients with metastatic neuroendocrine tumors. Clin Cancer Res 2004;10:6111–8.

[159] Dy GK, Thomas JP, Wilding G, et al. A phase I and pharmacologic trial of 2 schedules of the proteasome inhibitor PS-341 (Bortezomib, Velcade), in patients with advanced cancer. Clin Cancer Res 2005;11:3410–6.

[160] Davis NB, Taber DA, Ansari RH, et al. Phase II trial of PS-341 in patients with renal cell cancer: a University of Chicago phase II consortium study. J Clin Oncol 2004;22:115–9.

[161] Hamilton AL, Eder JP, Pavlick AC, et al. Proteosome inhibition with bortezomib (PS-341): a phase I study with pharmacodynamic endpoints using a day 1 and day 4 schedule in a 14-day cycle. J Clin Oncol 2005; 23:6107–16.

[162] Yang CH, Gonzalez-Angulo AM, Reuben JM, et al. Bortezomib (VELCADE) in metastatic breast cancer: pharmacodynamics, biological effects, and prediction of clinical benefits. Ann Oncol 2006;17: 813–7.

[163] Richardson PG, Barlogie B, Berenson J, et al. A phase 2 study of bortezomib in relapsed, refractory myeloma. N Engl J Med 2003;348:2609–17.

[164] Richardson PG, Sonneveld P, Schuster MW, et al. Bortezomib or high-dose dexamethasone for relapsed multiple myeloma. N Engl J Med 2005; 352:2487–98.

[165] Blaney SM, Bernstein M, Neville K, et al. Phase I study of the proteosome inhibitor bortezomib in pediatric patients with refractory solid tumors: a children's group study (ADVL0015). J Clin Oncol 2004;22:4804–9.

[166] Fisher RI, Bernstein SH, Kahl BS, et al. Multicenter phase II study of bortezomib in patients with relapsed or refractory mantle cell lymphoma. JClin Oncol 2006;24:4867–74.

[167] Gerecitano J, Goy A, Wright J, et al. Drug-induced cutaneous vasculitis in patients with non-Hodgkin lymphoma treated with the novel proteasome inhibitor bortezomib: a possible surrogate marker of response? Br J Hematol 2006;134:391–8.

[168] Agterof MJ, Biesma DH. Bortezomib-induced skin lesions. N Engl J Med 2005;352:2534.

[169] Min CK, Lee S, Kim YJ, et al. Cutaneous leucoclastic vasculitis (LV) following bortezomib

therapy in a myeloma patient; association with pro-inflammatory cytokines. Eur J Haematol 2006;76:265–8.

[170] Singhal S, Mehta J, Desikan R, et al. Antitumor activity of thalidomide in refractory multiple myeloma. N Engl J Med 1999;341:1565–71.

[171] Bartlett JB, Dredge K, Dalgfleish AG. The evolution of thalidomide and its IMID derivatives as anticancer agents. Nat Rev Cancer 2004;4:314–22.

[172] Moschella SL. Is there a role for tumor necrosis factor-alpha inhibitors especially thalidomide in dermatology? Skinmed 2005;4:19–32.

[173] Hall VC, El-Azhary RA, Bouwhuis S, et al. Dermatologic side effects in patients with multiple myeloma. J Am Acad Dermatol 2003;48:548–52.

[174] Le Nouail P, Viseaux V, Chaby G, et al [Drug reaction with eosinophilia and systemic symptoms (DRESS) following imatinib therapy]. Ann Dermatol Venereol 2006;133:686–8 [in French].

[175] Rajkumar SV, Gerz MA, Witzig TE. Life-threatening toxic epidermal necrolysis with thalidomide therapy for myeloma. N Engl J Med 2000;343:972–3.

[176] Bielsa I, Teixido J, Rivera M, et al. Erythroderma due to thalidomide: report of 2 cases. Dermatology 1994;189:179–81.

[177] Salafia A, Kharkar RD. Thalidomide and exfoliative dermatitis. Int J Lepr Other Mycobact Dis 1988;56:625.

[178] Horowitz SB, Stirling AL. Thalidomide-induced toxic epidermal necrolysis. Pharmacotherapy 1999;19:1177–80.

[179] Sharma RA, Steward WP, Daines CA, et al. Toxicity profile of the immunomodulatory thalidomide analogue, lenalidomide: phase I clinical trial of three dosing schedules in patients with solid malignancies. Eur J Cancer 2006;42:2318–25.

[180] Deng A, Harvey V, Sina B, et al. Interstitial granulomatous dermatitis associated with the use of tumor necrosis factor alpha inhibitors. Arch Dermatol 2006;142(2):198–202.

[181] Chu P, Connolly K, LeBoit PE. The histopathological spectrum of palisaded neutrophilic and granulomatous dermatitis in a patient with collagen vascular disease. Arch Dermatol 1994;130:1278–83.

[182] Ghobrial IM, Rajkumar SV. Management of thalidomide toxicity. J Support Oncol 2003;1:194–205.

[183] Singhal S, Mehta J. Peer viewpoint: management of thalidomide toxicity. J Support Oncol 2003;1:194–205.

[184] Skotnicki JS, Leone CL, Smith AL. Design, synthesis, and biological evaluation of C-42 hydroxyesters of rapamycin: the identification of CCI-779. Clin Cancer Res 2001;7:3749S–50S.

[185] Gibbons JJ, Discafanic C, Peterson R. The effect of CCI-779, a novel macrolide antitumor agent, on growth of tumor cells in vitro in nude mouse xenografts in vivo [a1000]. Proc Am Assoc Cancer Res 1999;40:301.

[186] Chan S, Scheulen ME, Johnston S, et al. Phase II study of temsirolimus (CCI-779), a novel inhibitor of mTOR, in heavily pretreated patients with locally advanced or metastatic breast cancer. J Clin Oncol 2005;23:5314–22.

[187] Witzig TE, Geyer SM, Ghobrial I, et al. Phase II trial of single-agent temsirolimus (CCI-779) for relapsed mantle cell lymphoma. J Clin Oncol 2005;23:5347–56.

[188] Atkins MB, Hidalgo M, Stadler WM, et al. Randomized phase II study of multiple dose levels of CCI-779, a novel mammalian target of rapamycin kinase inhibitor, in patients with advanced refractory renal cell carcinoma. J Clin Oncol 2004;22:909–18.

[189] Galanis E, Buckner Jesus Christ, Maurer MJ, et al. Phase II trial of temsirolimus (CCI-779) in recurrent glioblastoma multiforme: a north central treatment group study. J Clin Oncol 2005;23:5294–304.

[190] Raymond E, Alexandre J, Faivre S, et al. Safety and pharmacokinetics of escalated doses of weekly intravenous infusion of CCI-779, a novel mTOR inhibitor, in patients with cancer. J Clin Oncol 2004;22:2336–47.

[191] Kunzle N, Venetz JP, Pascual M, et al. Sirolimus-induced acneiform eruption. Dermatology 2005;211:366–9.

[192] Avastin package insert. South San Francisco, CA: Genentech Inc.

[193] Gordon MS, Margolin K, Talpaz M, et al. Phase I safety and pharmacokinetic study of recombinant human anti-vascular endothelial growth factor in patients with advanced cancer. J Clin Oncol 2001;19:843–50.

[194] Chen HX, Gore-Langton RE, Cheson BD. Clinical trials: referral resource: current clinical trials of the anti-VEGF monoclonal antibody bevacizumab. Oncology 2001;15:1019–26.

[195] Pegram MD, Reese DM. Combined biological therapy of breast cancer using monoclonal antibodies directed against HER2/neu protein and vascular endothelial growth factor. Semin Oncol 2002;29(Suppl 11):29–37.

[196] Gotlib V, Khaled S, Lapko I, et al. Skin rash secondary to bevacizumab in a patient with advanced colorectal cancer and relation to response [case reports]. Anti-Cancer Drugs 2006;17:1227–9.

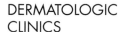

ELSEVIER
SAUNDERS

Dermatol Clin 26 (2008) 161–172

Radiation Therapy Toxicity to the Skin

T.J. FitzGerald, MD*, Maryann Bishop Jodoin, BS,
Gayle Tillman, MD, Jesse Aronowitz, MD, Richard Pieters, MD,
Susan Balducci, RN, NP, Joshua Meyer, MD,
M. Giulia Cicchetti, MD, Sidney Kadish, MD,
Shelagh McCauley, MD, Joanna Sawicka, MD,
Marcia Urie, PhD, Y.C. Lo, PhD, Charles Mayo, PhD,
Kenneth Ulin, PhD, Linda Ding, PhD, Maureen Britton, BSN,
Jiayi Huang, MD, Edward Arous, BS

*Department of Radiation Oncology and The Cancer Center, The University of Massachusetts Medical School,
UMass Memorial Health Care, 55 Lake Avenue N., Worcester, MA 01655, USA*

Radiation therapy is one of the core treatment strategies for the care of cancer patients. More than 60% of all cancer patients in North America are treated with radiation therapy as part of their treatment plan. Accordingly, understanding the short-term and long-term effects of radiation therapy to the skin is of importance to health care providers involved with these patients. With each passing year, there are more patients surviving their primary malignancy; therefore normal tissue toxicity is becoming of increasing relevance to those who care for these patients, from both an oncology and primary care perspective. Although modern technologies in radiation therapy may decrease dermal toxicity, it must be recognized that many patients were treated with less advanced treatment techniques and accelerated treatment delivery strategies. Understanding the evolution of treatment technology and the application of radiation therapy will aid health care providers in the evaluation and care of the cancer survivor.

Histology of the skin

The skin is composed of the epidermis and dermis. The epidermis is composed of stratified squamous epithelium, which in most regions of the body is no more than 2 mm in thickness, with many areas (eyelid and others) less thick. The cell population in the basal layer of the epidermis residing on the basement membrane undergoes division to replace cells at the surface. The cycle is thought to take 3 weeks, and is influenced by many factors, including various disease processes. The dermis resides beneath the epidermis, and can vary in thickness between a few millimeters to a centimeter. The portion of the dermis that contacts the epidermis is referred to as the papillary layer. This contains tissues such as lymphatic conduits, nerves, hair follicles, glandular tissue, and blood vessels embedded in a connective tissue stroma. The deeper portions of the dermis, which contains stroma, composed of elastic fibers and collagen, is referred to as the reticular layer. These structures sit upon subcutaneous tissue and other supportive cell structures, including adipose, nerves, and larger lymphatic and blood vessels. The vascular and nerve root connections in the dermis provide nutrients and support for the self-renewal process of the basal layer of the epidermis [1–6].

* Corresponding author.
E-mail address: fitzgert@ummhc.org
(T.J. FitzGerald).

0733-8635/08/$ - see front matter © 2008 Elsevier Inc. All rights reserved.
doi:10.1016/j.det.2007.08.005

derm.theclinics.com

History and evolution of radiation therapy in the care of the cancer patient

The discovery of radiography by Roentgen and radium by the Curies established the basis for radiation therapy. Within months of the discovery, radiographs were investigated by physicians, scientists, and curiosity seekers. Primitive radiograph tubes were quite bulky, and early investigators tested their function with fluoroscopy of their own hands. These investigators were the first to identify both erythema and epilation, thus suggesting their use for therapy. Multiple disease processes, both inflammatory and noninflammatory in origin, were treated with radiographs; however, continued unprotected use led to extraordinary consequences, including ulceration and gangrene of skin. Many of the first generation of radiographers required amputation, and many succumbed to squamous cell cancers, leukemia, and aplastic anemia (Marie Curie and her daughter, Irene) [7]. Many uses of radiation therapy were identified and published by 1910, including radium brachytherapy and orthovoltage teletherapy. Before the establishment of strategies to measure absorbed treatment dose, one of the first measures of radiation therapy was the use of erythema units, specifically the measure of how red the skin became from daily treatment. The single-fraction radiograph dose that induces erythema is approximately 500 centi-Gray units (cGy) [1,2,5,6,8].

For most patients the skin is an unintentional target of treatment. Improvements in teletherapy technique have improved acute and late effects to dermal surfaces. Until the introduction of megavoltage equipment (cobalt and linear accelerators) in the 1950s and 60s, orthovoltage energies (in the kilovoltage range), were used for radiotherapy. They are highly effective in treating tumors on the skin surface, but inadequate for treatment of tumors at depth (in the central aspect of the chest, abdomen, and pelvis). To deliver a tumoricidal radiation therapy dose to the target in the central aspect of the chest using orthvoltage radiography would necessitate delivery of two to three times the dose to the skin surfaces. Dermal surfaces received extremely high daily fractional and total treatment dose, resulting in severe acute and chronic dermal sequelae, including desquamation and chronic scarring. Maneuvers such as "filtration" (elimination of the least penetrating components of the radiographic beam) and "crossfiring" (the use of multiple intersecting beams) partially ameliorated the problem without improving depth dose. Megavoltage therapy offered the first true "skin sparing." By then, scientists could measure the dose absorbed by, rather than delivered to, tissue. Total absorbed dose is the sum of the doses transmitted by the primary beam and secondary scatter events. Biological effects in both clinical practice and laboratory research correlate with absorbed radiation dose, which is expressed as energy per unit mass of tissue. This correlation is consistent for gamma rays, fast neutrons, and electrons. The unit dose was originally referred to as a rad, which was defined as the energy absorption corresponding to 100 ergs/g. This unit has been replaced by the gray (Gy). One Gray is the equivalent of 100 rads. Because of limited backscatter, the dose to skin surface was considerably decreased for gamma rays generated by megavoltage equipment. This has further improved with the use of multifield therapy planning and higher therapy energies, thus further serving to decrease dose to skin surface [6]. Three-dimensional planning permits accurate delineation of skin contours and identifies tangential skin surfaces and skin folds, which would be vulnerable to radiation dose. Intensity modulation treatment techniques permit subsegment evaluation of dermal surfaces, and dynamic leaf motion serves to further decrease skin dose. There remains, however, a population of patients who were successfully treated with radiation therapy using older techniques and equipment, and who will bear the sequelae of treatment for a lifetime. It is therefore useful to document the methodology of treatment when evaluating its effects.

Radiation biology

There are many factors that influence the effects of radiation treatment on normal tissue function. Normal tissues vary greatly in their intrinsic sensitivity to radiation therapy. There are certain tissues that can tolerate extremely high doses of radiation therapy (bile duct), and others that can tolerate relatively little radiation therapy (bone marrow). The skin is a complex organ composed of tissues with a relatively rapid self-renewal potential, as well as support tissues with limited self-renewal potential. The dermis is composed of cells with intermediate radiation sensitivity. Therefore tissues within the skin are composed of cells that demonstrate both early and late response to radiation therapy. The dermal appendages, including hair and nails, likewise have varied sensitivity and self-renewal potential. The epithelial tissues of the skin are sensitive to radiation therapy with an alpha/beta ratio of 10, and hence sensitive to the effects of both daily dose fraction size and total dose. Other biological effects also influence sensitivity to treatment, however. The cell cycle remains an important issue for radiation sensitivity. Cells with rapid cell cycle kinetics, such as the epidermis, are more sensitive to treatment and demonstrate more acute effects during the course of treatment. This is because of the fact that both tumor and normal tissues are sensitive to radiation therapy in the G2M phase of the cell cycle, and are likely more resistant to therapy in DNA synthesis. The kinetics of healing with support of repopulation of stem cells from other skin surfaces outside of the radiation therapy treatment field results in relatively rapid healing of damage induced by radiography, largely generated through traditional inflammatory processes. Certain dermal structures such as glandular cells, basement membrane, elastic cells, and other support fibers have a more protracted response to radiography; therefore restoration of dermal lubrication, hair regrowth, and re-establishment of the complement of support fibers occurs at a more protracted pace [1–6,8].

Fractionation (daily treatment dose) is the most important aspect in determining both acute and late effects of radiation treatment. The earliest attempts at delivering radiation treatment against tumor targets consisted of long, protracted, single radiograph exposure to tumor targets. Although tumor response was documented, the effect upon normal tissues, including skin, was not acceptable with severe nonhealing injuries. Investigators at that time point began to evaluate the role of multiple treatment sessions over a more protracted time period. Enthusiasm was rapidly acquired for such an approach, because there was clear impact against tumor, with amelioration of sequelae identified with single-exposure treatments. From a biological perspective, fractionation provided significant advantage for sparing normal tissue. Repair, repopulation, regeneration, and reoxygenation are commonly referred to as the "four R's" of radiation biology, and each plays a significant role in support of normal tissue response to radiation treatment, as well as a traditional role in defining tumor response to radiation therapy [6].

Normal tissues repair radiation damage with varied capability. Certain cells in the body have limited to no capacity to repair radiation injury. These include bone marrow and sperm. Other cell systems appear to have more robust capacity to repair sublethal events. Bone and muscle are examples of these systems. Often the repair processes are clinically undetected because the damage to normal tissues is sublethal in nature; however, if the repair process were overwhelmed by single exposure treatment, the damage to normal tissue would be much more obvious. The balance in treatment fractionation is to deliver a tumoricidal dose of radiation, but not to consume the ability of the cell to repair sublethal events. Potentially lethal damage is a term used to describe the possible influence of radiation therapy effects in the recovery phase of management. This relates to alteration in post-therapy conditions, which may serve to influence normal tissue outcome. For example, if dermal tissues become secondarily infected at closure of radiation treatment, the system's ability to repair may be influenced by this event. During a protracted treatment course, repair kinetics often become stressed. The response to this phenomenon is to generate an inflammatory response to bring in stem cells from other dermal areas outside of the radiation therapy treatment field to aid in recovery. This is referred to as repopulation. This is an important aspect of self-renewal and healing, because we can draw upon resources from other body areas to heal. Treatments such as total skin radiation therapy for mycosis fungoides and total body radiation therapy for bone marrow transplant raise interesting questions for the concept of repopulation of skin, because treatment is directed to large volumes of the stem cell population. In both of these systems, fractionation of treatment is crucial in preserving normal tissue integrity. Kinetics of stem cell division are also increased through this process until healing is complete. This is referred to as regeneration, because cells are accelerated through the cell cycle to aid in repair processes. Tissues also reoxygenate because there is increased blood flow (erythema) in the treatment field. This aids in both tumor cell kill and healing of normal tissues [6].

Biology and response of normal tissue plays a crucial role in the response of skin to radiation therapy. The ability of the skin system to repair damage from therapy can be influenced by many factors, including general health, competing medical comorbidities, and concurrent or previous therapies. Repair can be influenced by chemo-therapy and genetic predisposition to less robust repair of injury (ataxia-telangietasia). Repopulation of stem cells can be influenced by previous or concurrent therapies, or by therapies that treat the majority of dermal stem cells, such as total skin radiation therapy and total body radiation therapy. Regeneration is influenced by previous therapies and perturbations in cell cycle kinetics. Reoxygenation is influenced by the integrity of the dermal structures of the host. For example, similar to surgery, radiation therapy to areas of the body without redundant dermal tissue (anterior tibia, sole of the foot, eyelid, and so on) often requires more protracted treatment courses because of the limited infrastructure associated with skin surfaces in those areas. Patients who have severe leg edema have compromise in dermal integrity and treating the lower extremity in these patients; hence treatment strategies, which promote a higher degree of daily injury, are often difficult in this cohort of patients because they are poorly oxygenated and thus heal poorly. Areas of previous graft placement often require protracted treatment strategies for similar reasons. One has to balance radiation treatment strategy of daily dose and treatment volume with the factors that influence response to injury in the management of patients. The biologic principals identified have clear influence in patient management.

Response of the skin to radiation therapy

Radiation therapy inhibits cells from dividing and producing daughter progeny. Often cells must go through three or four divisions for this effect to be visualized. In the acute phase of management, inhibition of mitosis of dermal stem cells appears 30 to 60 minutes after a single dose of 5 Gy, and is followed by a clear decrease in the proliferation of the stem cells along the basement membrane. Effects on the endothelium are identified at this level as well. One can see capillary dilatation within a few hours of treatment, and increased capillary permeability is identified. If radiation therapy is given in several protracted treatment doses (fractionated therapy), higher doses of radiation therapy are needed to produce the same effect because of the biologic principles identified, including repair, repopulation, regeneration, and reoxygenation. As treatment continues, a series of classic changes are identified in dermal tissue that are consistent with inflammatory response to injury. These consist of swelling and proliferation of capillary endothelial cells. In larger arteriole vessels, one begins to see thickening of the tunica intima as time goes on. The basal cells enlarge and demonstrate nuclear enlargement. Similar effects occur in maturing keratinocytes. These effects culminate in the moist desquamation phase, which often is visible 3 to 4 weeks after initiation of a relatively protracted phase of management. This is manifested as vascular dilatation and hyperemia, edema, and extravasation of blood cells [1,2,5]. Blisters may form as part of this process because fluid may coalesce into loculated areas. Similar changes are seen in support structures of the skin, and are exacerbated by the thinning and denudation of the epithelial layer of the skin. Hair follicles can be damaged at doses as low as 3 to 4 Gy. In the experience of the authors' department, patients have developed scalp alopecia with doses as low as 3 Gy (though this is unusual). Alopecia is not often visible until 2 to 4 weeks after the initiation of treatment, because hair follicles may adhere to strands of hair. Self-renewal of scalp hair is thought to take 3 weeks, although this can vary with environmental conditions. Hair appears to have varied sensitivity in the body, with the repopulation kinetics possibly influenced by its robust vascular supply. Hairs such as eyelashes and eyebrows appear to have a more delayed response and decreased repopulation ability. Glandular structures likewise appear to have delayed repopulation kinetics, because these are slowly dividing cells. This explains why xerosis remains a concern to patients long after therapy is completed. Nails appear sensitive to radiation therapy as well. If the nail matrix receives greater than 15 Gy, nail regrowth is compromised. Therefore, in patients treated with total skin radiation therapy, the nail beds (inferior to the cuticle) are often shielded at 14 to 15 Gy. Although skin ulceration is rare with modern therapy techniques, skin necrosis and ulceration can occur 2 to 3 month after completion of therapy, and are usually associated with soft tissue injury or infection. This may be of increasing importance in future patient care. In a similar manner to stereotactic treatment techniques for the central nervous system, hypofractionation techniques are now being employed for lesions in pulmonary parenchyma and the liver. If necrosis inhibits the repopulation and repair of the basement membrane, the skin surface will be susceptible to further injury. With injury to underlying blood vessels, the repair of the injury may take considerable time, and in rare circumstance, may require surgical repair with graft.

After the completion of treatment, there is a progressive decrease in the size and number of blood vessels, with a concomitant increase in fibrous tissue within the irradiated treatment area. The degree of fibrosis is influenced by treatment technique, type of treatment, total treatment dose, and daily treatment fraction. In more serious cases, the vasculature and soft connective tissue infrastructure continue to deteriorate and become susceptible to further injury with concurrent decrease in support cells and glandular tissue. Histologic evaluation reveals atrophy of the epidermis, with loss of dermal papillae. The basal layer reveals a marked decrease in cell number and mitoses. There is a thinning of the epidermis, a decrease in all vascular elements, and the presence of telangiectasia secondary to injury to the microvasculature [1,2,5]. Modern planning techniques using megavoltage energies have served to improve the clinical outcome for these patients. Prevention of untoward events should be the objective of advanced radiation therapy treatment technology.

Process improvements in radiation therapy support improved patient outcome

Advanced technology radiation therapy has generated a genuine opportunity to provide improved care for patients. Image-guided treatment platforms provide three-dimensional reconstruction of normal tissue and tumor objects. Skin rendering using three-dimensional planning computers is remarkably accurate, and can demonstrate skin folds and other areas of high risk of injury from treatment. Intensity modulation permits rapid motion of multileaf collimators, which can accommodate for multiple sloped surfaces of skin surface. Unlike previous treatment strategies that could not accommodate for multiple sloped surfaces, intensity modulation can adjust for these conditions and serve to decrease acute and presumably late dermal injury.

Fig. 1 is an example of the use of multileaf collimators for scalp epilation sparing for palliative management of patients who have central nervous system metastasis. Lateral field radiation therapy is used to treat the central nervous system. This is a straightforward technique appropriate for palliative management; however, this technique creates a tangential treatment surface at the level of the top of the skull. If one does not accommodate for this sloped surface, the radiation dose to this area is considerably higher both in daily and total dose. A one-step field within a field modification compensates for this surface, and facilitates the regrowth of hair to this region by creating a more uniform radiation dose distribution to the scalp surface. The evaluation of these late effects of the skin and appendages is important for patient outcome. Radiosurgery is altering the pattern of failure for patients who have metastasis to the central nervous system, and they may be living longer. Therefore, patient alopecia outcome may be improved with this technique.

Fig. 2 demonstrates improved radiation dose distribution to the skin surface for a patient who has head and neck cancer. These patients have multiple sloped surfaces both in the neck and jaw region. Oftentimes, skin demonstrates a moist breakdown at multiple tangential surfaces, with measurable dermal edema as a late effect at the

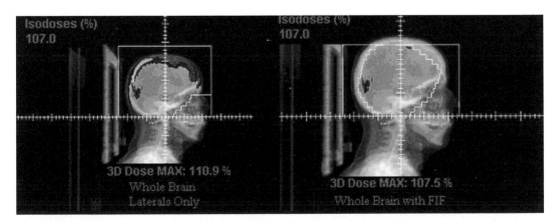

Fig. 1. A field-in-field technique (*right*) creating a more uniform dose distribution to scalp surface.

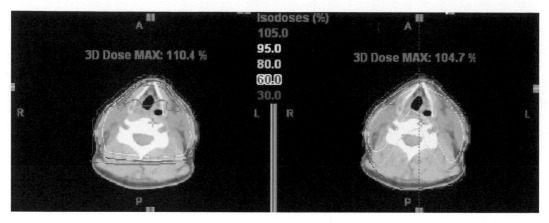

Fig. 2. Transversal views of isodose lines on same patient planed with conversional lateral beams (*left*) and intensity modulated radiation therapy (IMRT) technique (*right*).

level of the submental region. The degree of dermal skin reaction, including moist desquamation, is exacerbated by neoadjuvant and concurrent chemotherapy. Intensity modulation techniques permit adjustment to all of these surfaces. In the authors' experience, intensity modulation techniques result in less acute and late injury of the skin, with a near disappearance of submental dermal edema as a late effect of management. Although small segments of skin can actually receive a higher dose than anticipated, the volume of skin receiving this dose is minute in comparison to historical two-dimensional techniques.

The breast, chest wall, and supraclavicular regions likewise demonstrate improved outcome with intensity modulation techniques. The authors have demonstrated this improvement, especially with adjusting the planning target volume for intensity modulation [9,10]. The skin dose to the breast is markedly improved with this technique. The chest wall skin reaction for post-mastectomy patients is also improved using this technique. The slope of the supraclavicular fossa can create the potential for skin erythema and breakdown most often noted in areas of skin folds. Intensity modulation can also accommodate for this with bolus application techniques.

Perhaps the best improvement in outcome for patient care with intensity modulation is in the anal and vulva cancer patient population. In these patients the target volume includes multiple points of interest, including inguinal lymph nodes. Therefore the target volume includes areas of interest in the anterior and pelvic midplane. Two-dimensional and three dimensional techniques had to include multiple sloped surface

within the perineum. These patients are often treated with concurrent chemotherapy that may result in profound dermal injury during therapy, resulting in significant treatment interruption. Fig. 3 demonstrates a treatment plan using intensity modulation, which can adjust for the multiple sloped surfaces of the perineum. This has become a major improvement in patient care.

Multiple sloped surfaces are likewise encountered for extremity therapy. Patients who have sarcoma and other tumors of extremities have multiple steep-sloped surfaces, including areas in proximity to joint spaces. Fig. 4 demonstrates improved dosimetry to skin surface with intensity modulation. The authors' experience is that patients are having less skin erythema, dermal edema, and interstitial edema because of this technique. There are clinical situations that require augmenting the radiation dose to the skin surface. Such dose adjustments are made when normal tissue is drawn in close approximation to the original tumor site as part of the skin closure. Using image-guided objects to identify such areas serves to decrease the volume of skin receiving the prescription dose, thus improving patient outcome.

Improvements in treatment planning are having significant impact on patient outcome from primary radiotherapy. This is important because we are now encountering situations of retreatment. As patients survive their primary malignancy, we are asked to treat second cancers with increasing frequency. Often, especially in head and neck cancer, we need to bring the dose through previously irradiated sites. Improving initial techniques will likely make retreatment safer for patients moving forward. This will be

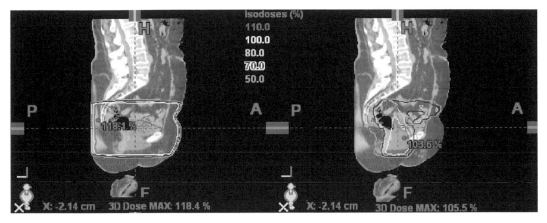

Fig. 3. Sagittal views of dose distributions from anterior–posterior pelvis plan (*left*), and IMRT plan (*right*).

an important area to study as requests for retreatment are increasing.

Drug–radiography interactions

Medications and chemotherapy appear to interact with radiation therapy via several mechanisms. Some medications can sensitize cells to the effects of radiation therapy, whereas some others appear to support the repair of dermal injury. Chemotherapy agents have been used in a concomitant basis with radiation therapy. Some have demonstrated an increase in both acute and late injury from radiation therapy. Actinomycin D, methotrexate, and doxorubicin are well-established in augmenting dermal reactions to radiation therapy as well as increasing reactions to

tissues of limited self-renewal potential. Although acute reactions are of concern, late injuries may be of more importance. The two events are not always related, however [11–15]. A phase 3 randomized trial evaluating the efficacy of mitoxantrone and cyclophosphamide delivered with radiation therapy inpatients with breast cancer has demonstrated an increase risk of subcutaneous fibrosis and breast atrophy in the patients receiving chemotherapy and radiation therapy on a concurrent basis [16,17]. Interestingly, both tetracycline and St. John's wort have been associated with similar events; however, there is little evidence supporting this claim [18,19]. Amifostine is the one medication associated with protection of dermal toxicity from radiation management. Topical steroids have been reported to decrease

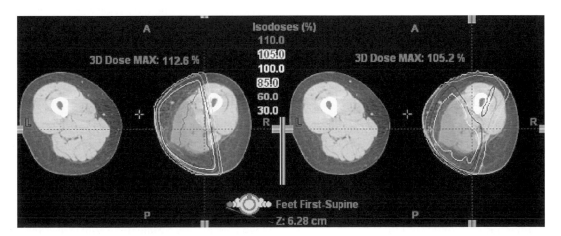

Fig. 4. Transversal views of the same patient. Conventional three-dimensional plan (*left*) versus an IMRT plan (*right*).

dermal reaction from radiation treatment, likely because of their anti-inflammatory effects [20]. There is one report indicating that gauze with granulocyte-macrophage colony stimulating factor (GM CSF) produces a similar effect, though the mechanism has not been established [21].

Radiation recall phenomenon is clinically described but poorly understood [22–24]. This phenomenon is characterized by the development of skin erythema and erosion in a radiation treatment precipitated by an unrelated drug. This eruption, similar to the skin changes observed during radiation therapy, occur several months after the completion of radiation therapy. Many chemotherapeutic agents and antibiotics have been associated with this phenomenon (Box 1). There is a case report associating statin medication with this phenomenon. The mechanism is thought to be either autoimmune, a result of inadequate stem cell function, or idiosyncratic drug sensitivity. Treatment is generally oral or topical steroids, supportive care, or other anti-inflammatory medication.

There have been anecdotal reports of bullous, necrotic, generalized skin eruptions secondary to radiation therapy [31–34]. Patients who have autoimmune disease such as systemic lupus erythematosus (SLE) and scleroderma are reported to have more acute and late complications from radiation management; however, these reports are scattered and anecdotal. Matched-pair analysis has not been able to validate this concern. Further work in this area is important because it could potentially aid oncologists in the treatment community when treating patients who have connective-tissue diseases such as scleroderma [31,34].

Box 1. Agents reported to precipitate radiation recall phenomenon

Antibiotics
Cefotetan [25]
Gatifloxacin [26]

Cytotoxics [15]
5-fluorouracil
Actinomycin D
Doxorubicin
Bleomycin
Capecitabine
Dacarbazine
Docetaxel
Edatrexate
Etoposide
Gemcitabine
Hydroxyurea
Melphalan
Methotrexate
Oxaliplatin
Paclitaxel
Tamoxifen [27]
Trimetraxate
Vinblastine

Other agents
Phentermine [28]
Ultraviolet light [29]
Simvastatin [30]
Interferon alpha-2b [15]
Tuberculosis treatment [15]

Secondary cutaneous malignancies as a consequence of cancer management

As both pediatric and adult patients survive their primary cancer, a new area of medicine is beginning to mature. Advising patients concerning risks and sequelae of management is under constant change and evaluation. Advising patients concerning risks of secondary malignancies is an important aspect of patient management and consent [35–44]. At this time, it remains difficult to determine if the development of second cancers is directly related to therapy or caused by predisposition of the host to the development of cancer [3,4]. Independent of the specific etiology of the event, it is clear that the predicted incidence of skin cancer in the population of patients successfully treated for a primary cancer appears higher than anticipated. Likewise, for patients treated for cancer at a relatively young age (Hodgkin's disease), the age of developing a cutaneous malignancy is younger than anticipated. There is evidence that these patients have an increased risk of developing melanoma in comparison to control populations. The role of radiation therapy is not established. This is often difficult to document, because dermal malignancies are not always coded as second malignancies caused by treatment. The relationship to the field of radiation therapy is often not part of the follow-up process; hence the data available for review are often incomplete. At the St. Jude medical center prior to 1986, four patients were evaluated for skin carcinoma (basal cell carcinoma) in areas that received previous radiation therapy [8]. The treatment sites were for acute lymphoblastic leukemia (central nervous system), Hodgkin's disease, and neuroblastoma. Three patients treated for squamous cell cancer of the skin had xeroderma pigmentosa. Before 1991, seven cases of basal cell carcinoma and three cases of squamous cell carcinoma were identified at the National Institute of Pediatrics in Mexico [44]. Five of the seven patients who had basal cell carcinoma had xeroderma pigment sum, one had basal cell nevus syndrome, and one developed tumor in a previous field of radiation therapy. One of the three patients who had squamous cell carcinoma had xeroderma pigmentosum. Radiation doses used for pediatric malignancies are in the low-to-intermediate range. If one assumes skin-sparing treatment strategies including megavoltage equipment, this raises an interesting question for the follow-up of these patients moving forward [8].

One population that has been studied for radiation-induced skin malignancies is a group of children treated in Israel from 1948 until 1960 for ringworm of the scalp. The mean scalp dose is 6.8 Gy. The relative risk of non-melanoma skin cancer is 4.2, with 98% of these cancers being basal cell carcinoma in the irradiated population. The mean interval of time between radiation treatment and the development of the malignancy is 21.6 years. The risk appears to increase as the age of exposure decreases. Chemotherapy appears to increase the risk as well in a manner not well understood. The risk of secondary epidermal malignancies generated from cancer therapy will require further study to better define the risk and identify preventative strategies moving forward [35–44].

Skin care for the radiation therapy patient

This is an important area for patient care. Symptoms associated with skin injury both during and after completion of radiation therapy are often visible and uncomfortable for patients. Patients largely prefer proactive management of problems during treatment, and often written instructions are very helpful for patients. Although cutaneous inflammation can be observed early in a traditional treatment course, often itching and skin discomfort occur during the third week of a treatment course as increase in blood flow is identified at this time point of treatment. As noted, the appearance of erythema is also driven by daily fraction size, dermal volume in the radiation therapy treatment field, and the degree of irregular dermal and subcutaneous contours within the radiation therapy treatment field. The skin can also become xerotic as glandular cells become less productive. Patients find moisturizers soothing because they decrease the degree of discomfort and improve dryness.

Skin reactions during treatment can vary from erythema to moist desquamation. Although the degree of injury does not follow a mathematical model, increased daily dose, increase volume of treatment, and tangential treatment plans contribute to acceleration and duration of injury. The patient and family are educated before starting treatment, and are taught self-care management. They are instructed to report redness and discomfort. Providers need to think of the area being treated and the potential of skin breakdown, often most noted in areas of skin folds (eg, perineal, axillary, and inframammary). The patient's skin status is evaluated at least once per week, and is graded on a 0 to 5 toxicity scale provided by the Radiation Therapy Oncology Group (RTOG). The patient is given written instructions that include gentle washing with warm water and mild soap such as Ivory (Proctor/Gamble, Cincinnati, Ohio), unscented Neutrogena (Neutrogena, Skillman, New Jersey), or unscented Dove (Unilever, London, United Kingdom). Ivory soap may result in increased dryness, however, because of the lack of moisturizers. Soaps should be unscented, pH balanced, and should not contain lanolin. Scalp care should include a gentle shampoo and pat dry without a hairdryer. Patients need to avoid gels, mousses, and hairspray. For comfort and moisture, several skin creams are recommended. They include Eucerin/Aquaphor (Beiersdorf, Hamburg, Germany), Lubriderm (Astra-Zenica, Westboro, Massachusetts), and Carasyn gel (Allegro Medical Supplies, Tempe, Arizona). These are applied after daily treatment, with use on weekends as well. Plain, unscented, lanolin-free hydrophilic cream may help decrease the extent of injury. It is important to note, however, that Aquaphore contains a small amount of lanolin, and the patient should discontinue its use if any untoward skin symptoms occur. A hydrocortisone 1% cream may be helpful in reducing itch (from increased blood flow) and discomfort. Fungal infections can occur in skin folds and need to be treated accordingly. Patients are instructed to avoid nonelectric razors, deodorants with metals, perfumed powders, and excessive heat or cold. Friction and chlorinated water may also add to skin irritation. Tape, underwire brassieres, and other tight garments can be sources of friction, and are to be avoided in areas receiving radiation. Along these lines, netting is preferred over tape to hold any wound dressings in place. Patients are advised to rinse with fresh water after exiting chlorinated water. Vitamin E oil may also be helpful in the perineum with sitz baths. If irritation increases with the use of vitamin E oil, patients should discontinue its use, because it can be a powerful contact allergen.

Skin reactions may progress after the treatment is complete, but will heal at a relatively rapid rate. The patient is instructed to continue with moisturizer. The treated area may remain hyperpigmented for several months or years after completion of therapy, depending on the patient's baseline skin color and ability to hyperpigment. Sun block (sun protection factor or SPF 30 or higher) with ultraviolet A and B protection is recommended for sun-exposed areas of skin treated with radiation.

After treatment, continued use of moisturizers is very reasonable, because cutaneous sebaceous glands have a relatively slow proliferative index and often require months to repopulate and return to function. With modern techniques, fibrosis and skin ulceration should be rare, unless treatment is delivered to site of previous injury or to dermal tissues of limited integrity [45].

Summary

Radiation therapy remains an integral component of the care and management of the cancer patient. Improvements in patient outcome and survival create accelerated awareness of the effect of therapy upon normal tissue. Cutaneous sequelae imposed by radiation therapy have undergone significant change over past decades. As process improvements have been made with both radiation therapy equipment and planning, fewer patients are experiencing acute or late changes to epidermal and dermal surfaces from radiation therapy. Optimal planning and treatment execution techniques have vastly improved the clinical outcome for patients with respect to skin tolerance. These process improvements are important. As advanced technology image platforms are incorporated into radiation therapy treatment plans, there exists significant interest in moving toward hypofractionation-based treatment strategies (fewer treatments at higher daily dose). Through cranial radiosurgery treatment mechanisms, the patterns of relapse for patients who

have disease in the central nervous system are changing, with fewer relapses now identified in the brain with careful application of these techniques. The current strategy is to apply similar radiosurgery applications with gating technology to the pulmonary and hepatic parenchyma moving forward. Historical experience with hypofractionation treatment strategies generated significant cutaneous sequelae. If we understand history, perhaps we will not be condemned to repeat this experience, especially as we incorporate more advanced treatment technologies and higher therapy energies into the treatment paradigm. Lessons learned from the initial experience with radiation therapy will help us avoid sequelae imposed on patients several decades ago as we move to accelerated treatment platforms. Technology improvements, appropriately applied, will help decrease sequelae imposed by therapy. The volume of therapy in the treatment field likewise influences outcome. Optimal planning helps to decrease the volume of high dose in the skin surface and decrease the volume of skin exposed to tangential radiography. Multileaf collimators permit dynamic adjustment to sloped surfaces, serving to decrease the risk of sequelae. Further improvements in technology and experience of practitioners will serve to improve outcome for patients. Radiation therapy will be used to vet new and improved targeted therapies as we move to design treatments to molecular-based targets. We have seen dermal consequence of epidermal growth factor receptor (EGFR)-targeted therapies that, in turn, have shown promise in head and neck cancer. Concurrent use of targeted therapies is expected in future protocols involving radiation therapy; therefore lessons learned from past experience may again improve outcome for patients. As more patients survive their primary oncology event, we need to constantly re-evaluate the impact of therapy on normal tissues to further improve patient outcome. Radiation therapy is entering a new phase of advanced technology treatment platforms. As we mature with our knowledge of advances in therapy technology, the patients we care for will be better served.

References

[1] Rubin P, Casarett G. Clinical radiation pathology, vol. 2. Philadelphia: WB Saunders; 1968.
[2] Farjardo L, Berthrong M, Anderson R. Radiation pathology—skin. New York: Oxford University Press; 2001. p. 411–20.

[3] Cleaver J. Defective repair of replication of DNA in xeroderma pigmentosum. Nature 1968;218:652–6.

[4] Anderson D, Taylor W, Falls H, et al. The nevoid basal cell carcinoma syndrome. Am J Hum Genet 1967;19:19–29.

[5] Cox JD, Ang KK. Radiation oncology: rationale-technique-results. 8th edition. St. Louis (MO): Mosby; 2003. p. 127–43.

[6] Hall E, Giaccia A. Radiobiology for the radiologist. 6th edition. Philadelphia: Lippincott Williams &Wilkins; 2006. p. 47–105.

[7] Matanoski G, Seltser P, Sartwell P, et al. The current mortality rates of radiologists and other physician specialists: specific causes of death. Am J Epidemiol 1975;101:199–210.

[8] Halperin E, Constine L, Tarbell N, et al. Pediatric radiation oncology. 4th edition. Philadelphia: Lippencott Williams & Wilkins; 2005. p. 514–5.

[9] Lo YC, Yasuda G, Fitzgerald TJ, et al. Intensity modulation for breast treatment using static multi-leaf collimators. Int J Radiat Oncol Biol Phys 2000;46(1):187–94.

[10] Mayo CS, Urie MM, Fitzgerald TJ. Hybrid IMRT plans—concurrently treating conventional and IMRT beams for improved breast irradiation and reduced planning time. Int J Radiat Oncol Biol Phys 2005;61(3):922–32.

[11] Aristizabal SA, Miller RC, Schlichtemeier AL, et al. Adriamycin-irradiation cutaneous complications. Int J Radiat Oncol Biol Phys 1977;2(3–4):325–31.

[12] Greco FA, Brereton HD, Kent H. Adriamycin and enhanced radiation reaction in normal esophagus and skin. Ann Intern Med 1975;85(3):294–8.

[13] Putnik K, Stadler C, Koelbl O. Enhanced radiation sensitivity and radiation recall dermatitis (RRD) after hypericin therapy—case report and review of literature. Radiat Oncol 2006;1:32.

[14] D'Angio GJ, Farber S, Maddock CL. Potentiation of x-ray effects by actinomycin-D. Radiology 1959;73:175–7.

[15] Toledano A, Garaud P, Serin D, et al. Concurrent administration of adjuvant chemotherapy and radiotherapy after breast-conserving surgery enhances late toxicities: long-term results of the ARCOSEIN multicenter randomized study. Int J Radiat Biol Phys 2006;65(2):324–32.

[16] Dubey A, Recht A, Come SE, et al. Concurrent CMF and radiation therapy for early stage breast cancer: results of a pilot study. Int J Radiat Oncol Biol Phys 1999;45(4):877–84.

[17] Vassilios E, Kouloulias JR, Kouvaris JD, et al. Impact on cytoprotective efficacy of intermediate interval between amifostine administration and radiotherapy: a retrospective analysis. Int J Radiat Oncol Biol Phys 2004;59(4):1148–56.

[18] Lin LC, Que J, Lin LK, et al. Zinc supplementation to improve mucositis and dermatitis in patients after radiotherapy for head-and-neck cancers: a double-blind, randomized study. Int J Radiat Oncol Biol Phys 2006;65(3):745–50.

[19] Xiao Z, Su Y, Yang S, et al. Protective effect of esculentoside A on radiation-induced dermatitis and fibrosis. Int J Radiat Oncol Biol Phys 2006;65(3):882–9.

[20] Boström A, Lindman H, Swartling C, et al. Potent corticosteroid cream (mometasone furoate) significantly reduces acute radiation dermatitis: results from a double-blind, randomized study. Radiother Oncol 2001;59(3):257–65.

[21] Kouvaris JR, Kouloulias VE, Plataniotis GA, et al. Dermatitis during radiation for vulvar carcinoma: prevention and treatment with granulocyte-macrophage colony-stimulating factor impregnated gauze. Wound Repair Regen 2001;9(3):187–93.

[22] Ristić B. Radiation recall dermatitis. Int J Dermatol 2004;43(9):627–31.

[23] Azria D, Magné N, Zouhair A, et al. Radiation recall: a well recognized but neglected phenomenon. Cancer Treat Rev 2005;31(7):555–70.

[24] Morris M, Powell S. Irradiation in the setting of collagen vascular disease: acute and late complications. J Clin Oncol 1997;15(7):2728–35.

[25] Ayoola A, Lee YJ. Recall dermatitis with cefotetan: a case study. Oncologist 2006;11(10):1118–20.

[26] Kang SK. Images in clinical medicine. Radiation recall reaction after antimicrobial therapy. N Engl J Med 2006;354(6):622.

[27] Singer EA, Warren RD, Pennanen MF, et al. Tamoxifen-induced radiation recall dermatitis. Breast J 2004;10(2):170–1.

[28] Ash RB, Videtic GM. Radiation recall dermatitis after the use of the anorexia phentermine in a patient with breast cancer. Breast J 2006;12(2):186–7.

[29] Scodan RL, Wyplosz B, Couchon S, et al. UV-light induced radiation recall dermatitis after a chemoradiotherapy organ preservation protocol. Eur Arch Otorhinolaryngol 2007;264(9):1099–102.

[30] Abadir R, Liebmann J. Radiation reaction recall following simvastatin therapy: a new observation. Clin Oncol (R Coll Radiol) 1995;7(5):325–6.

[31] Gold D, Miller R, Peterson I, et al. Radiotherapy for malignancy in patients with scleroderma: the Mayo clinic experience. Int J Radiat Oncol Biol Phys 2007;67(2):559–67.

[32] Chen A, Obedian E, Hafty B, et al. Breast-conserving therapy in the setting of collagen vascular disease. Cancer J 2001;7(6):475–6.

[33] Ross J, Hussey D, Mayr N, et al. Acute and late reactions to radiation therapy in patients with collagen vascular diseases. Cancer 1993;71(11):3744–52.

[34] Phan C, Mindrum M, Silverman M, et al. Matched-control retrospective study of the active and late complications in patients with collagen vascular diseases treated with radiation therapy. Cancer J 2003;9(6):461–6.

[35] Ron E, Preston DL, Mabuschi K, et al. Skin tumor risk among atomic-bomb survivors in Japan. Cancer Causes Control 1998;9:393–401.

[36] Ron E, Modan B, Preston D, et al. Radiation-induced skin carcinomas of the head and neck. Radiat Res 1991;125:318–25.

[37] Shore RE. Radiation-induced skin cancer in humans. Med Pediatr Oncol 2001;36:549–54.

[38] Olsen JH, Garwicz S, Hertz H, et al. Second malignant neoplasms after cancer in childhood or adolescence. Br Med J 1993;307:1030–6.

[39] Boice JD, Day N, Andersen A, et al. Second cancers following radiation treatment for cervical cancer. An international collaboration among cancer registries. J Natl Cancer Inst 1985;74:955–75.

[40] Wong FL, Boice JD, Abramson D, et al. Cancer incidence after retinoblastoma: radiation dose and sarcoma risk. JAMA 1997;278:1262–7.

[41] Van Leewen FE, Klokman WJ, van't Veer MB, et al. Long-term risk of second malignancy in survivors of Hodgkin's disease treated during adolescence or young adulthood. J Clin Oncol 2000;18: 487–97.

[42] Baird EA, McHenry PM, Mackie RM. Effect of maintenance chemotherapy in childhood on numbers of melanocytic naevi. Br Med J 1992;305: 799–801.

[43] Metayer C, Lynch CF, Clarke A, et al. Second cancers among long-term survivors of Hodgkin's disease diagnosed in childhood and adolescence. J Clin Oncol 18:2435–43.

[44] De la Luz Orozco-Cavarrubias M, Tamoyo-Sanchez L, Duran -McKinster C, et al. Malignant cutaneous tumors in children: twenty years of experience in a large pediatric hospital. J Am Acad Dermatol 1994;30:243–9.

[45] Bruner D, Haas M, Gosselin-Acomg T. Radiation oncology nursing practice and education. 3rd edition. Pittsburgh: Oncology Nursing Society (ONS); 2005.

ELSEVIER
SAUNDERS

Dermatol Clin 26 (2008) 173–182

DERMATOLOGIC
CLINICS

Index

Note: Page numbers of article titles are in **boldface** type.

0733-8635/08/$ - see front matter © 2008 Elsevier Inc. All rights reserved.
doi:10.1016/S0733-8635(08)00128-3

derm.theclinics.com

Moving?

Make sure your subscription moves with you!

To notify us of your new address, find your **Clinics Account Number** (located on your mailing label above your name), and contact customer service at:

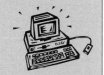

E-mail: elspcs@elsevier.com

800-654-2452 (subscribers in the U.S. & Canada)
407-345-4000 (subscribers outside of the U.S. & Canada)

Fax number: 407-363-9661

Elsevier Periodicals Customer Service
6277 Sea Harbor Drive
Orlando, FL 32887-4800

*To ensure uninterrupted delivery of your subscription, please notify us at least 4 weeks in advance of move.